T0259574

Psychopharmacology

Guest Editors

HARSH K. TRIVEDI, MD
KIKI D. CHANG, MD

CHILD AND ADOLESCENT PSYCHIATRIC CLINICS OF NORTH AMERICA

www.childpsych.theclinics.com

Consulting Editor
HARSH K. TRIVEDI, MD

October 2012 • Volume 21 • Number 4

SAUNDERS an imprint of ELSEVIER, Inc.

W.B. SAUNDERS COMPANY
A Division of Elsevier Inc.

Elsevier Inc. ● 1600 John F. Kennedy Boulevard ● Suite 1800 ● Philadelphia, Pennsylvania 19103-2899

http://www.childpsych.theclinics.com

CHILD AND ADOLESCENT PSYCHIATRIC CLINICS OF NORTH AMERICA Volume 21, Number 4
October 2012 ISSN 1056–4993, ISBN-13: 978-1-4557-4922-5

Editor: Joanne Husovski
Developmental Editor: Donald Mumford

Child and Adolescent Psychiatric Clinics of North America (ISSN 1056-4993) is published quarterly by Elsevier Inc., 360 Park Avenue South, New York, NY 10010-1710. Months of issue are January, April, July, and October. Business and Editorial Offices: 1600 John F. Kennedy Boulevard, Suite 1800, Philadelphia, PA 19103-2899. Periodicals postage paid at New York, NY and additional mailing offices. Subscription prices are $297.00 per year (US individuals), $453.00 per year (US institutions), $150.00 per year (US students), $343.00 per year (Canadian individuals), $546.00 per year (Canadian institutions), $190.00 per year (Canadian students), $408.00 per year (international individuals), $546.00 per year (international institutions), and $190.00 per year (international students). International air speed delivery is included in all *Clinics* subscription prices. All prices are subject to change without notice. **POSTMASTER:** Send address changes to *Child and Adolescent Psychiatric Clinics of North America*, Elsevier Health Sciences Division, Subscription Customer Service, 3251 Riverport Lane, Maryland Heights, MO 63043. **Customer Service: 1-800-654-2452 (U.S. and Canada); 314-447-8871 (outside U.S. and Canada). Fax: 314-447-8029. E-mail: JournalsCustomer Service-usa@elsevier.com (for print support) or journalsonlinesupport-usa@elsevier.com (for online support).**

Reprints. For copies of 100 or more of articles in this publication, please contact the Commercial Reprints Department, Elsevier Inc., 360 Park Avenue South, New York, New York 10010-1710 Tel.: (212) 633-3812; Fax: (212) 462-1935, e-mail: reprints@elsevier.com.

Child and Adolescent Psychiatric Clinics of North America is covered in *MEDLINE/PubMed (Index Medicus), ISI, SSCI, Research Alert, Social Search, Current Contents,* and *EMBASE/Excerpta Medica.*

Printed and bound by CPI Group (UK) Ltd, Croydon, CR0 4YY

Transferred to digital print 2012

Contributors

CONSULTING EDITOR

HARSH K. TRIVEDI, MD
Associate Professor of Psychiatry, Vanderbilt University School of Medicine; Executive Medical Director and Chief-of-Staff, Vanderbilt Psychiatric Hospital, Nashville, Tennessee

CONSULTING EDITOR EMERITUS

ANDRÉS MARTIN, MD, MPH

FOUNDING CONSULTING EDITOR

MELVIN LEWIS, MBBS, FRCPSYCH, DCH

GUEST EDITORS

HARSH K. TRIVEDI, MD
Associate Professor of Psychiatry, Vanderbilt University School of Medicine; Executive Medical Director and Chief-of-Staff, Vanderbilt Psychiatric Hospital, Nashville, Tennessee

KIKI D. CHANG, MD
Stanford Pediatric Bipolar Disorders Program, Department of Psychiatry, Professor of Psychiatry and Behavioral Sciences, Division of Child and Adolescent Psychiatry, Stanford University School of Medicine, Stanford, California

AUTHORS

KIKI D. CHANG, MD
Stanford Pediatric Bipolar Disorders Program, Department of Psychiatry, Professor of Psychiatry and Behavioral Sciences, Division of Child and Adolescent Psychiatry, Stanford University School of Medicine, Stanford, California

CHRISTINE J. CHOE, MD
Assistant Professor of Psychiatry, Department of Psychiatry, University of Texas Southwestern Medical Center, Dallas, Texas

NANCY L. CLOAK, MD
Staff Psychiatrist, Oregon Center for Clinical Investigations; Private Practice, Portland, Oregon

SUCHETA CONNOLLY, MD
Institute for Juvenile Research (MC 747), Director, Department of Psychiatry, Pediatric Stress and Anxiety Disorders Clinic, Professor of Clinical Psychiatry, University of Illinois at Chicago, Chicago, Illinois

PAUL E. CROARKIN, DO
Division of Child and Adolescent Psychiatry, Department of Psychiatry and Psychology, Mayo Clinic, Rochester, Minnesota

MELISSA P. DELBELLO, MD, MS
Division of Bipolar Disorders Research, Department of Psychiatry and Behavioral Neuroscience, University of Cincinnati College of Medicine, Cincinnati, Ohio

RASIM S. DILER, MD
Assistant Professor, Western Psychiatric Institute and Clinic, University of Pittsburgh School of Medicine, Pittsburgh, Pennsylvania

GRAHAM J. EMSLIE, MD
Professor of Psychiatry, Department of Psychiatry and Pediatrics, University of Texas Southwestern Medical Center; Division Chief, Department of Psychiatry, Children's Medical Center, University of Texas Southwestern Medical Center, Dallas, Texas

JEAN A. FRAZIER, MD
Robert M. and Shirley S. Siff Chair in Autism, Professor of Psychiatry and Pediatrics, Co-Director, Child and Adolescent NeuroDevelopment Initiative (CANDI); Vice Chair & Director, Division of Child and Adolescent Psychiatry, Department of Psychiatry, University of Massachusetts Memorial Health Care, University of Massachusetts Medical School, Worcester, Massachusetts

GEORGINA GARCIA, MD
Assistant in Psychiatry, Department of Psychiatry, Boston Children's Hospital; Instructor, Harvard Medical School, Boston, Massachusetts

BENJAMIN I. GOLDSTEIN, MD, PhD
Assistant Professor, Departments of Psychiatry and Pharmacology, Sunnybrook Health Sciences Centre, University of Toronto Faculty of Medicine, Toronto, Ontario

JOSEPH GONZALEZ-HEYDRICH, MD
Associate in Psychiatry and Chief, Psychopharmacology Clinic, Department of Psychiatry, Boston Children's Hospital; Assistant Professor, Harvard Medical School, Boston, Massachusetts

BRETT A. KOPLIN, MD
Division of Child and Adolescent Psychiatry, Department of Psychiatry and Psychology, Mayo Clinic, Rochester, Minnesota

CHRISTOPHER J. KRATOCHVIL, MD
Assistant Vice Chancellor for Clinical Research, Professor of Psychiatry and Pediatrics, Chief Medical Officer UneHealth, Departments of Psychiatry and Pediatrics, University of Nebraska Medical Center, Omaha, Nebraska

GRACE E. LOGAN, BA
Department of Psychiatry, Boston Children's Hospital, Boston, Massachusetts

ANN E. MALONEY, MD
Assistant Professor, Department of Psychiatry, Child and Adolescent NeuroDevelopment Initiative (CANDI), University of Massachusetts Memorial Health Care, University of Massachusetts Medical School, Worcester, Massachusetts

TARYN L. MAYES, MS
Faculty Associate of Psychiatry, Department of Psychiatry, University of Texas Southwestern Medical Center, Dallas, Texas

ROBERT K. MCNAMARA, PhD
Division of Bipolar Disorders Research, Department of Psychiatry and Behavioral
Neuroscience, University of Cincinnati College of Medicine, Cincinnati, Ohio

RAFAEL PELAYO, MD
Associate Professor, Stanford Sleep Medicine Center, Stanford University School
of Medicine, Stanford, California

TODD E. PETERS, MD
Assistant Professor, Department of Psychiatry, Division of Child and Adolescent
Psychiatry, Vanderbilt Psychiatric Hospital, Vanderbilt University School of Medicine,
Nashville, Tennessee

PAULINE S. POWERS, MD
Professor of Psychiatry and Behavioral Medicine, Department of Pediatrics; Director,
Center for Eating and Weight Disorders, College of Medicine, University of South Florida,
Tampa, Florida

ROBERTO SASSI, MD, PhD
Assistant Professor, Department of Psychiatry and Behavioural Neurosciences,
McMaster University Faculty of Health Sciences, Hamilton, Ontario

MATTHEW SIEGEL, MD
Assistant Professor of Psychiatry, Department of Psychiatry, Tufts University School
of Medicine, Boston, Massachusetts; Director, Developmental Disorders Program, Spring
Harbor Hospital, Westbrook, Maine; Clinical Investigator, Center for Outcomes Research
and Evaluation, Maine Medical Center Research Institute, Portland, Maine

MANPREET K. SINGH, MD, MS
Assistant Professor of Psychiatry and Behavioral Sciences, Division of Child and
Adolescent Psychiatry, Stanford University School of Medicine, Stanford, California

JEFFREY R. STRAWN, MD
Division of Bipolar Disorders Research, Department of Psychiatry and Behavioral
Neuroscience, University of Cincinnati College of Medicine, Cincinnati, Ohio

OLIVER STROEH, MD
Child and Adolescent Psychiatry Residency Training Director, Assistant Professor of
Psychiatry, Vanderbilt University School of Medicine, Nashville, Tennessee

COSIMA SWINTAK, MD
Division of Child and Adolescent Psychiatry, Department of Psychiatry and Psychology,
Mayo Clinic, Rochester, Minnesota

HARSH K. TRIVEDI, MD
Associate Professor of Psychiatry, Vanderbilt University School of Medicine; Executive
Medical Director and Chief-of-Staff, Vanderbilt Psychiatric Hospital, Nashville, Tennessee

BRIGETTE VAUGHAN, MSN, APRN-BC, NP
Department of Psychiatry, University of Nebraska Medical Center, Omaha, Nebraska

CHRISTOPHER A. WALL, MD
Division of Child and Adolescent Psychiatry, Department of Psychiatry and Psychology,
Mayo Clinic, Rochester, Minnesota

LAUREN J. YAKUTIS, BA
Research Coordinator, Department of Psychiatry, Child and Adolescent
NeuroDevelopment Initiative (CANDI), University of Massachusetts Medical School,
Worcester, Massachusetts

KIN YUEN, MD, MS
Stanford Sleep Medicine Center, Stanford University School of Medicine, Stanford,
California

Contents

SECTION 1: PSYCHOPHARMACOLOGY

The issue of prescribing psychotropic medications is one that stirs much emotion and debate among parents and providers alike. This article is presented as a primer on the appropriate and judicious use of psychotropic medications in youth. Rather than focusing on any specific class of medications or on any clinical condition, the article presents best practices as well as key clinical pearls regarding the art and science of psychopharmacology in youth.

This article is a review of several of the most concerning side effects of psychotropic medications in children and adolescents. An emphasis is placed on review of the prevalence, presentation, monitoring, and evidence-based management of these side effects.

Increasing evidence from retrospective and prospective studies is beginning to validate criteria to identify individuals at high risk for developing bipolar disorder or schizophrenia. In parallel, intervention trials are evaluating the efficacy and tolerability of pharmacologic and nonpharmacologic approaches for the treatment of subthreshold and possibly prodromal presentations in these high-risk populations with the ultimate objective of mitigating illness progression. This article reviews current evidence for candidate interventions for high-risk individuals to guide future research in this rapidly emerging field. A clinical vignette describing antidepressant-induced manic symptoms in an adolescent with a family history of bipolar disorder is provided.

Little is known about the neurobiological effects of psychotropic medications used in the treatment of children and adolescents diagnosed with a psychiatric disorder. This review provides a synopsis of the literature demonstrating the neural effects associated with exposure to psychotropic medication in youth using multimodal neuroimaging. The article concludes by illustrating how, taken together, these studies suggest that pharmacological interventions during childhood do indeed affect brain structure and function in a detectable manner, and the effects appear to be ameliorative.

This article provides an overview of where psychiatric pharmacogenomic testing stands as an emerging clinical tool in modern psychotropic prescribing practice, specifically in the pediatric population. This practical discussion is organized around the state of psychiatric pharmacogenomics research when choosing psychopharmacologic interventions in the most commonly encountered mental illnesses in youth. As with the rest of the topics on psychopharmacology for children and adolescents in this publication, a clinical vignette is presented, this one highlighting a clinical case of a 16 year old genotyped during hospitalization for recalcitrant depression.

SECTION 2: DISEASES

Anxiety is an innate emotion that all humans experience, especially during early childhood in periods of significant growth and development. Treatment strategies exist for anxiety disorders that cause significant dysfunction and impairment in youth. This article provides a current overview of the literature on psychopharmacologic management of pediatric anxiety disorders. Potential side effects and complications of psychotropic medications are reviewed. The treatment of anxiety disorders in patients with comorbid conditions is explored, addressing the impact on treatment course and pharmacologic recommendations. A clinical vignette describing a 10-year-old boy with increasing anxiety is presented describing in-hospital and outpatient treatment and therapies.

This article reviews the assessment and treatment for depression in children and adolescents, emphasizing the implementation of evidence-based treatments into clinical care. Past trials of antidepressant medications are reviewed, as well as the clinical use of antidepressants and pharmacologic strategies for refractory illness or in the context of comorbid conditions. Clinicians who treat youth now have a body of empiric research to help guide treatment decisions; however, personalized treatment based on associated symptoms, comorbid conditions, contextual factors, and psychiatric history is essential. Further research is needed in the pharmacologic treatment of depressed youth, including expanding the study of non-SSRI antidepressants, augmentation and adjunctive strategies, and treatment in patients with comorbid conditions.

CHILD AND ADOLESCENT PSYCHIATRIC CLINICS

Preface

Better and Safer Pharmacotherapy for Youth with Psychiatric Illness

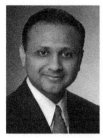 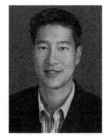

Harsh K. Trivedi, MD   Kiki D. Chang, MD
Guest Editors

Welcome to the Pediatric Psychopharmacology issue of the *Child and Adolescent Psychiatric Clinics of North America*. It has been 6 years since the last review and in that time there have been significant advances in the field. While there is clearly much more to be learned in this arena, in this issue we collect from the wisdom of leading researchers in the field to benefit clinicians and academicians alike in their quest to provide better and safer interventions for youth with psychiatric illnesses.

The topic of pediatric psychopharmacology is one that stirs much emotion and debate among parents and providers alike. Drs Stroeh and Trivedi begin this issue with a thoughtful primer on the appropriate and judicious use of psychotropic medications in youth. Their approach to conducting a comprehensive psychiatric evaluation, developing a treatment plan, and preventing polypharmacy provides a strong foundation from which to build this issue. Dr Gonzalez-Heydrich's group then presents a comprehensive review of medication adverse effects and provides valuable insights into their management.

Two rapidly advancing areas in the field are interventions for youth at high risk for serious psychopathology and pharmacogenomics. Dr McNamara and colleagues highlight the progress that has been made in identifying and treating children and

Child Adolesc Psychiatric Clin N Am 21 (2012) xiii–xv
http://dx.doi.org/10.1016/j.chc.2012.07.013
childpsych.theclinics.com

adolescents who are at risk for developing schizophrenia and bipolar disorder. The potential for prevention is tantalizing, but questions remain as to the best pharmacologic approach to these youth. Biological markers to guide these and other treatments would be enormously helpful to the clinician, and Dr Wall and colleagues describe the current state of pharmacogenomics in providing clues regarding treatment response and adverse effects. This tool is already becoming clinically useful and should become even more so in the decade to come.

The next series of articles focuses on specific clinical conditions in youth. Drs Peters and Connelly review the evidence base for the psychopharmacologic treatment of anxiety disorders and discuss how to incorporate treatment within the context of common comorbid conditions. Dr Emslie's group educates us about depression in youth and management of both acute and treatment refractory presentations of the illness. Drs Powers and Cloak then review medications used for obesity and eating disorders. They also present data on investigational agents currently under review. Drs Pelayo and Yuen present an overview of sleep disorders with important nonpharmacologic considerations to ascertain before the initiation of a medication trial. The empirical evidence for pharmacologic treatment in early onset psychosis and schizophrenia is then explored by Dr Frazier's group, including analysis of important findings from the Treatment of Early-Onset Schizophrenia Study.

Drs Goldstein, Sassi, and Diler present a review of the evidence base for psychopharmacologic treatment of bipolar disorder in youth. Their balanced approach reviews data from all bipolar research groups to help the reader distill clinically relevant takeaway points. Dr Kratchovil's group reports on the pharmacotherapy of attention-deficit/hyperactivity disorder. Their ability to synthesize nearly 80 years of research and provide clinical direction is appreciated. Next, Dr Siegel reviews the evidence-based treatment options for autism spectrum disorders. This is a quickly developing topic and his ability to divide treatments by core target symptoms will be useful for the clinician.

Finally, we end with a review and synthesis regarding the effects of the medications discussed here on the developing human brain. Drs Singh and Chang summarize the extant neuroimaging data as it pertains to pharmacologic neural effects in youth. While studies are establishing the utility of psychotropic medications in improving the quality of life and decreasing morbidity and mortality in children, there is still rightfully the concern of long-term adverse effects to the brain as well as the body. Understanding these effects, including beneficial ones, of psychotropic medications will help clinicians to weigh the risks and benefits of such interventions better in the future.

We wish to commend the authors for their valued contributions to this issue. The psychopharmacology issue of *Child and Adolescent Psychiatric Clinics of North America* is always highly anticipated and commonly referenced. We thank them for sharing their expertise, for helping us to make meaning of the hundreds of studies that they reviewed, and for providing key insights on translating the science into clinical practice.

We wish to sincerely thank Joanne Husovski at Elsevier for her guidance, her perseverance, and her support as we worked to get this issue just right. Her ability to think about article structure and to create article templates that facilitate the communication of information and her steadfast clarity about the importance of clinical application of the data were quite helpful.

Last, thank-you to the readership of *Child and Adolescent Psychiatric Clinics of North America* for turning to this issue on psychopharmacology as you think about how to manage the clinical care of your patients. We hope that you are pleased with the final product.

Harsh K. Trivedi, MD
Vanderbilt Psychiatric Hospital
1601 23rd Avenue South
Nashville, TN 37212, USA

Kiki D. Chang, MD
Stanford Pediatric Bipolar Disorders Program
Stanford University School of Medicine
Department of Psychiatry, 401 Quarry Road
Stanford, CA 94305, USA

E-mail addresses:
harsh.k.trivedi@vanderbilt.edu (H.K. Trivedi)
kchang88@stanford.edu (K.D. Chang)

Appropriate and Judicious Use of Psychotropic Medications in Youth

Oliver Stroeh, MD[a],*, Harsh K. Trivedi, MD[a,b]

KEYWORDS

- Psychotropic • Medication • Psychopharmacology • Youth • Appropriate
- Judicious • Treatment

KEY POINTS

- Before any treatments with psychotropic medications can be considered, it is paramount to have an accurate understanding of a youngster's presentation, of the presence of pertinent signs and symptoms, and of the resulting diagnostic formulation of the case.
- It is vital that a parent or guardian understand the formulation and have ample opportunity to receive psychoeducation as well as ask questions about the findings.
- Even after clinical gains are made, such that response or remission of the target symptoms is achieved, clinical assessment with direct observation of the youngster should continue on a regular basis.
- Nonspecificity of symptoms plus the issue of comorbidity in psychiatric conditions make diagnosis difficult, because each condition may work uniquely, additively, synergistically, or contradictorily to produced the observed behavior or symptom.

ASSESSING THE YOUNGSTER

The key element to the appropriate and judicious use of psychotropic medications in youth is a high-quality comprehensive psychiatric evaluation. Before any treatment decisions can be considered, it is paramount to have an accurate understanding of a youngster's presentation, of the presence of pertinent signs and symptoms, and of the resulting diagnostic formulation of the case. It is vital that a parent or guardian understand the formulation and have ample opportunity to receive psychoeducation as well as ask questions about the findings. Having a common understanding and

Funding Sources: Dr Stroeh—None. Dr Trivedi—Consulting Editor, *Child and Adolescent Psychiatric Clinics of North America*.
Conflict of Interest: None.
[a] Vanderbilt University School of Medicine, 1601 23rd Avenue South, Nashville, TN 37212-3139, USA; [b] Vanderbilt Psychiatric Hospital, Vanderbilt University School of Medicine, 1601 23rd Avenue South, Nashville, TN 37212-3139, USA
* Corresponding author.
E-mail address: oliver.stroeh@vanderbilt.edu

being on the same page aids in building a sound therapeutic alliance to facilitate all subsequent conversations regarding treatment.

Understanding Development

When assessing children, a commonly encountered question is what constitutes atypical or abnormal behavior? Is hearing voices of an imaginary friend abnormal in a 6-year-old child? How about the same presentation in a 17-year-old teenager who has a family history of schizophrenia? When first hearing of a youngster's problems, it is important to keep a developmental perspective. Notions of typical and atypical are functions of each individual child's progress across multiple developmental lines. To make appropriate diagnoses, a solid understanding of normative development is needed to differentiate which symptoms are concerning and which are simply normal variants. Although outside the scope of the article, there are excellent review articles available regarding normal child development.[1,2] Because children can vary substantially along developmental lines, it is important to obtain information from parents and other informants (such as pediatricians and school teachers) about developmental history, whether there has been any regression, and the time course of any current developmental concerns.

Beyond understanding development to understand a patient's presentation, providers can also use this same developmental sensitivity to select more effective strategies to facilitate communication and information gathering.[3] For example, understanding that a particular 7-year-old boy is temperamentally shy and timid allows an interviewer to use both play and displacement. Instead of a more direct interaction that may lead a patient to shut down, an interviewer can use toy animals and engage in play. Using displacement to explore why the duckling is feeling sad, a child may provide valuable insights that may not otherwise be elicited.

Putting Nonspecific Symptoms into Context

Youth commonly present with nonspecific chief complaints, such as withdrawn behavior, impulsivity,[4] aggression,[5] and irritability. Several different diagnoses could each independently account for a particular symptom or behavior. Does a youngster's irritability stem from a major depressive episode, a hypomanic or manic episode, a generalized anxiety, or an attention-deficit/hyperactive state or is it a consequence of oppositional or defiant behavior? Such symptom nonspecificity reflects a limitation of the current nosologic system of classification and also speaks to the possibility of neurobiologic overlap of what are termed separate psychiatric diagnoses at this time. The difficulty with such nonspecificity is that it creates the potential for bias in the diagnostic method. Without using objective measures and without using a thorough approach to differential diagnosis, even seasoned clinicians may develop a tendency to diagnose youth more often with one particular diagnosis.

Adding to the complexity of nonspecificity of symptoms is the issue of comorbidity in psychiatric conditions.[6,7] Comorbidities, such as an adolescent with both a mood disorder and attention-deficit/hyperactivity disorder (ADHD), make diagnosis difficult because each condition may work uniquely, additively, synergistically, or contradictorily to produce the observed behavior or symptom. Furthermore, if only one diagnosis is recognized during an evaluation, the existence of a comorbidity may hamper subsequent treatment. For example, consider the case of a child who starts taking atomoxetine for ADHD. If the comorbid diagnosis of a mood disorder was missed, the implemented treatment plan may have deleterious effects on the child.

Thus, a fundamental point is that when treatment does not work to desired outcomes, it is imperative to first review the diagnostic formulation. Have the correct diagnoses been considered? Could it be possible that a child actually has a different diagnosis or has an additional comorbid diagnosis? Such a review may prove more valuable than attempting to simply augment with another medication due to partial response.

Incorporating the Use of Rating Scales

Rating scales can be helpful in teasing apart similar behaviors, ensuring that comorbid conditions are appropriately deciphered, and determining whether a patient is making gains in treatment. These instruments can complement information gathered during a clinical interview and from collaterals. They may also get a patient or parent to provide information about topic that may not be discussed as easily in a clinical interview. Likewise, there are times when a child, parent, or even provider questions what effect a particular treatment has had. Serial administration of specific rating scales can provide objective measures to track response to treatment and can guide subsequent treatment decisions. Rating scales include standardized measures, such as screening questionnaires, and structured or semistructured diagnostic interviews. See **Table 1** for a review of commonly used rating scales.

Table 1 Standardized screening tools and rating scales	
General screening	• Child behavior checklist www.aseba.org • Pediatric symptom checklist http://psc.partners.org
Anxiety symptoms	• Screen for Childhood Anxiety Related Disorders (SCARED) http://psychiatry.pitt.edu/research/tools-research/assessment-instruments • Multidimensional Anxiety Scale for Children (MASC) www.mhs.com
ADHD symptoms	• Vanderbilt ADHD Diagnostic Parent Rating Scale http://www2.massgeneral.org/schoolpsychiatry/screening_adhd.asp#Vanderbilt • SNAP-IV rating scale–revised www.adhd.net/ • Connors Rating Scales–Revised www.pearsonassessments.org
Bipolar disorder/mania symptoms	• Young Mania Rating Scale (YMRS) www.atlantapsychiatry.com/forms/ymrs.pdf • Kiddie Schedule for Affective Disorders and Schizophrenia (K-SADS) http://psychiatry.pitt.edu/research/tools-research/ksads-pl
Depressive symptoms	• Children's Depression Inventory www.pearsonassessments.org • Reynolds Adolescent Depression Scale, Second Edition (RAD-2) www.parinc.com
Obsessive-compulsive symptoms	• Children's Yale-Brown Obsessive Compulsive Scale (CY-BOCS) www.thereachinstitute.org/files/documents/cybocs.pdf
Psychosis	• Kiddie Schedule for Affective Disorders and Schizophrenia (K-SADS) http://psychiatry.pitt.edu/research/tools-research/ksads-pl

Adapted from Trivedi HK, Kershner JD, editors. Practical child and adolescent psychiatry for pediatrics and primary care. Cambridge (UK): Hogrefe and Huber; 2009.

Using Multiple Informants for Collateral

Incorporated into the life of an average youngster are several potential sources for rich clinical information. Because children often present differently in different environments, it is helpful to obtain collateral from pediatricians, teachers, school counselors, coaches, and other individuals who have regular contact with a patient. With the consent of a parent or guardian, collaterals can provide information to facilitate the diagnostic process, longitudinal information regarding clinical symptoms and functioning, and serial feedback of a patient's response to any initiated treatments or interventions.

Ordering the Medical Work-up and Consulting Colleagues

There are times when diagnostic questions cannot be answered through a clinical interview and collateral information alone. In such cases, it is important to consider whether further testing or additional consultation may complement the current formulation of a patient's case.

Medical causes of psychiatric symptoms must be ruled out before considering psychiatric diagnoses. Even in cases where a psychosocial stressor is readily identifiable, it is prudent to consider medical causes. Consider the case of a short 16-year-old girl with an atypical and distinctive physical appearance who presents with depressive symptoms in the context of her parents' divorce. It is important to determine whether she has had long-standing poor school performance and a history of primary amenorrhea. Concern about Turner syndrome warrants a referral to a gynecologist and a geneticist. Depending on the case, consultation with a patient's pediatrician or other appropriate specialist (eg, neurologist, gastroenterologist, or endocrinologist) can be helpful.

Medical screening studies (eg, liver function tests, urine tests, and electrocardiograms) may also help identify concerns regarding a potential medical cause. For example, a 4-year-old child presenting with irritability, loss of appetite, fatigue, abdominal pain, constipation, and learning difficulties would benefit from a lead level to rule out lead poisoning.

There are also cases where psychological testing or neuropsychological testing may be helpful. Consider the case of a 16-year-old girl with history of sexual trauma and posttraumatic stress disorder who presents with disorganized behavior and auditory hallucinations. Psychologic testing would be helpful in determining whether her disorganization and hallucination are secondary to an underlying psychotic process or an anxiety disorder.

DEVELOPING THE TREATMENT PLAN
Identifying a Target of Treatment

The identification of discrete target symptoms or behaviors is a critical step in the development of any treatment plan. Often, parents and providers are defining success of the treatment based on different criteria or expectations. This can lead to situations where a provider identifies in an improvement in mood or better concentration, but the patient and family report that the medication has provided little benefit because the patient's tics have worsened.

Because the response of the target symptom to any initiated treatment defines the success or failure of the treatment, the target symptom should be chosen thoughtfully and carefully. It should be chosen in a collaborative process and should involve the input of the youngster, his or her family, psychiatrist, and possibly other key members of the youngster's treatment team as well. Ideally, the target symptom should be one that is easily recognized by the patient and parent. Also, it should be one that has clinical significance.

By helping a patient and family identify an appropriate target symptom, a psychiatrist can increase the likelihood of attaining symptomatic relief and clinically meaningful change. Within this context, it is important that all parties are on the same page regarding what is defined as improvement. For a student who is removed from class daily due to impulsivity and aggression, it may be unrealistic to expect him to sit in his seat all day or that he will not have an occasional anger episode. It is helpful to provide the patient and the family appropriate expectations of what the treatment can and cannot do. Likewise, it is imperative with many psychiatric illnesses for patients and families to understand that medication is only one piece of the treatment plan.

Developing a Comprehensive Treatment Plan

Biosocial formulation

The process of creating a comprehensive treatment plan is greatly facilitated by first completing a comprehensive psychiatric assessment. Developing a biopsychosocial formulation is helpful in understanding the potential roles that biologic treatments, psychological treatments, and social supports have in patient recovery. Increasingly, studies have concluded that combined treatment with both therapy and medication can lead to more favorable outcomes relative to psychotherapy or psychopharmacologic treatment alone.[8,9] In some instances, a combination of medication and therapy may be complementary rather than additive or synergistic.

Psychosocial interventions

Psychosocial interventions are another form of treatment that all mental health providers should consider when drafting a treatment plan. Such interventions may pertain to the systems in which youngsters live and in which their symptoms and struggles are amplified. For instance, when working with a 13-year-old boy who has previously undiagnosed ADHD or a previously unrecognized learning disability, advocate for the implementation a 504 plan or an individualized education plan. While working with an 8-year-old girl with posttraumatic stress disorder symptoms, the psychiatrist might write a letter requesting that the girl's family be released from the apartment lease given the unsafe conditions of the apartment building and the likely role of the daily presence of actual danger in the young girl's persistent active symptomatology. In addition to potentially resulting in beneficial clinical outcomes that are magnitudes greater than the effort invested by the psychiatrist, such interventions may also adjust the youngster's circumstances so as to increase the likelihood that any implemented psychopharmacologic treatment may lead to additional clinical improvement.

Other potential psychosocial interventions that a psychiatrist might consider could be less formal but result in positive change of equally great scope. When working with a shy isolative 9-year-old boy, the psychiatrist could encourage the boy and his family to enroll him in activities at the local YMCA. The psychiatrist similarly could recommend that a 16-year-old socially awkward girl who loves animals but struggles with depressed mood, low self-esteem, and feelings of worthlessness volunteer at a local animal shelter. Such interventions can be remarkably and invaluably therapeutic and in a manner that is more normative and less potentially stigmatizing than either psychotherapy or pharmacotherapy.

Feasability of interventions

In drafting a treatment plan and in considering potential interventions of different modalities, the feasibility and availability of the different modalities need to be considered. Such practical and logistical parameters fundamentally affect the implementation of an individual treatment plan and, therefore, should be taken into account in the drafting thereof. In the case of psychotherapy, practical limitations of time, cost, and the availability of therapists may make psychotherapy difficult to implement or sustain.

If multiple treatment providers are involved in a patient's care, it is imperative that they agree on and follow one comprehensive treatment plan. There also needs to be a good working relationship among members of the treatment team and avenues for regular communication regarding a patient's care. It is also important that patient and family understand what the role is of each provider. It is not uncommon for families to assume that saying something to one provider (for example, the therapist) is the same as every provider having access to that information. It is particularly important to make sure that patients and parents clearly understand that they must contact the prescriber for any concerns regarding medications as well as any side effects or clinical deterioration that may occur. Likewise, all members of a treatment team need to understand each other's role and facilitate clear and effective communication in a patient's best interest.

Establishing the Pretreatment Baseline

Before initiating treatment, the provider should work with the youngster and the family to establish a pretreatment baseline with respect to the identified target symptom. In general, such a baseline facilitates the assessment of the effects, whether positive or negative, of subsequently initiated treatment. An established pretreatment baseline is particularly important for those target symptoms that occur less predictably or less frequently. The establishment of a baseline before the initiation of a psychopharmacologic treatment might prevent premature termination of the trial of a potentially efficacious medication.

A pretreatment symptom or behavior baseline can be established by various means. A provider can determine a baseline by having the patient or family document various parameters of the identified target symptom or behavior (eg, any precipitating contexts, the intensity of the experienced symptom, and the frequency with which the symptom or behavior occurs over time). Likewise, many of the standardized tools listed in **Table 1** can be used to establish a quantitative pretreatment symptom baseline.

Laying out the Game Plan

Identification of treatment goals

Before the initiation of any psychopharmacologic treatment, there should be a discussion regarding initial target medication doses and the anticipated frequency of dose increases. Discussion might also include the identification of anticipated goals regarding symptom reduction as well as definitions of treatment outcomes. In cases with severe symptoms at the outset of treatment, the provider might consider specifically noting that partial response may be the realistic expectation of treatment and, therefore, might represent success. It usually is also helpful to discuss anticipated next steps should the initial treatment steps not result in the desired or expected clinical outcomes.

Discussion of adverse medication effects

An important topic that also warrants discussion before the initiation of a psychopharmacologic treatment is possible adverse effects. Consistent with the principle of informed consent, the risks, benefits, and alternatives of any proposed treatments should be reviewed. It is important to explicitly outline that adverse effects are possible. Although perhaps obvious, it is also important to inform patients and families that understanding of medications and their adverse effects is ever-changing. As exemplified by the recent Food and Drug Administration (FDA) warning regarding the potential for QTc prolongation with higher doses of citalopram,[10] there may be potential adverse effects that only the future will disclose. It is also good practice to review with patients and parents whether the treatment selections are FDA approved or are used off-label. Once informed consent is obtained from a parent and, if applicable, assent from the youngster, it should be documented in the youngster's chart.

To be able to recognize the emergence of any potential adverse effects, a thorough review of systems should be documented before the initiation of any new psychopharmacologic treatments. Drug-specific parameters (eg, establishment of the baseline frequency and intensity of suicidal ideation before the initiation of a selective serotonin reuptake inhibitor) should also be explored and documented before the initiation of a psychopharmacologic agent. Some standardized tools have been developed to facilitate assessments for drug-specific adverse effects (eg, the Abnormal Involuntary Movements Scale to determine the presence of involuntary movements in those individuals taking antipsychotics). Certain medications also warrant baseline serum drug tests (eg, obtaining fasting glucose levels and fasting lipid panels before the initiation of any atypical antipsychotics or obtaining baseline renal function and thyroid function tests before the initiation of lithium).

Review of pre-existing medication regimen

If a youngster is already taking a regimen of medications, a final step before the initiation of a new pharmacologic agent is a review of the youngster's pre-existing medication regimen. The provider should ensure that the new medication considered does not have any significant adverse interactions with other medications the patient might be taking. The youngster's regimen should also be reviewed for any redundancy of psychopharmacologic mechanism of action. Duplicate agents or those without any identified benefit should be tapered and discontinued before the initiation of any new medications, thereby reducing the risk of adverse effects secondary to polypharmacy and increasing the likelihood that a youngster is able to tolerate the new agent.

Evidence-Based Selection of Medication

Although new medications are introduced every few months, the importance of selecting evidence-based treatments cannot be overstated. Nearly all new psychotropic medications are introduced having been researched only on adult subjects. Furthermore, nearly all medications are approved with sufficient evidence stating only that they are as good as another medication already on the market and with which it is likely that providers have greater experience using in children, not to mention that most phase 3 clinical trials likely miss potentially significant rare side effects due to testing a limited number of subjects. Combining each of these facts with the knowledge that several evidence-based options for youth already exist for certain disorders, the preference to select evidence-based treatments that have a track record for safety in children is a clear one given the off-label nature of most prescribing in children.

Limiting the Total Number of Medications

As a general rule, it is important to limit the total number of medications to improve compliance with treatment, to decrease risk of drug-drug interactions, and to limit medication side effects. When starting a medication, it is important to start one medication at a time, giving preference to target symptoms that are the highest priority to resolve. Likewise, for whichever medication is started, it is important that the dosage of that medication is fully optimized before medications from the same class are added to the medication regimen. Lastly, whenever considering the addition of a medication, it is important to review all current medications to determine if other medications can be stopped.

Giving the Treatment a Chance to Work

Once a medication trial is begun, it is imperative that the plan be advanced in a deliberate manner. Although it is important not to titrate the medication at a rate in excess of what a patient can tolerate, moving too slowly is equally problematic because patients and families may give up on the medication trial before therapeutic dosages are reached. Titrating a dose at an efficient rate requires that a provider see the patient often enough to guide the titration and ensure the patient's safety (eg, in accordance with FDA recommendations, a patient started on a selective serotonin reuptake inhibitor should be seen weekly for the first month and so on[11]).

Monitoring for Efficacy and Adverse Effects

Just as standardized tools can be used in the process of diagnosis, they can also be used to serially monitor a youngster's response to initiated and/or adjusted treatment. The use of standardized assessment tools also decreases the likelihood that patients or providers might misconstrue the absence of change in symptomatic domains outside that of target symptoms as demonstrative of treatment inefficacy. Regularly monitoring for adverse effects tends to be as important as monitoring for benefits. Studies indicate that the most thorough way to assess for adverse effects is to regularly conduct a complete review of systems.[12,13]

If a patient reports an adverse effect, provider and patient should discuss whether the treatment plan should be adjusted. A candid discussion should take place to determine whether the adverse effect is tolerable or, even if tolerable, whether it is prudent to continue treatment. For those adverse effects that seem less severe, the provider may adopt a wait-and-see approach given that the adverse effects may subside in intensity or spontaneously resolve.

Maintaining Gains Made

Even after clinical gains are made such that response or remission of the target symptoms is achieved, diligence is required to maintain current gains. Clinical assessment with direct observation of the youngster should continue on a regular basis. Monitoring provides opportunities for potential medication dose adjustments and potential tapering of the medication after a period of stability. As youth grow and develop, they may require higher doses of medication (eg, as a result of greater total body mass) or lower doses of medication (eg, as a result of decreased rates of metabolism or excretion or of further cerebral development and maturation). Furthermore, achievement and progress in other areas of treatment (eg, therapy with successful development of skills that the youngster might use to better regulate emotions) may lead patient and provider to decide that less medication is required. Regular appointments also better ensure regular assessment for potential adverse effects, including those adverse effects that might increase in probability with duration of treatment (eg, tardive dyskinesia with antipsychotic medications).

Facilitating Earlier Psychiatric Consultation

In what may initially seem a paradoxic statement, one of the most important points is facilitation of earlier psychiatric consultation. Too often, referral for psychiatric evaluation is only considered in the context of a significant worsening of clinical status, such as onset of suicidal ideation, or when a patient or family is beginning to lose hope and turn to medications "as a last resort." It is important for providers to inform patients and families that waiting for symptoms to become more severe may decrease the probability of response or remission of symptoms. Furthermore, this delay may ironically place a youngster at greater risk of developing side effects because symptoms of greater severity may require medications at higher doses than might have been necessary when symptoms were less severe. Finally, the emotional valence that frequently accompanies the Hail Mary approach (which can include discouragement, desperation, and hopelessness of patient and family alike) represents a challenging therapeutic hurdle and one that places a family in the difficult position of making some of the most important decisions at a time when they are in the deepest midst of their crisis.

REFERENCES

1. Trivedi HK, Peters TE. Birth, childhood, and adolescence. In: Wedding D, Stuber ML, editors. Behavior and medicine. 5th edition. Cambridge (UK): Hogrefe and Huber; 2010. p. 31–46.
2. A development framework. In: Martin A, Volkmar FR, editors. Lewis's child and adolescent psychiatry. 4th edition. Philadelphia: Wolters Kluwer/Lippincott Williams & Wilkins; 2007. p. 252–301.
3. Greenspan SI. Chronological age and phase appropriate illustrations for each observational category. In: The clinical interview of the child. 3rd edition. Washington, DC: American Psychiatric Publishing, Inc; 2003. p. 75–98.
4. Halperin JM, Matier K, Bedi G, et al. Specificity of inattention, impulsivity, and hyperactivity to the diagnosis of attention-deficit hyperactivity disorder. J Am Acad Child Adolesc Psychiatry 1992;31:190–6.
5. Vitiello B, Stoff DM. Subtypes of aggression and their relevance to child psychiatry. J Am Acad Child Adolesc Psychiatry 1997;36:307–15.
6. Biederman J, Newcorn J, Sprinch S. Comorbidity of attention deficit hyperactivity disorder with conduct, depressive, anxiety, and other disorders. Am J Psychiatry 1991;148:564–77.
7. Angold A, Costello EJ, Erkanli A. Comorbidity. J Child Psychol Psychiatry 1999; 40:57–87.
8. Walkup JT, Albano AM, Piacentini J, et al. Cognitive behavioral therapy, sertraline, or a combination in childhood anxiety. N Engl J Med 2008;359(26):2753–66.
9. March J, Silva S, Petrycki S, et al, Treatment for Adolescents With Depression Study (TADS) Team. Fluoxetine, cognitive-behavioral therapy, and their combination for adolescents with depression: Treatment for Adolescents with Depression Study (TADS) randomized controlled trial. JAMA 2004;292(7):807–20.
10. Celexa (citalopram hydrobromide): Drug safety communication—abnormal heart rhythms associated with high doses. In: Safety information. 2011. Available at: http://www.fda.gov/Safety/MedWatch/SafetyInformation/SafetyAlertsforHuman MedicalProducts/ucm269481.htm. Accessed March 20, 2012.
11. Medication guide about using antidepressants in children and teenagers. In: Drug Safety. 2005. Available at: http://www.fda.gov/downloads/drugs/drugsafety/./UCM 161646.pdf. Accessed March 15, 2012.
12. Greenhill LL, Vitiello B, Fisher P, et al. Comparison of increasingly detailed elicitation methods for the assessment of adverse effects in pediatric psychopharmacology. J Am Acad Child Adolesc Psychiatry 2004;43:1488–96.
13. Greenhill LL, Vitiello B, Riddle MA, et al. Review of safety assessment methods used in pediatric psychopharmacology. J Am Acad Child Adolesc Psychiatry 2003;42:627–33.

Management of Psychotropic Medication Side Effects in Children and Adolescents

Georgina Garcia, MD[a,c,]*, Grace E. Logan, BA[a],
Joseph Gonzalez-Heydrich, MD[a,b,c]

KEYWORDS

- Treatment of side effects • Antidepressants • Citalopram • SSRI • Antipsychotics
- Mood Stabilizers • Stimulants • Suicide

KEY POINTS

- Side effects due to psychopharmacologic treatment in children and adolescents range from the common adverse symptoms of headache, gastrointestinal (GI) distress, weight changes, and sleep disturbances to the more rarely reported but serious adverse cardiovascular, suicidal, and hypersensitivity events.
- Frequent monitoring and assessment of children and adolescents using standardized screening measures should occur in the context of increased risk for suicidality with antidepressants and antiepileptic drugs (AEDs).
- Metabolic screening panels should be obtained at strict time points for children and adolescents initiated on antipsychotic agents.
- The small number of prospective large-scale studies in children and adolescents affects practitioners' ability to clinically interpret the risk of serious adverse events and the long-term effects of psychopharmacologic agents.

Funding sources: Dr Garcia, Nil; Grace Logan, Nil; and Dr Gonzalez-Heydrich, Tommy Fuss Foundation, the Al Rashed Family, Seaside Therapeutics, Pfizer Inc, Glaxo-SmithKline, and Johnson & Johnson.
Conflicts of interest: Dr Garcia, Nil; Grace Logan, Nil; and Dr Gonzalez-Heydrich, Previously a consultant to Abbott Laboratories, Pfizer Inc, Johnson & Johnson (Janssen, McNeil Consumer Health), Novartis, Parke-Davis, Glaxo-SmithKline, AstraZeneca, and Seaside Therapeutics; has been a speaker for Abbott Laboratories, Pfizer Inc, Novartis, and Bristol-Meyers Squibb; and has received grant support from Abbott Laboratories, Pfizer Inc, Johnson & Johnson (Janssen, McNeil Consumer Health), Akzo-Nobel/Organon, and the National Institute of Mental Health.
Disclosures statement: The authors/editors have identified the following professional or financial affiliations for themselves or their spouse/partner: Georgina Garcia, MD, is an employee at Children's Hospital Boston; Grace Logan, BA, is an employee at Children's Hospital Boston; Joseph Gonzalez-Heydrich, MD, has received industry funded research or been a consultant/speaker to the following: Tommy Fuss Foundation, the Al Rashed Family, Seaside Therapeutics, Pfizer Inc., Glaxo-SmithKline, Abbott Laboratories, Pfizer Inc, Johnson & Johnson (Janssen, McNeil Consumer Health), Novartis, Parke-Davis, AstraZeneca, Bristol-Meyers Squibb, Akzo-Nobel/Organon, and the National Institute of Mental Health.
^a Department of Psychiatry, Boston Children's Hospital, 300 Longwood Avenue, Hun 129, Boston, MA 02115, USA; ^b Psychopharmacology Clinic, Department of Psychiatry, Boston Children's Hospital, 300 Longwood Avenue, Hun 129, Boston, MA 02115, USA; ^c Harvard Medical School, Boston, MA, USA
* Corresponding author.
E-mail address: georgina.garcia@childrens.harvard.edu

Child Adolesc Psychiatric Clin N Am 21 (2012) 713–738
http://dx.doi.org/10.1016/j.chc.2012.07.012
1056-4993/12/$ – see front matter © 2012 Elsevier Inc. All rights reserved.

childpsych.theclinics.com

INTRODUCTION

Over the past 20 years there has been an explosion in the use of psychotropic medication in children in the United States. Unfortunately, there are few prospective double-blind placebo-controlled trials in children to guide clinicians in the safety and management of antidepressants, mood stabilizers stimulants, and antipsychotics. Children and adolescents represent a heterogeneous group in clinical presentation of psychiatric symptoms, response to medications, and expression of side effects. As more youth have been exposed to psychotropic medications, there has been an increasing awareness of the impact of side effects, specifically complex ones, such as suicide and metabolic syndrome. In an effort to expand the knowledge base, several large-scale prospective studies have been designed, such as Treatment for Adolescents with Depression (TADS); Multimodal Treatment Study of Children with Attention Deficit Hyperactivity Disorder (MTA); Nonrandomized Second-Generation Antipsychotic Treatment Indications, Effectiveness, and Tolerability in Youth (SATIETY); Treatment of Adolescent Suicide Attempters (TASA); and Treatment of Early-Onset Schizophrenia Spectrum Disorders (TEOSS).

An evidence-based review of the published literature on the side effects of psychotropic medications on children and adolescents is provided. Due to the large scope of side effects, some of the most commonly presenting side effects are focused on and the rare but serious effects where controversy still exists around monitoring and management (eg, suicidality and metabolic syndrome) are highlighted. Emphasis is placed on the presentation of side effects, prevalence, treatment, and management of the adverse effects associated with psychotropic medication.

ANTIDEPRESSANTS

Depression and anxiety are 2 of the most debilitating illnesses for children and adolescents in the United States, leading to an increase in the use of antidepressants (**Table 1**). Some of the most common side effects noted in the adult literature include sexual side effects, headache, nausea, weight gain, and sedation.[1] A study comparing differences in antidepressant side effects by age group found that children may be more susceptible to certain side effects, such as activation and vomiting.[2] Due to the unique vulnerabilities to certain side effects, the recent black box warnings and recommended treatment and management of cardiotoxicity and suicidality are discussed. Common somatic complaints in children (ie, headache, weight gain, and GI distress) are also discussed.

Cardiotoxicity

The risk of cardiotoxicity in the use of selective serotonin reuptake inhibitors (SSRIs) was recently highlighted by a Food and Drug Administration (FDA) advisory warning in 2011 due to the dose-dependent increase in the risk of QTc prolongation in the use of citalopram, as shown in **Table 1**.[3] The mechanism of action is postulated to be via the metabolite didesmethylcitalopram, which causes inhibition of K^+ and Ca^{2+} channels in the heart, resulting in QTc prolongation.[4,5] The effect of citalopram is generally seen within 24 hours of ingestion but has been described in one case report to occur delayed as much as 32 hours.[5] At this time, the FDA does not recommend the use of citalopram above 40 mg and above 20 mg for patients with hepatic impairment, older than 60 years of age, or taking a cytochrome P450 2C19 (CYP2C19) inhibitory agent or poor CYP2C19 metabolizers. Changes in QTc have been reported with the use of fluoxetine, sertraline, paroxetine, bupropion, venlafaxine, and trazodone.[6]

Before initiating antidepressants in children, practitioners need to assess for cardiovascular risk, including in children with known cardiac disease, family history of early

Table 1
Antidepressant medications and their side effects

Class	Generic Name (Trade Names)	Common Side Effects	Rare and/or Serious Side Effects
Azapirone	Buspirone (Buspar)	Changes in cognition Dry mouth Sedation Headache Dizziness Excitement Extrapyramidal reactions GI discomfort Increase in prolactin and growth hormones Parasthesias	Hypersensitivity reaction Tachycardia/palpitations Serotonin syndrome if combined with other serotonin potentiating agents or monoamine oxidase inhibitors (MAOIs)
MAOs Reversible MAO-A Irreversible MAO Selective inhibitor MAO-B	Moclobemide (Aurorix, Manerix) Isocarboxazid (Enerzer, Marplan, Marplon) Phenelzine (Nardil, Nardelzine) Tranylcypromine (Parnate, Jatrosom) Selegiline transdermal system (Emsam)	Sedation Insomnia Excitement Headache Dry mouth Extrapyramidal effects (ie, tremor) Orthostatic hypotension Tachycardia GI discomfort Weight gain Sexual dysfunction	Cardiac arrhythmia ECG changes Mania Seizures Serotonin syndrome (when mixed with other serotonin potentiating drugs or foods) Withdrawal/discontinuation syndrome
Noradrenergic specific serotonergic agent	Mirtazapine (Remeron)	Sedation Headache Dry mouth Blurred vision Constipation GI discomfort Weight gain Sexual dysfunction	Cardiac arrhythmia ECG changes Mania Serotonin syndrome mania Seizures Serotonin syndrome (when mixed with other serotonin potentiating drugs)
Norepinephrine dopamine reuptake inhibitor	Bupropion (Wellbutrin)	Insomnia Excitement Headache Dry mouth Blurred vision Constipation Sweating GI discomfort Dermatitis, rash Weight loss Sexual dysfunction	Cardiac arrhythmia ECG changes Hypersensitivity reactions Mania Seizures (increased risk with purging) Withdrawal/discontinuation syndrome

(continued on next page)

Table 1
(continued)

Class	Generic Name (Trade Names)	Common Side Effects	Rare and/or Serious Side Effects
Serotonin-2 antagonist/ reuptake inhibitor	Trazodone (Desyrel)	Sedation Insomnia Excitement Headache Hyponatremia Dry mouth Extrapyramidal effects (ie, tremor) Orthostatic hypotension GI discomfort Weight gain Sexual dysfunction/ priapism	Abnormal bleeding Cardiac arrhythmia ECG changes Mania Seizures Serotonin syndrome (when mixed with other serotonin potentiating drugs or foods) Suicidality Withdrawal/ discontinuation syndrome
Serotonin-norepinephrine reuptake inhibitor	Venlafaxine (Effexor) Duloxetine (Cymbalta)	Sedation Insomnia Excitement Headache Hyponatremia Confusion Dry mouth Sweating Hypertension Orthostatic hypotension GI discomfort Sexual dysfunction	Abnormal bleeding Cardiac arrhythmia ECG changes Mania Seizures Serotonin syndrome (when mixed with other serotonin potentiating drugs) Suicidality Withdrawal/ discontinuation syndrome
SSRI	Citalopram (Celexa) Escitalopram (Lexapro) Fluvoxamine (Luvox, Luvox CR) Fluoxetine (Prozac, Sarafem, Symbyax) Paroxetine (Paxil, Prexeva) Sertraline (Zoloft)	Sedation Insomnia Excitement Headache Dry mouth Blurred vision Extrapyramidal effects (ie, tremor) Hyponatremia Orthostatic hypotension Tachycardia GI discomfort Weight gain Sexual dysfunction	Abnormal bleeding Cardiac arrhythmia ECG changes (Qtc prolongation) Mania Serotonin syndrome mania Seizures Serotonin syndrome (when mixed with other serotonin potentiating drugs) Suicidality Withdrawal/ discontinuation syndrome

(continued on next page)

Table 1 (continued)			
Class	Generic Name (Trade Names)	Common Side Effects	Rare and/or Serious Side Effects
SSRI plus 5-HT1a agonist	Vilazodone (Viibryd)	Sedation Insomnia Excitement Headache Dry mouth Blurred vision Extrapyramidal effects (ie, tremor) Hyponatremia Orthostatic hypotension Tachycardia GI discomfort Weight gain Sexual dysfunction	Abnormal bleeding Cardiac arrhythmia ECG changes Hypersensitivity reactions Seizures Suicidality Mania Serotonin syndrome (when mixed with other serotonin potentiating drugs) Withdrawal/ discontinuation syndrome
Tricyclic antidepressants	Amitriptyline (Elavil, Endep, Vanatrip) Clomipramine (Anafranil) Desipramine (Norpramin, Pertofrane) Doxepin (Silenor, Sinequan, Adapin) Imipramine (Tofranil) Nortriptyline (Aventyl, Pamelor) Protriptyline (Vivactil) Trimipramine (Surmontil)	Sedation Insomnia Excitement Headache Anticholinergic effects Extrapyramidal effects Orthostatic hypotension GI discomfort Weight gain Sexual dysfunction ECG changes (including prolongation of QT interval)	Cardiac arrhythmia Hypersensitivity reactions Seizures Mania Withdrawal/ discontinuation syndrome

cardiac disease, electrolyte imbalances due to disease (eg, bulimia or anorexia) or medications (eg, potassium-lowering diuretics), or concurrent use of medications that may prolong the QTc or those taking medications that impair metabolism of the prescribed antidepressant (eg, CYP2C19 inhibitors when citalopram is prescribed). If any of these cardiovascular risk factors is identified and an antidepressant is prescribed, it is recommended to obtain an ECG and/or electrolyte monitoring prior to treatment per FDA recommendation and after initiation of medication.[3,6] If a patient has a prolonged QTc, providers may preferentially choose escitalopram over citalopram due to its lower dose-dependent impact on QTc prolongation.[3] If patients are at risk of an electrolyte imbalance, they should be assessed at baseline and periodically for potassium and magnesium levels.[3]

Suicidality

Suicide is the third leading cause of death in youths in the United States and a leading cause of death in other countries.[7] The relationship between suicide and the use of antidepressants has been a safety concern since the 1990s and received critical attention in 2004 when the FDA issued a black box warning regarding antidepressants and the risk of suicide.[8] The black box warning was initially issued for children and adolescents and extended in 2006 to young adults ages 18 to 25 years.[9] The warning extends to all medications used in the treatment of depression/anxiety, not just SSRIs. There were no completed suicides in any of the analyzed clinical trials; however, the pediatric age group was found to have a higher risk of suicidal thoughts or actions while taking an antidepressant than while taking placebo.[8,10] This risk seems age specific because older patients seem to have a lower risk of suicidality while on antidepressants compared with young adults.[9–12] These findings are contrary to a head-to-head study of fluoxetine and venlafaxine indicating that the use of these medications can reduce suicidal thoughts.[13] Similarly, a 27-year longitudinal study from 5 academic institutions with prospective assessments found that antidepressants were associated with a reduction in the risk of suicide attempts of suicide by 20%.[14]

The mechanism connecting increased suicidality and antidepressants is unclear, but drug-induced disinhibition (DID), or activation syndrome, has been hypothesized to contribute to self-harm behavior. Antidepressants can cause moderate agitation, insomnia, irritability, hyperarousal, aggressivity, restlessness, impulsivity, social withdrawal, hypomania/mania, psychosis, or disinhibition.[15–17] It can often be managed by reducing the antidepressant dose or stopping the antidepressant but rarely requires additional medication. When the symptoms of DID or activation syndrome are severe and/or they continue after stopping the antidepressants, they are thought to constitute what is variously termed, antidepressant-induced mania, switching, or treatment-emergent mania.[18–20] Some of these symptoms can be difficult to distinguish from antidepressant-induced akathisia, which may similarly respond to dose reduction or switching antidepressants and rarely requires antiparkinsonian agents or β-blockers. To distinguish antidepressant-induced mania or treatment-emergent mania from DID/activation, it has been recommended to observe for changes in mood/state from depressive to euphoric with symptoms of grandiosity, pressured speech/thoughts, and hypersexuality.[21] Additional studies are required with clear definitions of changes in mood state as opposed to activation to elucidate the impact on suicidality.

When interpreting the literature and developing best clinical practice, clinicians must weigh the proved efficacy in meta-analysis of antidepressants in the treatment of depression against the FDA's warning of the potential increased risk of suicide in treating children and adolescents (**Table 2**).[22] Providers should assess for risk factors associated with suicide, including female gender, family history of suicide, higher rate of depression, greater number of suicide attempts, acute stressful events (eg, illness, war, and trauma), chronic adversity, bullying, poverty, and negative family relationships.[23–27] Prescribers need to monitor for any increase in their patients' impulses or suicidal ideation at distinct intervals (see **Table 2**). Given the complex interaction between biologic, psychological, and social factors, clinicians should also be aware of the successful use of adjunctive treatments to antidepressants, such as cognitive behavioral therapy, which has been found to give some protection from suicidal acts and can aid in the reduction of depressive symptoms.[23,28–31]

Common Somatic Side Effects

Headache, GI distress, and weight gain are commonly reported side effects of antidepressants that may have an impact on medication compliance.[32] A recent study by Andersen and colleagues[33] of claims data for 40,017 patients in the United States identified headache and nausea as 2 of the most common complaints reported in adults and adolescents.

Table 2
Black box warnings issued by the FDA indicating potential serious side effects for common psychotropic medications

Generic drug name	Serious Risks	Monitoring Recommendations	Issue Date
Antidepressants	Increased risk of suicidal thoughts or behavioral	Children and adolescents should be monitored for changes in thoughts and behavior.[a]	2004 (Children and adolescents), 2006 (young adults)
AEDs	Increased risk of suicidal thoughts or behavioral	Children and adolescents should be monitored for changes in thoughts and behavior[a]	2008
Citalopram	QT-interval prolongation at doses >40 mg	Patients with QT syndrome, congestive heart failure, bradyarrhythmias, or predisposition to hypokalemia or hypomagnesemia should be monitored via ECG if requiring treatment with citalopram.	2011, revised in 2012
Lamotrigine	Stevens-Johnson syndrome Aseptic meningitis Increased risk of suicidal thoughts or behavior	Patients should be advised of the risk and know to monitor the early warning signs of a hypersensitivity reaction. If suspected cause of aseptic meningitis, lamotrigine should be discontinued. Providers should be aware that in a few cases of aseptic meningitis, underlying autoimmune disorders were also identified. Children and adolescents should be monitored for changes in thoughts and behavior.[a]	2006, 2010, 2008
Stimulant agents and atomoxetine	Cardiovascular events	Children with serious heart conditions or vulnerable to increases in blood pressure/heart rate should avoid these medications. Blood pressure/heart rate should be monitored in all children with ADHD prescribed these agents.	2009, revised in 2011

[a] Monitoring should occur weekly for weeks 1–4 of treatment, biweekly during weeks 5–8, monthly after the first 2 months, and within 1 week after dose adjustment.

Alterations in norepinephrine and serotonin can have an impact on pain transmission in the central nervous system and are implicated in the causes of headaches.[34] For this reason, several studies have explored the use of antidepressants in the treatment of migraines.[34,35] A 2005 Cochrane review, however, found that compared with placebo, SSRIs were not effective in the treatment of migraines.[36] The frequency and severity of headache can sometimes be reduced by switching to another antidepressant, especially one with a different mechanism. If a patient cannot be easily switched to another antidepressant, however, the headache may still be treated with the addition of a medication with an antimigraine effect. For this reason, amitriptyline may be considered as either an antidepressant alternative or adjunctive medication because it has been extensively studied and found effective for the treatment of migraines in adults and children.[36]

GI distress is also a commonly reported side effect experienced by approximately 15% to 24% of pediatric patients taking antidepressants.[2,32] GI side effects are generally understood as a consequence of the high density of serotonin receptors within the GI tract being stimulated by the higher levels of serotonin after SSRI blockade.[1,2] Several strategies have been recommended to reduce GI side effects, including initiating antidepressants at low doses. Providers may also recommend either divided doses or taking medication with food.[37] Patients presenting with severe nausea, vomiting, and anorexia should be evaluated with laboratory panels to assess for pancreatitis. Pancreatitis is a rare but serious side effect that has been associated with the use of SSRIs.[38,39] It is generally not recommended to screen for liver and pancreatic enzymes when treating children and adolescents with antidepressants unless there is an identified risk factor (eg, cystic fibrosis or patients taking immunomodulators or monoamine oxidase inhibitors) or persistent GI symptoms are present.[40,41]

A systematic chart review of children and adolescents taking SSRIs reported a 9% weight gain.[32] It seems that changes in weight and depressive symptoms are linked but that the causal direction is not clear. Antidepressants have been hypothesized to contribute to weight gain via changes in serotonin 5-HT_{2c} receptor activity having an impact on appetite regulation.[42,43] Conversely, weight loss due to anhedonia or withdrawal symptoms and weight gain due to overeating are core symptoms of depression, and identified changes in weight can also represent treatment or remission of symptoms. Fava[44] found in a double-blind study of paroxetine, sertraline, and fluoxetine that 25.5% of the patients on paroxetine had an increase in weight. Bupropion, a norepinephrine-dopamine reuptake inhibitor, has been shown in multiple studies to result in dose-dependent 2.4-lb to 10-lb weight loss.[45–47] Mirtazapine has serotoninergic and noradrenergic impact, which has a significant H_2 receptor blocking effect that has been found to increased weight gain compared with placebo.[48–50] A recent meta-analysis and several longitudinal mental health studies have identified obesity as a risk factor for developing depression.[51–53] Due to the complex relationship between weight gain, depression, and medication, clinicians should tailor their treatments to each patient's predisposition to weight gain, premorbid body habitus, gender, coping skills, and previous responses to medications prior to initiating antidepressant therapy.

ANTIPSYCHOTICS

Despite the ongoing debate about the use of antipsychotic medications in children, the prescribing of these medications continues to rise (**Table 3**).[54–56] Antipsychotics are FDA approved for the treatment of schizophrenia, mood stabilization, and autism in children. A recent comparison of first-generation versus second-generation

Table 3
Antipsychotic medications and their side effects

Class	Generic Name (Trade Names)	Common Side Effects	Rare and/or Serious Side Effects
First-generation antipsychotics	• Chlorpromazine (Largactil, Thorazine) • Fluphenazine (Moditen, Prolixin, Modecate) • Haolperidol (Haldol) • Loxapine (Loxapac, Loxitane) • Methotrimeprazine (Nosinan, Nizinan, Levoprome) • Molindone (Moban) • Pericyazine (Neuleptil) • Perphenazine (Trilafon) • Pimozide (Orap) • Thioridazine (Mellaril)	• Drowsiness • Sedation • Insomnia • Agitation • Parkinsonism • Akathisia • Hypotension • ECG changes • Sexual dysfunction • Galactorrhea • Weight gain • Hyperglycemia • Hyperlipidemia • Photosensitivity • Rash • Pigmentation (lenticular or skin) • Pigmentary retinopathy • Hepatic disorder	• Blood dyscrasias • Dystonias • Neuroleptic malignant syndrome • Seizures • Tardive dyskinesia • Qtc prolongation • Suicide • Increased morbidity in elderly patients with dementia • Hypersensitivity reaction (asenapine)
Second-generation antipsychotics	• Asenapine (Saphris) • Clozapine (Clozaril) • Iloperidone (Fanapt) • Lurasidone (Latuda) • Olanzapine (Zyprexa) • Risperidone (Risperdal) • Paliperidone (Invega) • Quetiapine (Seroquel) • Ziprasidone (Geodon)		
Third-generation antipsychotics	• Aripiprazole (Abilify)		

antipsychotics has found minimal differences between side effects and discontinuation rates.[57] For this reason, this article does not differentiate between first-generation and second-generation antipsychotics and focuses on movement disorders and metabolic syndrome as both can have significant and persistent long-term impact on children and adolescents.

Movement Disorders

The development of antipsychotic-induced movement disorders should be considered in the treatment of children. Extrapyramidal side effects (EPS) can encompass dystonia, tardive dyskinesia, akathisia, and bradykinesia/drug-induced parkinsonism. EPS symptoms are caused by D_2 receptor antagonism in the nigrostriatal pathway that can cause sustained contractions, repetitive motions (most often of the small muscles of the neck, jaw, and tongue), restlessness, tremor, akinesia, and rigidity. The prevalence in adolescents in a cross-sectional study found that patients suffered from the following: parkinsonism (25.8%), tardive dyskinesia (39.8%), and akathisia

(11.8%). In the United Kingdom, the Pediatric Atypical Antipsychotic Monitoring Safety study reported a 3% prevalence of EPS.[58] The risk of developing movement disorders has been related to length of exposure to the antipsychotic, suggesting an increased sensitization of D_2 receptors.[59] Although it has been reported that second-generation antipsychotics cause fewer movement disorders than typical antipsychotics, several randomized controlled trials have had conflicting results indicating a need for further studies.[60–62]

Providers should monitor patients on antipsychotics with a standardized movement rating scale (eg, Abnormal Involuntary Movement Scale or Barnes Akathisia Rating Scale) at regular intervals. Also, clinicians should be aware of both exacerbation of movements due to withdrawal of the antipsychotic or rebound due to switching to an antipsychotic with lower affinity for receptors.[63] Neuroleptic-induced EPS can be treated with anticholinergic agents, benzodiazepines, β-blockers, vitamin E, switching antipsychotic agents, benzodiazepines, amantadine, or naloxone.[64–66]

Metabolic Syndrome

Metabolic syndrome was first identified nearly 50 years ago when it was described by the World Health Organization and the National Cholesterol Education Program Adult Treatment Panel. Metabolic syndrome has been increasingly studied in the past 10 years due in part to concern over the increases in psychotropic prescribing practices and polypharmacy in the United States.[54,56] The National Health and Nutrition Examination Survey, from 1999 to 2002, reported that the rate of metabolic syndrome varies from 2% to greater than 9% depending on the diagnostic criteria applied.[67]

Metabolic syndrome has been previously described with great variability as multiple metabolic syndrome, syndrome X, and insulin resistance syndrome by the National Cholesterol Education Program, World Health Organization, International Diabetes Federation, National Institute of Health Pediatric Metabolic Syndrome Working Group, and American Diabetes Association. The key components of metabolic syndrome include changes in weight, blood pressure, cholesterol, and glucose intolerance (**Table 4**). There is a complex relationship between metabolic syndrome and obesity, indicating that it may be a bidirectional relationship with significant impact on cardiovascular morbidity and mortality.[68–70] Weight gain and obesity have been associated with an increase in elevated blood pressure, coronary artery disease, dyslipidemia, colorectal cancer, insulin resistance, type 2 diabetes mellitus, and inflammatory responses.[70,71] Metabolic syndrome is also a risk factor for the development of polycystic ovarian syndrome, obstructive sleep apnea, inflammation, smoking, endothelial dysfunction, and abnormal liver tests.[67] The relationship between antipsychotic use and the increased risk of insulin resistance, weight gain, type 2 diabetes, and dyslipidemia has been well documented in multiple pediatric studies.[72–76] Given that antipsychotics have been found effective in the treatment of psychiatric disorders, it is of critical importance that practitioners understand the risks of treatment and monitor patients carefully for metabolic syndrome.[55,76–79]

Treatment and management of children and adolescents with antipsychotics should include the following key components: review and identification of risk factors, regular monitoring of metabolic markers, and identification of potential modifiers to the development of metabolic syndrome (ie, lifestyle and polypharmacy). When risk factors pertaining to weight gain are present at baseline, practitioners should preferentially avoid medications that have consistently been associated with weight gain (clozapine, olanzapine, and risperidone) and preferentially choose medications, such as aripiprazole.[69,72,76,80–82] In patients with known cardiovascular risks, providers may choose to avoid ziprazidone, which has been associated with an increased risk of prolonged

Table 4
The International Diabetes Federation[a] pediatric definition of metabolic syndrome and additional risk factors identified by the Adult Treatment Panel III and the World Health Organization

Pediatric Risk Factors and Clinical Parameters Defined by IDF[a]	Clinical Cutoff Scores Defined for Children and Adolescents by IDF[a] (ages 10–<16)	Clinical Cutoff Scores Defined for Adolescents (ages ≥16) and Adults by IDF[a]
Obesity[a,b,c]	Central/abdominal obesity, waist: hip ratio, or BMI	Waist circumference ≥90th percentile	Waist circumference: male, ≥94 cm; female, ≥80 cm
Glucose metabolism impairment[a,b,c]	Increased fasting glucose, decreased glucose tolerance	Fasting plasma glucose ≥5.6 mmol/L (100 mg/dL) or T2DM	Fasting plasma glucose ≥5.6 mmol/L (100 mg/dL) or T2DM
Dyslipidemia[a,b,c]		Triglyceride levels ≥1.7 mmol/L (150 mg/dL)	Triglyceride levels ≥1.7 mmol/L (150 mg/dL)
Decreased HDL cholesterol[a,b]		HDL cholesterol <1.03 mmol/L (40 mg/dL)	HDL cholesterol: male, <1.03 mmol/L (40 mg/dL); female, <1.29 mmol/L (50 mg/dL), or specific treatment for low HDL
Hypertension[a,b,c]	Elevated systolic or diastolic pressure	Systolic pressure ≥130 mm Hg, diastolic pressure ≥85 mm Hg	Systolic pressure ≥130 mm Hg, diastolic pressure ≥85 mm Hg
Additional Risk Factors and Clinical Parameters Defined by the ATP-III[c] and WHO for Adults		**Clinical Cutoff Scores Defined by Adult Consensus Guidelines**	
Insulin resistance[b]	Hyperinsulinemia	Insulin resistance as measured by the homeostatic model assessment and/or the quantitative insulin sensitivity check index	
Microalbuminemia[b]	Urinary albumin excretion rate, albumin: creatine ratio	Urinary albumin excretion rate ≥20 μg/min or albumin: creatine ratio ≥3.4 mg/mmol	
Inflammation[c]	Increased cytokine and CRP release	Elevated CRP	
Hypercoagulability[c]	Increased plasma plasminogen activator inhibitor type 1 or fibrinogen	Elevated thrombotic state ± elevated inflammatory markers	

Abbreviations: ATP-III, Adult Treatment Panel III; CRP, C-reactive protein; IDF, International Diabetes Federation; T2DM, type 2 diabetes mellitus; WHO, World Health Organization.

[a] IDF defines metabolic syndrome for ages 10–<16 as 3 of the above child and adolescent risk factors co-occurring. *Data from* Zimmet P, Alberti KG, Kaufman F, et al. IDF Consensus Group. The metabolic syndrome in children and adolescents—an IDF consensus report. Pediatr Diabetes 2007;8:299–306.

[b] WHO defines metabolic syndrome in adults as 2 of the above risk factors co-occurring with T2DM or glucose metabolism impairment/insulin resistance. *Data from* Grundy SM, Brewer HB, Cleeman JI, et al. NHLBI/AHA Conference Proceedings. Circulation 2004;109:433–8.

[c] ATP-III defines metabolic syndrome in adults as 3 out of 5 of the above co-occurring risk factors. *Data from* Grundy SM, Brewer HB, Cleeman JI, et al. NHLBI/AHA Conference Proceedings. Circulation 2004;109:433–8.

Qtc interval.[72,79,82] Patients at risk for dyslipidemia may not be candidates for olanzapine or risperidone, which have been associated with clinically significant negative effects on lipid profiles.[72,76] The authors recognize that no consistent guidelines around monitoring practices exist, although this article summarizes the evidence-based guidelines proposed for metabolic monitoring (**Table 5** as possible best clinical practice guidelines.

MOOD STABILIZERS

As a class of agents, mood stabilizers represent the most pharmacokinetically heterogeneous medication treatment for children and adolescents (**Table 6**). As a result, the literature has been sparse in controlled head-to-head trials and large trials of efficacy and safety in children. What has been published in the literature has been predominantly on the use of AEDs in adult populations and in children with epilepsy. In an effort to consolidate the literature, the black box warnings for suicidality and anticonvulsant hypersensitivity syndrome are discussed because of their generalizability to most mood stabilizers. Additionally, lithium and renal toxicity are addressed because of their increasing importance in response to the concerns about suicidality and metabolic syndrome with the use of antipsychotics as mood stabilizers.

Suicidality

In 2008, an FDA scientific advisory committee reviewed and analyzed 199 placebo-controlled trials of 11 AEDs and released a warning about the significant association between the use of antiepileptic medications and suicidality.[83] They reported the risk of patients taking AEDs was twice the risk of suicide (0.43%) compared with placebo (0.22%).[83] It is estimated that 25% to 50% of patients with bipolar disorder report suicide attempts during treatment and that the lifetime risk of suicide is approximately 15 times higher than in the general population.[84-86] This warning was particularly concerning because epidemiologic studies have shown that patients with epilepsy have a 5-fold higher rate of suicide than the general population.[87] One cohort of 44,300 patients with epilepsy treated with AEDs found a 3-fold increased risk of self-harm/suicidal behavior.[88] Another cohort study, of more than 5 million patients from the United Kingdom who had used AEDs, found that patients with epilepsy or bipolar disorder did not have an increase in suicide-related events but that there was an increased risk in patients with depression.[89] A 30-year observational study at 5 institutions in the United States found that the risk of suicide attempts or suicide was not associated with the use of AEDs.[90] The only clear conclusion that can be made of the literature at this time is that more prospective, controlled trials with the use of AEDs using evidence-based measures of suicide and parasuicidal behavior are required to clarify the relationship between the use of AEDs and suicide. In the interim, providers should screen all patients taking AEDs for increased suicidality because 2 of the more frequent diagnostic categories are associated with a marked increased risk for suicide.

Anticonvulsant Hypersensitivity Syndrome

The first cases of a hypersensitivity reaction to anticonvulsants were reported in 1950. It has been identified in the literature as antiepileptic hypersensitivity syndrome (AHS), drug hypersensitivity syndrome (DHS), and drug reaction with eosinophilia and systemic symptoms.[91-93] It was first recognized as a response to aromatic AEDs but since then has been expanded to include other classifications of medications. The mechanism of AHS is an immune reaction to the toxic metabolites of the (typically) aromatic anticonvulsant leading to cell death. AHS is characterized by fever,

Table 5
Recommended metabolic screening and assessments for children and adolescents using atypical antipsychotics

Recommended Screening Parameters	Recommended Reference	Recommended Assessment Schedule[a,b]
Fasting plasma glucose	≤5.6–6.1[c] mmol/L[a]	Baseline; 3 mo, 6 mo, and 12 mo; then, annually
Fasting insulin	≤100 pmol/L[a]	Baseline; 3 mo, 6 mo, and 12 mo; then, annually
OGTT		*When fasting plasma glucose = 5.6–6.1 or fasting insulin levels >100 pmol/L[a]*
Waist circumference	Percentile	Baseline; 1 mo, 2 mo, 3 mo, 6 mo, 9 mo, and 12 mo; then annually
Height (cm)	Percentile	Baseline; 1 mo, 2 mo, 3 mo, 6 mo, 9 mo, and 12 mo; then, annually
Weight (kg)	Percentile	Baseline; 1 mo, 2 mo, 3 mo, 6 mo, 9 mo, and 12 mo; then, annually
BMI (kg/m^2)	Percentile	Baseline; 1 mo, 2 mo, 3 mo, 6 mo, 9 mo, and 12 mo; then, annually
Blood pressure (mm Hg)	Percentile	Baseline; 1 mo, 2 mo, 3 mo, 6 mo, 9 mo, and 12 mo; then, annually
Fasting total cholesterol	<5.2 mmol/L[a]	Baseline; 3 mo, 6 mo, and 12 mo; then, annually
Fasting LDL-C	<3.35 mmol/L[a]	Baseline; 3 mo, 6 mo, and 12 mo; then, annually
Fasting HDL-C	≥1.05 mmol/L[a]	Baseline; 3 mo, 6 mo, and 12 mo; then, annually
Fasting triglycerides	<1.5 mmol/L[a]	Baseline; 3 mo, 6 mo, and 12 mo; then, annually
Neurologic testing: Abnormal Involuntary Movement Scale, Simpson Angus Scale, Extrapyramidal Symptom Rating Scale, Barnes Akathisia Rating Scale		Baseline; 1 mo, 2 mo, 3 mo, 6 mo, 9 mo, and 12 mo; then, annually
AST		Baseline; 6 mo and 12 mo; then, annually
ALT		Baseline; 6 mo and 12 mo; then, annually
TSH		Baseline; 6 mo and 12 mo; then, annually
Prolactin		Baseline; 3 mo and 12 mo; then, annually
ECG		*Unknown*
Pharmacogenetics		*Unknown*

Abbreviations: HDL-C, high-density lipoprotein cholesterol; LDL, low-density lipoprotein cholesterol; OGTT, oral glucose tolerance test; TSH, thyroid-stimulating hormone.

[a] *Data from* Pringsheim T, Panagiotopoulos C, Davidson J, et al. CAMESA Guideline Group. Evidence-based recommendations for monitoring safety of second generation antipsychotics in children and youth. J Can Acad Child Adolesc Psychiatry 2011;20:218–33. Although CAMESA does not recommend specific monitoring guidelines after month 12, it is standard practice to monitor annually thereafter.

[b] *Data from* Correll CU. Antipsychotic use in children and adolescents: minimizing adverse effects to maximize outcomes. J Am Acad Child Adolesc Psychiatry 2008;47:9–20.

[c] *Data from* IDF Consensus Group International Diabetes Federation. The IDF consensus worldwide definition of the metabolic syndrome. International Diabetes Federation (IDF), 2006. www.idf.org/webdata/docs/IDF_Meta_def_final.pdf. Accessed August 23, 2012.

Table 6
Mood stabilizers and their side effects

Class	Generic Name (Trade Names)	Common Side Effects	Rare and/or Serious Side Effects
Lithium carbonate	Lithium (Carbolith, Cibalith-S, Eskalith, Lithane, Lithobid)	Drowsiness Fatigue Cognitive blunting Muscle weakness Incoordination GI discomfort Hypothyroidism Hyperparathyroidism Bradycardia ECG changes Pruritis Acne Blurred vision	Renal toxicity Blood dyscrasias Discontinuation syndrome Lithium toxicity Fetal malformations
Anticonvulsants	Carbamazepine (Carbatrol, Epitol, Equitro, Tegretol) Gabapentin (Fanatrex, Gabarone, Gralise, Neurontin, Nupetin) Lamotrigine (Lamictal) Oxcarbazepine (Trileptal) Pregabalin (Lyrica) Topiramate (Topamax, Topiragen) Valproate (Depacon, Depakote, Depakene, Stavzor) Zonisamide (Zonegran)	Sedation Cognitive blunting Restlessness/agitation Anxiety Anticholinergic side effects Abdominal discomfort Nausea Vomiting Weight changes ($\pm$) Dizziness Edema Liver enzyme elevations Menstrual disturbances Sexual dysfunction Dose-dependent decreases in platelets and absolute neutrophil count	Blood dyscrasias Severe bone marrow suppression Hepatic toxicity Hyponatremia Nephrolithiasis Occular side effects Osteopenia/osteoporosis Reduced growth rate Rash/hypersensitivity syndrome Stevens-Johnson syndrome Metabolic acidosis

eosinophilia, rash, lymphadenopathy, coagulopathy, and internal organ involvement. In severe cases, AHS can progress to Stevens-Johnson syndrome or toxic epidermal necrosis. The onset of AHS classically begins with initiation of the medication and differs in onset by drug and is not related to a dosage or serum concentration of anticonvulsants.[93] AHS is reported to occur in approximately 1 in 1000 to 1 in 10,000 exposures.[92,94] Mansur and colleagues[95] reported on 31 patients who presented with AHS in response to the following agents: carbamazepine (48.38%), phenytoin (35.48%), lamotrigine (9.6%), and combined valproic acid and lamotrigine (6.45%).

Due to the heterogeneous presentation of AHS, clinicians should be vigilant for the key symptoms present in almost all cases: fever, rash, and organ failure/hepatotoxicity.[91] Treatment of AHS is generally discontinuation of offending agent, supportive management (antihistamines, topical corticosteroids, and proton pump inhibitors), and avoidance of hepatotoxic medications, such as nonsteroidal anti-inflammatory drugs. The use of corticosteroids, plasmapheresis, and intravenous immunoglobulin has not been studied in case-controlled studies and the risks versus benefits reviewed carefully due to their ability to worsen symptoms.[91,92] Due to the cross-reactivity between aromatic AEDs, providers need to be conscious when choosing alternative medication and their charts should be labeled with an allergy to phenytoin, carbamazepine, phenobarbital, primidone, and lamotrigine.[91] Lamotrigine rechallenge has been cited in the literature in a case series of 27 cases with an 85% success rate and in a meta-analysis of 48 published cases with an 85% success rate.[96]

Renal Toxicity

The increased diagnosis and treatment of pediatric bipolar disorder has resulted in an increase in the use of anticonvulsants and lithium.[97,98] One study looking at prescriptive practice from 1991 to 1998 reported a 73% increase in the use of mood stabilizers.[98] Due to the increased awareness of the side effects of mood stabilizers in children, in particular the concern of metabolic syndrome and antipsychotics, there seems to be a resurgence of interest in lithium. Lithium is FDA approved for the treatment of children 12 years and older for bipolar disorder but is often avoided by practitioners due to the concern for renal damage, hypothyroidism, hyperparathyroidism, and weight gain. Lithium causes damage to the sodium channels in the renal collecting tubes, resulting in nephrogenic diabetes insipidus.[99] Few longitudinal studies have been completed in children looking at the long-term impact of these side effects. Recently, McKnight and colleagues[100] published a meta-analysis encompassing 5988 abstracts and 385 studies from 1966 to 2010, concluding an absolute risk of renal failure of 0.5% (18/3369 patients).

It is recommended that prior to initiation providers should check the following—serum urea nitrogen, creatinine, thyroid function, calcium level, white blood count, and weight (measured body mass index [BMI])—and obtain an ECG.[100–102] There is little consensus on the frequency of repeating lithium levels, renal function, thyroid function, weight (BMI), and calcium levels, but best clinical practice indicates between 3 and 6 months for each with the addition of ECG annually unless clinically indicated.[100–102] Practioners should also be aware of any concomitant treatment with diuretics, nonsteroidal anti-inflammatory drugs, angiotensin-converting enzyme inhibitors, or other medications that could reduce renal excretion of lithium.[101]

STIMULANTS

Attention-deficit/hyperactivity disorder (ADHD) has an impact on approximately 4% to 10% of children in the United States (**Table 7**).[103] Although stimulant products have been extensively studied for efficacy and tolerability, there has been an increased public concern about the long-term side effects with the use of stimulants. Many of the short-term side effects, such as GI discomfort and tics, are easily ameliorated by discontinuation, lowering dosage, or switching medications. For this reason, emphasis is placed on the risk of cardiotoxicity and long-term growth deficits. Sleep disturbances are reviewed because they are a common side effect that has an impact on tolerance and compliance across all stimulants.

Insomnia

Sleep disturbance is one of the most common side effects reported with the treatment of ADHD. The rates of sleep disturbances in ADHD reported in the literature range from 25% to 50%, as compared to 7% in controls.[104] Children with ADHD reportedly have more difficulties with initiating and maintaining sleep, nocturnal awakenings, parasomnias, early morning awakenings, restless leg syndrome, obstructive sleep apnea, and enuresis.[105–107]

Despite the myriad complex factors involved in the management of sleep disturbances in the treatment of ADHD, there are several strategies that can be used to reduce sleep disturbances. The first recommendation is careful assessment and

Table 7
Stimulant and nonstimulant medications and their side effects

Class	Generic Name (Trade Names)	Common Side Effects	Rare and/or Serious Side Effects
Amphetamine products	Dextroamphetamine (Dexedrine, Dextrostat) Methamphetamine (Desoxyn) Dextroamphetamine/ amphetamine salts (Adderall) Lisdexamfetamine (Vyvanse)	Activation/restlessness Anticholinergic symptoms Anxiety Delayed growth Insomnia Irritability GI symptoms Headache Mood symptoms Rebound depression Sexual dysfunction Social withdrawal Tics/Tourette exacerbation Uticaria	Cardiovascular (tachycardia, hypertension/ hypotension, palpitations) Exacerbate psychosis or mania Lower seizure threshold (not usually significant, can be used cautiously in patients with epilepsy)
Methylphenidate products	Methylphenidate (Ritalin, Methylin, Metadate CD, Concerta, Biphentin) Methylphenidate transdermal system (Daytrana) Dexmethylphenidate (Focalin/Focalin XR)	Activation/restlessness Anticholinergic symptoms Anxiety Contact sensitization/ dermatitis with transdermal Delayed growth Insomnia Irritability GI symptoms Headache Mood symptoms Rebound depression Social withdrawal Tics/Tourette exacerbation Upper respiratory infections/ inflammation	Cardiovascular (tachycardia, hypertension/ hypotension, palpitations) Exacerbate psychosis/ or mania Blood dyscrasias, leukopenia Lower seizure threshold (not usually significant, can be used cautiously in patients with epilepsy)
Selective norepinephrine reuptake inhibitor	Atomoxetine (Strattera)	Anticholinergic symptoms Appetite/weight loss GI symptoms Headache Insomnia Mood symptoms	Hypertension/ hypotension Suicide Hepatic injury
α_2-Adrenergic agonist	Clonidine (Catapres, Kapvay) Guanfacine (Tenex, Intuniv)	Anxiety Agitation/delirium Dermatologic Dry mouth Headache Hypotension GI symptoms Insomnia Sedation Sexual side effects Sleep disturbances	Bradycardia Cardiovascular complications possible when used with psychostimulants Hypotension/rebound hypertension Hypotension $\pm$ syncope Mania

documentation of premorbid sleep disturbances because children with ADHD are at 5-fold increased risk of disturbances. Unfortunately, assessments of adverse reactions to methylphenidate treatments have failed to find any personal or clinical characteristics of patients that might indicate patients at risk of sleep disturbances.[108] If there is identification of a de novo sleep disturbance in a child who has shown clinical improvement with treatment, switching to a longer-acting or shorter-acting medication within the same classification is reasonable. In terms of switching stimulants, several studies have compared dosing strategies of twice daily with 3 times a day with inconclusive results.[109–111] Comparisons of long-acting osmotic release and transdermal formulations of methylphenidate did not show worsening of sleep and indicate that premorbid sleep disturbances are stronger indicators of sleep disturbances in children.[112,113] If a patient has minimal improvement switching stimulants, the use of atomoxetine or the addition of melatonin may be considered reasonable and safe.[114,115]

Cardiotoxicity

Stimulants increase noradrenergic and dopaminergic transmission, leading to an increase in sympathomimetic activity, which can have an impact on heart rate and blood pressure. As a result, the FDA released a black box warning on the use of stimulants and their potential cardiovascular risk.[116] Initial studies and reviews looking at the impact of placebo-controlled trials of methylphenidate reported an increase in heart rate and blood pressure in children.[117–119] More recently, the MTA published a prospective trial on cardiovascular effects in 579 children over a 10-year period and found that "stimulant treatment did not increase the risk of prehypertension or hypertension," but "stimulants had a persistent adrenergic effect on heart rate during treatment."[120] Adult literature on stimulants has found that although the use of methylphenidate has shown an increase in sudden death or ventricular arrhythmia, there does not seem to be a dose-dependent association and there may not be a causal relationship.[121] Similarly, one retrospective large cohort study of young and middle-aged adults and their use of stimulants reported no increase in serious cardiovascular events.[122]

Before initiating stimulant treatment, practitioners should review with their patients and families a complete family history of cardiac events, including syncopal episodes, hypertension, ECG abnormalities, sudden cardiac death, and cardiomyopathies. If clinically indicated, providers may request an ECG to assess for any signs of abnormalities, but it is not required.[123] Routine monitoring of heart rate and blood pressure is recommended every 6 months in the United Kingdom.[124]

Physical Growth

Emerging evidence on the effects of stimulant and nonstimulant agents on physical growth have resulted in critical questions for clinicians and parents initiating psychopharmacologic interventions for youth with ADHD. Several retrospective and observational analyses in the past decade have provided evidence that mild deficits to height and weight occur with stimulant use.[125–131] Yet controversy remains in the clinical significance of such deficits due to a lack of long-term prospective trials. Based on the available body of evidence, psychopharmacology continues to be the supported first-line treatment for ADHD because the documented effects to stature are mild and transient.[127,132–135] The MTA study provides perhaps the most significant source of prospective data to guide clinicians in assessing the potential impact of stimulant medication on a child's growth. Post hoc analyses of the trial's anthropometric outcomes suggest a 2-cm decline in height associated with stimulant use.[136] Although retrospective cohorts seem to undergo attenuation in growth rate deceleration and suppression within a limited range of follow-up, longer-term effects into adulthood need to be elucidated via prospective assessment.

The mechanisms underlying the pathophysiology of medication-induced growth suppression in ADHD remain unknown, with various theories accounting for these delays in growth, as outlined in a 2008 review by Faraone and Buitelaar.[132] Stimulant agents produce direct effects on the dopaminergic pathway, which in turn affect the expression of growth hormone.[132] Additionally, a theory of developmental delay in the etiology of ADHD has been proposed, suggesting a potential mechanism of delayed physical growth mirroring the theorized delay in cortical development.[132]

Proper assessment and management of changes to stature over the course of medication therapy should include scheduled height and weight monitoring conducted by a patient's psychopharmacologist. Specifically, patients should have their BMI calculated and a z score used to assess for changes in weight.[63,69] Whether children who present with delays in growth should discontinue medication or pursue a drug holiday has incurred some debate in the literature.[132]

SUMMARY

This review of the side effects and monitoring of psychotropics in children and adolescents has highlighted the limitations in interpreting the literature for application to clinical practice. Specifically, it is difficult to compare and contrast studies based on the wide variability in sample sizes, study population, and short time frames typical in phase III studies. There is also a lack of standardization for screening and monitoring of side effects/adverse events. Monitoring of these side effects/adverse events is complex in the context of a developmentally diverse population that has variable levels of expressing themselves in terms of distress and behaviors (ie, mania, suicide, and psychosis). The development of new medications and increased use of psychotropic medications in the pediatric population has resulted in limited data on side effects. In the monitoring of rare side effects/adverse events, the number of cases identified may not rise above the detection level until more children are exposed to the medication than is typical in the premarketing studies conducted to gain FDA approval. In these instances, the literature is reduced to case reports and meta-analysis of diverse publications. Unfortunately, clinicians are often forced to review the adult literature and extrapolate the data to children and adolescents.

Child and adolescent psychiatrists are constantly at the frontier of understanding pediatric mental health disorders. This review emphasizes the upsurge in the use of psychotropics in a dynamic environment with evolving symptom definition, diagnostic criteria of complex side effect syndromes (ie, suicidality and metabolic syndrome), and measurement of symptom contribution to the development of such syndromes. There is a need for further consensus around specific symptom criteria (ie, obesity) and clear cutoff levels for physical markers of developing pathology. Future studies using these defined criteria in controlled randomized trials could be designed to carefully assess the risks versus benefits of psychotropic modalities. Once the risk factors are identified, improved screening tools can be developed and guidelines around screening and monitoring can be further developed and disseminated for clinicians.

REFERENCES

1. Goethe JW, Woolley SB, Cardoni AA, et al. Selective serotonin reuptake inhibitor discontinuation: side effects and other factors that influence medication adherence. J Clin Psychopharmacol 2007;27(5):451–8.

2. Safer DJ, Zito JM. Treatment-emergent adverse events from selective serotonin reuptake inhibitors by age group: children versus adolescents. J Child Adolesc Psychopharmacol 2006;16(1–2):159–69.
3. FDA. 2012. Available at: http://www.fda.gov/Drugs/DrugSafety/ucm297391.htm. Accessed March 28, 2012.
4. Boeck V, Overo KF, Svendsen O. Studies on acute toxicity and drug levels of citalopram in the dog. Acta Pharmacol Toxicol (Copenh) 1982;50(3):169–74.
5. Tarabar AF, Hoffman RS, Nelson L. Citalopram overdose: late presentation of torsades de pointes (TdP) with cardiac arrest. J Med Toxicol 2008;4(2):101–5.
6. McNally P, McNicholas F, Oslizlok P. The QT interval and psychotropic medications in children: recommendations for clinicians. Eur Child Adolesc Psychiatry 2007;16(1):33–47.
7. Gibbons RD, Mann JJ. Strategies for quantifying the relationship between medications and suicidal behaviour: what has been learned? Drug Saf 2011;34(5):375–95.
8. FDA. Public Health Advisory: Antidepressant Use in Children, Adolescents, and Adults. 2004. Available at: http://www.fda.gov/Safety/MedWatch/SafetyInformation/SafetyAlertsforHumanMedicalProducts/ucm155489.htm. Accessed February 27, 2012.
9. FDA. Antidepressant Use in Children, Adolescents, and Adults. 2006. Available at: http://www.fda.gov/Drugs/DrugSafety/InformationbyDrugClass/UCM096273. Accessed February 27, 2012.
10. Hammad TA, Laughren T, Racoosin J. Suicidality in pediatric patients treated with antidepressant drugs. Arch Gen Psychiatry 2006;63(3):332–9.
11. Carpenter DJ, Fong R, Kraus JE, et al. Meta-analysis of efficacy and treatment-emergent suicidality in adults by psychiatric indication and age subgroup following initiation of paroxetine therapy: a complete set of randomized placebo-controlled trials. J Clin Psychiatry 2011;72(11):1503–14.
12. Olfson M, Marcus SC, Shaffer D. Antidepressant drug therapy and suicide in severely depressed children and adults: a case-control study. Arch Gen Psychiatry 2006;63(8):865–72.
13. Gibbons RD, Brown CH, Hur K, et al. Suicidal thoughts and behavior with antidepressant treatment: reanalysis of the randomized placebo-controlled studies of fluoxetine and venlafaxine. Arch Gen Psychiatry 2012;69(6):580–7.
14. Leon AC, Solomon DA, Li C, et al. Antidepressants and risks of suicide and suicide attempts: a 27-year observational study. J Clin Psychiatry 2011;72(5):580–6.
15. Carlson GA, Mick E. Drug-induced disinhibition in psychiatrically hospitalized children. J Child Adolesc Psychopharmacol 2003;13(2):153–63.
16. Goodman WK, Murphy TK, Storch EA. Risk of adverse behavioral effects with pediatric use of antidepressants. Psychopharmacology (Berl) 2007;191(1):87–96.
17. Walkup J, Labellarte M. Complications of SSRI treatment. J Child Adolesc Psychopharmacol 2001;11(1):1–4.
18. Faedda GL, Baldessarini RJ, Glovinsky IP, et al. Treatment-emergent mania in pediatric bipolar disorder: a retrospective case review. J Affect Disord 2004;82(1):149–58.
19. Henry C, Sorbara F, Lacoste J, et al. Antidepressant-induced mania in bipolar patients: identification of risk factors. J Clin Psychiatry 2001;62(4):249–55.
20. Truman CJ, Goldberg JF, Ghaemi SN, et al. Self-reported history of manic/hypomanic switch associated with antidepressant use: data from the Systematic

Treatment Enhancement Program for Bipolar Disorder (STEP-BD). J Clin Psychiatry 2007;68(10):1472–9.

21. Kowatch RA, Youngstrom EA, Danielyan A, et al. Review and meta-analysis of the phenomenology and clinical characteristics of mania in children and adolescents. Bipolar Disord 2005;7(6):483–96.

22. Bridge JA, Iyengar S, Salary CB, et al. Clinical response and risk for reported suicidal ideation and suicide attempts in pediatric antidepressant treatment: a meta-analysis of randomized controlled trials. JAMA 2007;297(15):1683–96.

23. Brent DA, Greenhill LL, Compton S, et al. The Treatment of Adolescent Suicide Attempters study (TASA): predictors of suicidal events in an open treatment trial. J Am Acad Child Adolesc Psychiatry 2009;48(10):987–96.

24. Jones L. Responding to the needs of children in crisis. Int Rev Psychiatry 2008; 20(3):291–303.

25. Parker G, Brotchie H. Gender differences in depression. Int Rev Psychiatry 2010;22(5):429–36.

26. Restifo K, Bogels S. Family processes in the development of youth depression: translating the evidence to treatment. Clin Psychol Rev 2009;29(4):294–316.

27. Thapar A, Collishaw S, Pine DS, et al. Depression in adolescence. Lancet 2012; 379(9820):1056–67.

28. Goodyer I, Dubicka B, Wilkinson P, et al. Selective serotonin reuptake inhibitors (SSRIs) and routine specialist care with and without cognitive behaviour therapy in adolescents with major depression: randomised controlled trial. BMJ 2007; 335(7611):142.

29. March J, Silva S, Petrycki S, et al. Fluoxetine, cognitive-behavioral therapy, and their combination for adolescents with depression: Treatment for Adolescents With Depression Study (TADS) randomized controlled trial. JAMA 2004;292(7): 807–20.

30. Stanley B, Brown G, Brent DA, et al. Cognitive-behavioral therapy for suicide prevention (CBT-SP): treatment model, feasibility, and acceptability. J Am Acad Child Adolesc Psychiatry 2009;48(10):1005–13.

31. Vitiello B, Brent DA, Greenhill LL, et al. Depressive symptoms and clinical status during the Treatment of Adolescent Suicide Attempters (TASA) Study. J Am Acad Child Adolesc Psychiatry 2009;48(10):997–1004.

32. Wilens TE, Biederman J, Kwon A, et al. A systematic chart review of the nature of psychiatric adverse events in children and adolescents treated with selective serotonin reuptake inhibitors. J Child Adolesc Psychopharmacol 2003;13(2):143–52.

33. Anderson HD, Pace WD, Libby AM, et al. Rates of 5 common antidepressant side effects among new adult and adolescent cases of depression: a retrospective US claims study. Clin Ther 2012;34(1):113–23.

34. Smitherman TA, Walters AB, Maizels M, et al. The use of antidepressants for headache prophylaxis. CNS Neurosci Ther 2011;17(5):462–9.

35. Punay NC, Couch JR. Antidepressants in the treatment of migraine headache. Curr Pain Headache Rep 2003;7(1):51–4.

36. Moja PL, Cusi C, Sterzi RR, et al. Selective serotonin re-uptake inhibitors (SSRIs) for preventing migraine and tension-type headaches. Cochrane Database Syst Rev 2005;(3):CD002919.

37. Murphy TK, Segarra A, Storch EA, et al. SSRI adverse events: how to monitor and manage. Int Rev Psychiatry 2008;20(2):203–8.

38. Norgaard M, Jacobsen J, Gasse C, et al. Selective serotonin reuptake inhibitors and risk of acute pancreatitis: a population-based case-control study. J Clin Psychopharmacol 2007;27(3):259–62.

39. Spigset O, Hagg S, Bate A. Hepatic injury and pancreatitis during treatment with serotonin reuptake inhibitors: data from the World Health Organization (WHO) database of adverse drug reactions. Int Clin Psychopharmacol 2003;18(3): 157–61.
40. Birmaher B, Brent D, Bernet W, et al. Practice parameter for the assessment and treatment of children and adolescents with depressive disorders. J Am Acad Child Adolesc Psychiatry 2007;46(11):1503–26.
41. Dodd S, Malhi GS, Tiller J, et al. A consensus statement for safety monitoring guidelines of treatments for major depressive disorder. Aust N Z J Psychiatry 2011;45(9):712–25.
42. Harvey BH, Bouwer CD. Neuropharmacology of paradoxic weight gain with selective serotonin reuptake inhibitors. Clin Neuropharmacol 2000;23(2):90–7.
43. Sussman N. Venlafaxine XR therapy for major depression and anxiety disorders. The clinical implications that its advantages pose. Postgrad Med 1999; 106(Suppl 6):31–6.
44. Fava M. Weight gain and antidepressants. J Clin Psychiatry 2000;61(Suppl 11): 37–41.
45. Croft H, Houser TL, Jamerson BD, et al. Effect on body weight of bupropion sustained-release in patients with major depression treated for 52 weeks. Clin Ther 2002;24(4):662–72.
46. Harto-Truax N, Stern WC, Miller LL, et al. Effects of bupropion on body weight. J Clin Psychiatry 1983;44(5 Pt 2):183–6.
47. Weisler RH, Johnston JA, Lineberry CG, et al. Comparison of bupropion and trazodone for the treatment of major depression. J Clin Psychopharmacol 1994; 14(3):170–9.
48. Goodnick PJ, Goldstein BJ. Selective serotonin reuptake inhibitors in affective disorders—I. Basic pharmacology. J Psychopharmacol 1998;12(3 Suppl B): S5–20.
49. Montgomery SA. Efficacy and safety of the selective serotonin reuptake inhibitors in treating depression in elderly patients. Int Clin Psychopharmacol 1998; 13(Suppl 5):S49–54.
50. Smith WT, Glaudin V, Panagides J, et al. Mirtazapine vs. amitriptyline vs. placebo in the treatment of major depressive disorder. Psychopharmacol Bull 1990;26(2):191–6.
51. Herva A, Laitinen J, Miettunen J, et al. Obesity and depression: results from the longitudinal Northern Finland 1966 Birth Cohort Study. Int J Obes (Lond) 2006; 30(3):520–7.
52. Patten SB, Williams JV, Lavorato DH, et al. Major depression, antidepressant medication and the risk of obesity. Psychother Psychosom 2009;78(3):182–6.
53. Patten SB, Williams JV, Lavorato DH, et al. Weight gain in relation to major depression and antidepressant medication use. J Affect Disord 2011;134(1–3): 288–93.
54. Comer JS, Olfson M, Mojtabai R. National trends in child and adolescent psychotropic polypharmacy in office-based practice, 1996-2007. J Am Acad Child Adolesc Psychiatry 2010;49(10):1001–10.
55. Findling RL, Drury SS, Jensen PS. Practice parameter for the use of atypical antipsychotic medications in children. J Am Acad Child Adolesc Psychiatry 2011. http://www.aacap.org/galleries/PracticeParameters/Atypical_Antipsychotic_ Medications_Web.pdf. Accessed August 23, 2012.
56. Mojtabai R, Olfson M. National trends in psychotropic medication polypharmacy in office-based psychiatry. Arch Gen Psychiatry 2010;67(1):26–36.

57. Naber D, Lambert M. The CATIE and CUtLASS studies in schizophrenia: results and implications for clinicians. CNS Drugs 2009;23(8):649–59.
58. Rani FA, Byrne PJ, Murray ML, et al. Paediatric atypical antipsychotic monitoring safety (PAMS) study: pilot study in children and adolescents in secondary- and tertiary-care settings. Drug Saf 2009;32(4):325–33.
59. Laita P, Cifuentes A, Doll A, et al. Antipsychotic-related abnormal involuntary movements and metabolic and endocrine side effects in children and adolescents. J Child Adolesc Psychopharmacol 2007;17(4):487–502.
60. Caroff SN, Hurford I, Lybrand J, et al. Movement disorders induced by antipsychotic drugs: implications of the CATIE schizophrenia trial. Neurol Clin 2011; 29(1):127–48, viii.
61. Correll CU, Leucht S, Kane JM. Lower risk for tardive dyskinesia associated with second-generation antipsychotics: a systematic review of 1-year studies. Am J Psychiatry 2004;161(3):414–25.
62. Miller DD, Caroff SN, Davis SM, et al. Extrapyramidal side-effects of antipsychotics in a randomised trial. Br J Psychiatry 2008;193(4):279–88.
63. Correll CU. Assessing and maximizing the safety and tolerability of antipsychotics used in the treatment of children and adolescents. J Clin Psychiatry 2008;69(Suppl 4):26–36.
64. Simpson GM. The treatment of tardive dyskinesia and tardive dystonia. J Clin Psychiatry 2000;61(Suppl 4):39–44.
65. Soares KV, McGrath JJ. The treatment of tardive dyskinesia—a systematic review and meta-analysis. Schizophr Res 1999;39(1):1–16 [discussion 17–8].
66. van Harten PN, Tenback DE. Tardive dyskinesia: clinical presentation and treatment. Int Rev Neurobiol 2011;98:187–210.
67. Cook S, Auinger P, Li C, et al. Metabolic syndrome rates in United States adolescents, from the National Health and Nutrition Examination Survey, 1999-2002. J Pediatr 2008;152(2):165–70.
68. D'Adamo E, Santoro N, Caprio S. Metabolic syndrome in pediatrics: old concepts revised, new concepts discussed. Pediatr Clin North Am 2011;58(5): 1241–55, xi.
69. Maayan L, Correll CU. Weight gain and metabolic risks associated with antipsychotic medications in children and adolescents. J Child Adolesc Psychopharmacol 2011;21(6):517–35.
70. Steinberger J, Daniels SR, Eckel RH, et al. Progress and challenges in metabolic syndrome in children and adolescents: a scientific statement from the American Heart Association Atherosclerosis, Hypertension, and Obesity in the Young Committee of the Council on Cardiovascular Disease in the Young; Council on Cardiovascular Nursing; and Council on Nutrition, Physical Activity, and Metabolism. Circulation 2009;119(4):628–47.
71. Jerrell JM, McIntyre RS. Adverse events in children and adolescents treated with antipsychotic medications. Hum Psychopharmacol 2008;23(4):283–90.
72. Correll CU, Manu P, Olshanskiy V, et al. Cardiometabolic risk of second-generation antipsychotic medications during first-time use in children and adolescents. JAMA 2009;302(16):1765–73.
73. De Hert M, Vancampfort D, Correll CU, et al. Guidelines for screening and monitoring of cardiometabolic risk in schizophrenia: systematic evaluation. Br J Psychiatry 2011;199(2):99–105.
74. Panagiotopoulos C, Ronsley R, Kuzeljevic B, et al. Waist circumference is a sensitive screening tool for assessment of metabolic syndrome risk in children treated with second-generation antipsychotics. Can J Psychiatry 2012;57(1):34–44.

75. Pringsheim T, Panagiotopoulos C, Davidson J, et al. Evidence-based recommendations for monitoring safety of second generation antipsychotics in children and youth. J Can Acad Child Adolesc Psychiatry 2011;20(3):218–33.
76. Seida JC, Schouten JR, Boylan K, et al. Antipsychotics for children and young adults: a comparative effectiveness review. Pediatrics 2012;129(3):e771–84.
77. Battista M, Murray RD, Daniels SR. Use of the metabolic syndrome in pediatrics: a blessing and a curse. Semin Pediatr Surg 2009;18(3):136–43.
78. Ho J, Panagiotopoulos C, McCrindle B, et al. Management recommendations for metabolic complications associated with second generation antipsychotic use in children and youth. J Can Acad Child Adolesc Psychiatry 2011;20(3):234–41.
79. Vitiello B, Correll C, van Zwieten-Boot B, et al. Antipsychotics in children and adolescents: increasing use, evidence for efficacy and safety concerns. Eur Neuropsychopharmacol 2009;19(9):629–35.
80. De Hert M, Dobbelaere M, Sheridan EM, et al. Metabolic and endocrine adverse effects of second-generation antipsychotics in children and adolescents: a systematic review of randomized, placebo controlled trials and guidelines for clinical practice. Eur Psychiatry 2011;26(3):144–58.
81. Rummel-Kluge C, Komossa K, Schwarz S, et al. Head-to-head comparisons of metabolic side effects of second generation antipsychotics in the treatment of schizophrenia: a systematic review and meta-analysis. Schizophr Res 2010; 123(2–3):225–33.
82. Stigler KA, Potenza MN, McDougle CJ. Tolerability profile of atypical antipsychotics in children and adolescents. Paediatr Drugs 2001;3(12):927–42.
83. FDA. Suicidal Behavior and Ideation and Antiepileptic Drugs. 2008. Available at: http://www.fda.gov/Drugs/DrugSafety/PostmarketDrugSafetyInformationforPatients andProviders/ucm100190.htm. Accessed February 27, 2012.
84. Dennehy EB, Marangell LB, Allen MH, et al. Suicide and suicide attempts in the Systematic Treatment Enhancement Program for Bipolar Disorder (STEP-BD). J Affect Disord 2011;133(3):423–7.
85. Harris KM, McLean JP, Sheffield J, et al. The internal suicide debate hypothesis: exploring the life versus death struggle. Suicide Life Threat Behav 2010;40(2): 181–92.
86. Rihmer Z, Gonda X. The effect of pharmacotherapy on suicide rates in bipolar patients. CNS Neurosci Ther 2012;18(3):238–42.
87. Kalinin VV. Suicidality and antiepileptic drugs: is there a link? Drug Saf 2007; 30(2):123–42.
88. Andersohn F, Schade R, Willich SN, et al. Use of antiepileptic drugs in epilepsy and the risk of self-harm or suicidal behavior. Neurology 2010;75(4):335–40.
89. Arana A, Wentworth CE, Ayuso-Mateos JL, et al. Suicide-related events in patients treated with antiepileptic drugs. N Engl J Med 2010;363(6):542–51.
90. Leon AC, Solomon DA, Li C, et al. antiepileptic drugs for bipolar disorder and the risk of suicidal behavior: a 30-year observational study. Am J Psychiatry 2012;169(3):285–91.
91. Bessmertny O, Pham T. Antiepileptic hypersensitivity syndrome: clinicians beware and be aware. Curr Allergy Asthma Rep 2002;2(1):34–9.
92. Knowles SR, Shapiro LE, Shear NH. Anticonvulsant hypersensitivity syndrome: incidence, prevention and management. Drug Saf 1999;21(6):489–501.
93. Kumari R, Timshina DK, Thappa DM. Drug hypersensitivity syndrome. Indian J Dermatol Venereol Leprol 2011;77(1):7–15.
94. Hebert AA, Ralston JP. Cutaneous reactions to anticonvulsant medications. J Clin Psychiatry 2001;62(Suppl 14):22–6.

95. Mansur AT, Pekcan Yasar S, Goktay F. Anticonvulsant hypersensitivity syndrome: clinical and laboratory features. Int J Dermatol 2008;47(11):1184–9.

96. Aiken CB, Orr C. Rechallenge with lamotrigine after a rash: a prospective case series and review of the literature. Psychiatry (Edgmont) 2010;7(5):27–32.

97. Lekhwani M, Nair C, Nikhinson I, et al. Psychotropic prescription practices in child psychiatric inpatients 9 years old and younger. J Child Adolesc Psychopharmacol 2004;14(1):95–103.

98. Najjar F, Welch C, Grapentine WL, et al. Trends in psychotropic drug use in a child psychiatric hospital from 1991-1998. J Child Adolesc Psychopharmacol 2004;14(1):87–93.

99. Elbe D, Savage R. How does this happen? Part I: mechanisms of adverse drug reactions associated with psychotropic medications. J Can Acad Child Adolesc Psychiatry 2010;19(1):40–5.

100. McKnight RF, Adida M, Budge K, et al. Lithium toxicity profile: a systematic review and meta-analysis. Lancet 2012;379(9817):721–8.

101. Gerrett D, Lamont T, Paton C, et al. Prescribing and monitoring lithium therapy: summary of a safety report from the National Patient Safety Agency. BMJ 2010; 341:c6258.

102. Nicholson J, Fitzmaurice B. Monitoring patients on lithium—a good practice guideline. Psychiatrist 2002;26:348–51.

103. Hammerness PG, Perrin JM, Shelley-Abrahamson R, et al. Cardiovascular risk of stimulant treatment in pediatric attention-deficit/hyperactivity disorder: update and clinical recommendations. J Am Acad Child Adolesc Psychiatry 2011;50(10):978–90.

104. Ivanenko A, Johnson K. Sleep disturbances in children with psychiatric disorders. Semin Pediatr Neurol 2008;15(2):70–8.

105. Corkum P, Tannock R, Moldofsky H. Sleep disturbances in children with attention-deficit/hyperactivity disorder. J Am Acad Child Adolesc Psychiatry 1998;37(6):637–46.

106. Day HD, Abmayr SB. Parent reports of sleep disturbances in stimulant-medicated children with attention-deficit hyperactivity disorder. J Clin Psychol 1998;54(5):701–16.

107. Ring A, Stein D, Barak Y, et al. Sleep disturbances in children with attention-deficit/hyperactivity disorder: a comparative study with healthy siblings. J Learn Disabil 1998;31(6):572–8.

108. Sonuga-Barke EJ, Coghill D, Wigal T, et al. Adverse reactions to methylphenidate treatment for attention-deficit/hyperactivity disorder: structure and associations with clinical characteristics and symptom control. J Child Adolesc Psychopharmacol 2009;19(6):683–90.

109. Corkum P, Panton R, Ironside S, et al. Acute impact of immediate release methylphenidate administered three times a day on sleep in children with attention-deficit/hyperactivity disorder. J Pediatr Psychol 2008;33(4):368–79.

110. Kent JD, Blader JC, Koplewicz HS, et al. Effects of late-afternoon methylphenidate administration on behavior and sleep in attention-deficit hyperactivity disorder. Pediatrics 1995;96(2 Pt 1):320–5.

111. Stein MA, Blondis TA, Schnitzler ER, et al. Methylphenidate dosing: twice daily versus three times daily. Pediatrics 1996;98(4 Pt 1):748–56.

112. Faraone SV, Glatt SJ, Bukstein OG, et al. Effects of once-daily oral and transdermal methylphenidate on sleep behavior of children with ADHD. J Atten Disord 2009;12(4):308–15.

113. Kim HW, Yoon IY, Cho SC, et al. The effect of OROS methylphenidate on the sleep of children with attention-deficit/hyperactivity disorder. Int Clin Psychopharmacol 2010;25(2):107–15.

114. Sangal RB, Owens J, Allen AJ, et al. Effects of atomoxetine and methylphenidate on sleep in children with ADHD. Sleep 2006;29(12):1573–85.
115. Weiss MD, Wasdell MB, Bomben MM, et al. Sleep hygiene and melatonin treatment for children and adolescents with ADHD and initial insomnia. J Am Acad Child Adolesc Psychiatry 2006;45(5):512–9.
116. FDA. Stimulant Medications used in Children with Attention-Deficit/Hyperactivity Disorder—Communication about an Ongoing Safety Review. 2009. Available at: http://www.fda.gov/safety/medwatch/safetyinformation/safetyalertsforhumanmedical products/ucm166667.htm. Accessed February 27, 2012.
117. Findling RL, Biederman J, Wilens TE, et al. Short- and long-term cardiovascular effects of mixed amphetamine salts extended release in children. J Pediatr 2005;147(3):348–54.
118. Rapport MD, Moffitt C. Attention deficit/hyperactivity disorder and methylphenidate. A review of height/weight, cardiovascular, and somatic complaint side effects. Clin Psychol Rev 2002;22(8):1107–31.
119. Samuels JA, Franco K, Wan F, et al. Effect of stimulants on 24-h ambulatory blood pressure in children with ADHD: a double-blind, randomized, crossover trial. Pediatr Nephrol 2006;21(1):92–5.
120. Vitiello B, Elliott GR, Swanson JM, et al. Blood pressure and heart rate over 10 years in the multimodal treatment study of children with ADHD. Am J Psychiatry 2012;169(2):167–77.
121. Schelleman H, Bilker WB, Kimmel SE, et al. Methylphenidate and risk of serious cardiovascular events in adults. Am J Psychiatry 2012;169(2):178–85.
122. Habel LA, Cooper WO, Sox CM, et al. ADHD medications and risk of serious cardiovascular events in young and middle-aged adults. JAMA 2011;306(24): 2673–83.
123. Pliszka S. Practice parameter for the assessment and treatment of children and adolescents with attention-deficit/hyperactivity disorder. J Am Acad Child Adolesc Psychiatry 2007;46(7):894–921.
124. Sever P. New hypertension guidelines from the National Institute for Health and Clinical Excellence and the British Hypertension Society. J Renin Angiotensin Aldosterone Syst 2006;7(2):61–3.
125. Dura-Trave T, Yoldi-Petri ME, Gallinas-Victoriano F, et al. Effects of osmotic-release methylphenidate on height and weight in children with Attention-Deficit Hyperactivity Disorder (ADHD) following up to four years of treatment. J Child Neurol 2012;27(5):604–9.
126. Poulton A, Cowell CT. Slowing of growth in height and weight on stimulants: a characteristic pattern. J Paediatr Child Health 2003;39(3):180–5.
127. Spencer TJ, Faraone SV, Biederman J, et al. Does prolonged therapy with a long-acting stimulant suppress growth in children with ADHD? J Am Acad Child Adolesc Psychiatry 2006;45(5):527–37.
128. Swanson J, Arnold LE, Kraemer H, et al. Evidence, interpretation, and qualification from multiple reports of long-term outcomes in the Multimodal Treatment study of Children With ADHD (MTA): part I: executive summary. J Atten Disord 2008;12(1):4–14.
129. Swanson J, Greenhill L, Wigal T, et al. Stimulant-related reductions of growth rates in the PATS. J Am Acad Child Adolesc Psychiatry 2006;45(11): 1304–13.
130. Swanson JM, Elliott GR, Greenhill LL, et al. Effects of stimulant medication on growth rates across 3 years in the MTA follow-up. J Am Acad Child Adolesc Psychiatry 2007;46(8):1015–27.

131. Swanson JM, Hinshaw SP, Arnold LE, et al. Secondary evaluations of MTA 36-month outcomes: propensity score and growth mixture model analyses. J Am Acad Child Adolesc Psychiatry 2007;46(8):1003–14.

132. Faraone SV, Buitelaar J. Comparing the efficacy of stimulants for ADHD in children and adolescents using meta-analysis. Eur Child Adolesc Psychiatry 2010; 19(4):353–64.

133. Goldman RD. ADHD stimulants and their effect on height in children. Can Fam Physician 2010;56(2):145–6.

134. Spencer TJ, Kratochvil CJ, Sangal RB, et al. Effects of atomoxetine on growth in children with attention-deficit/hyperactivity disorder following up to five years of treatment. J Child Adolesc Psychopharmacol 2007;17(5):689–700.

135. Vitiello B. Understanding the risk of using medications for attention deficit hyperactivity disorder with respect to physical growth and cardiovascular function. Child Adolesc Psychiatr Clin N Am 2008;17(2):459–74, xi.

136. Swanson J, Arnold LE, Kraemer H, et al. Evidence, interpretation, and qualification from multiple reports of long-term outcomes in the Multimodal Treatment Study of children with ADHD (MTA): Part II: supporting details. J Atten Disord 2008;12(1):15–43.

Interventions for Youth at High Risk for Bipolar Disorder and Schizophrenia

Robert K. McNamara, PhD[a], Jeffrey R. Strawn, MD[a],
Kiki D. Chang, MD[b], Melissa P. DelBello, MD, MS[a],*

KEYWORDS

- Bipolar disorder • Mania • Schizophrenia • Psychosis • Pediatric • Adolescent
- Prevention • Clinical staging

KEY POINTS

- There have been some promising findings in evaluating SGA medications, antidepressants, LCn-3 fatty acids, and cognitive-behavioral therapy in patients at high risk for developing psychosis.
- Potential iatrogenic effects of antidepressant and psychostimulant medications, lack of efficacy of mood-stabilizer medications for prodromal mood symptoms, and adverse cardiometabolic effects associated with SGA medications highlight the urgent need to identify and evaluate evidence-based treatments for youth at high risk for BP.
- Preliminary evidence endorses the adoption of a clinical staging approach for treating youth at risk for developing mania or psychosis, beginning with low-risk first-line interventions, including psychosocial or LCn-3 fatty acids.

OVERVIEW

Bipolar disorder (BP) and schizophrenia (SZ) are chronic and typically recurring illnesses with significant psychosocial morbidity and excess premature mortality. Increasing evidence from retrospective and prospective studies is beginning to elucidate prodromal criteria to identify individuals that are at high risk (also termed ultra high risk) for developing mania, and by definition, BP-I or SZ. In general, high-risk criteria involve having a first-degree relative with BP or SZ, a history of subthreshold mood or psychotic symptoms, and being in the age range most frequently associated with the initial onset of BP or SZ (ie, adolescence). Although ongoing research is seeking

[a] Division of Bipolar Disorders Research, Department of Psychiatry and Behavioral Neuroscience, University of Cincinnati College of Medicine, 260 Stetson Street, Cincinnati, OH 45267, USA;
[b] Stanford Pediatric Bipolar Disorders Program, Department of Psychiatry, Stanford University School of Medicine, 401 Quarry Road, Stanford, CA 94305, USA
* Corresponding author. Department of Psychiatry, University of Cincinnati College of Medicine, 260 Stetson Street, Suite 3200, ML 559, Cincinnati, OH 45219.
E-mail address: delbelmp@ucmail.uc.edu

Child Adolesc Psychiatric Clin N Am 21 (2012) 739–751
http://dx.doi.org/10.1016/j.chc.2012.07.009
1056-4993/12/$ – see front matter © 2012 Elsevier Inc. All rights reserved.

to validate and refine these criteria, there is also increasing experimental interest in developing and evaluating interventions that can be delivered before the initial onset of manic or psychotic symptoms to slow or prevent illness progression in high-risk populations. Additionally, potential negative effects associated with conventional pharmacologic interventions used to treat comorbid symptoms in the prodromal stage indicate a need for alternative treatment approaches. In this article, we summarize evidence for potential interventions for high-risk individuals and highlight associated ethical and safety considerations.

BP is typically characterized by recurrent episodes of mania and depression, and interepisode periods of euthymia. In the United States, lifetime prevalence estimates of BP are 1% for BP-I, 1.1% for BP-II, and 2.4% for subthreshold BP (4.4% total).[1] The initial onset of BP typically occurs during adolescence,[2] with a lifetime prevalence of adolescents having BP-I or II in the United States of 2.5%.[3] Family and twin studies indicate that the cause of BP involves genetic and environmental factors, and having a first-degree relative with BP or unipolar depression substantially increases the risk for developing BP compared with the general population.[4] Untreated patients with BP typically exhibit progressive increases in the frequency and severity of manic and depressive episodes over time, and mood-stabilizers and second-generation antipsychotics (SGAs) are widely prescribed for the treatment and secondary prevention of mood episodes in patients with BP.

Mood symptoms commonly exhibited by children and adolescents before the initial onset of mania include syndromal and subsyndromal major depressive disorder (MDD); anxiety; and episodic subsyndromal manic symptoms (sleep disturbances, anger or irritability, increased energy, and rapid mood fluctuations termed "cyclotaxia").[5–8] For example, Strober and Carlson[9] found that 20% of adolescents with MDD developed BP-I over 3 to 4 years, especially if they had a family history of BP, rapid symptom onset, or psychosis. Furthermore, a prospective study found that 38% of children and adolescents initially diagnosed with subsyndromal BP symptoms (BP not otherwise specified), and 25% diagnosed with BP-II, transitioned to BP-I during the 4-year follow-up.[10] Cognitive symptoms, particularly deficits in concentration and attention, also frequently precede the initial onset of mania. Indeed, the high rate of comorbid attention-deficit/hyperactivity disorder (ADHD) in pediatric BP, as high as 98%, and lower age at onset of mania in patients with comorbid ADHD, are consistent with ADHD being a prodromal feature in a subset of patients.[11] One research group has proposed criteria for individuals at high risk for developing BP-I (termed "bipolar at-risk"), which included having a first-degree relative with BP-I, a history of subthreshold mania, MDD, or rapid mood fluctuations (cyclothymia), and being younger than age 25 years.[12] Using these criteria, they found that 23% of help-seeking patients meeting these high-risk criteria transitioned to threshold mania within an average follow-up period of 265 days compared with 0.7% of patients not meeting BP at-risk criteria.[12] Other groups have proposed high-risk criteria based on the presentation of prodromal clinical features, ADHD, and other putative risk factors and endophenotypes.[8,13]

SZ is a progressive psychiatric disorder with a lifetime prevalence rate of approximately 1%, and is typically characterized by positive (delusions, hallucinations, incoherent speech) and negative (apathy, depression) symptoms and cognitive impairments (memory, attention). Concordance rates among monozygotic twins indicates genetic and nongenetic factors play a pathogenic role, and males are at greater risk of developing SZ.[14] The initial onset of psychosis typically occurs in late adolescence or early adulthood, and first-episode psychotic patients are typically prescribed SGA medications. The initial onset of psychosis is frequently preceded by a prodromal period of approximately 1 to 5 years, which is associated with subthreshold psychotic symptoms, negative symptoms, MDD, cognitive impairments, and impaired social and occupational functioning.[15] Although there is currently no consensus regarding high-risk criteria, ultra-high-risk criteria have been more extensively evaluated and require attenuated psychotic symptoms (defined using PANNS scores), transient psychosis, or schizotypal personality disorder or a first-degree relative with Diagnostic and Statistical Manual (DSM)-IV psychotic disorder.[16] A recent meta-analysis of 27 prospective studies of 2502 high-risk patients found a consistent and increasing risk of psychosis transition over 3 years.[17] It is also important to note that transition to psychosis does not equate with transition to SZ, and a recent meta-analysis of 23 prospective studies of 2182 high-risk patients found that only a small percentage of high-risk patients (15.7%) who transition to psychosis subsequently receive a formal diagnosis of SZ.[18]

EMPIRIC EVIDENCE FOR ETHICAL ISSUES

Although establishing effective and safe early intervention strategies is of critical importance for minimizing the significant morbidity and mortality associated with the progression of mood and psychotic disorders, there are several ethical dilemmas that the field needs to consider. First, the consequences of labeling children and adolescents with a "prodromal" diagnosis need to be deliberated, as illustrated by the controversy surrounding whether a diagnosis of "Risk Syndrome of Psychosis," which consists of subthreshold or attenuated positive psychotic symptoms that are sufficiently distressing or disabling to the patient, should be added to DSM-V.[19]

Second, because the initial onset of mania and psychosis most frequently occurs during adolescence, a developmental period associated with rapid and dynamic changes in regressive (ie, synaptic pruning) and progressive (ie, myelination) cortical maturational processes,[20] understanding the long-term impact of pharmacologic medications on brain developmental trajectories represents an important consideration, particularly in view of preclinical evidence that psychotropic medications significantly alter normal brain development.[21–23]

Third, early intervention studies need to better assess the short- and long-term impact of standard of care treatment strategies for prodromal symptomatology (eg, depression, inattention, and hyperactivity). Antidepressant and psychostimulant medications used for these early manifestations of incipient mania may hasten illness progression in high-risk youth.

Lastly, SGA medications, which may be efficacious for the treatment of mood and subthreshold psychotic symptoms in high-risk youth, are frequently associated with significant treatment-emergent weight gain and obesity, metabolic syndrome, and elevated cardiovascular risk factors in adolescent patients.[24]

Together, these data highlight potential risks associated with the use of pharmacologic medications for the treatment of prodromal symptoms in high-risk individuals, and endorse the adoption of a clinical staging model.[8,25] The clinical staging model proposes that interventions with lower risks (including psychosocial therapy) may be appropriate for the treatment of subthreshold symptoms in earlier stages of the illness, whereas those with greater risks are reserved for threshold symptoms emerging at later stages.[25]

TREATMENT OF BP IN THE PRESENCE OF COMORBID CONDITIONS

MDD frequently precedes the initial onset of mania and is commonly treated with antidepressant medications regardless of the risk for developing BP. However, an emerging body of evidence suggests that treatment with antidepressants may precipitate or exacerbate suicidality and manic symptoms and possibly reduce the age at onset of mania.[26]

An epidemiologic study found that peripubertal children (age 10–14 years) exposed to antidepressants were at highest risk for manic conversion,[27] and another study found that children who received prior antidepressant treatment had an earlier onset of BP than never exposed children.[28] A retrospective study found that five of six (83%) adolescent/young adult patients transitioning to mania were previously treated with a selective serotonin reuptake inhibitor antidepressant.[12] Additionally, in a cohort of 52 children and adolescents with or at high risk for BP, 50% had experienced antidepressant-induced mania, and 26% experienced new-onset suicidal ideation within 1 month of starting an antidepressant.[29] In a small (n = 9) prospective open-label treatment trial, more than 50% of youth at high risk for BP experienced new manic symptoms or suicidality after treatment with paroxetine or paroxetine plus divalproex.[30]

Together, these data highlight the potential vulnerability of youth at high risk for BP to serious psychiatric side effects of antidepressant medications. Of additional concern is that these medications may cause "kindling" toward an earlier onset of mania than otherwise would have occurred.[31] It is possible that such side effects as mania or suicidality may create a type of neurobiologic "scar" that accelerates the development of mania in response to psychosocial stress,[32] although retrospective data have not supported this acceleration model of mania onset.[33] Furthermore, MDD is also a common feature of the psychosis prodrome,[15] and preliminary evidence suggests that antidepressants may be protective against the development of psychosis in high-risk patients.[34,35] Therefore, additional prospective research is needed to evaluate the risks and benefits associated with antidepressant treatment in youth at risk for BP and SZ.

Cognitive symptoms, particularly deficits in concentration and attention, also frequently precede the initial onset BP and SZ, and are commonly initially treated with psychostimulant medications, including methylphenidate or amphetamine (AMPH) derivatives. Although the role of early treatment with psychostimulants in the pathoetiology of mania or psychosis is poorly understood, acute treatment with psychostimulants may produce clinical features that are analogous to idiopathic mania, and repeated AMPH treatment is associated with psychotogenic effects in a subset of individuals.[36] Moreover, the incremental increase in psychomotor responses (ie, increased eye-blink rate, arousal, euphoria) observed in healthy control subjects after repeated AMPH treatment is not exhibited by first-episode manic or psychotic patients,[37] and may reflect presensitization in response to prior exposure to psychostimulants or stress.[38] Adolescents with BP and a history of stimulant exposure before the onset of BP may have an earlier age at onset of mania than those without prior stimulant exposure, independent of co-occurring ADHD.[39] Thus, psychostimulants may share similar problematic psychiatric effects with antidepressants in youth at high-risk for BD and SZ.[26] Although controlled trials have found that treatment with psychostimulants are effective and largely safe for treating ADHD symptoms in BP youth in conjunction with mood-stabilizers,[40–42] it is not clear that such treatment is either safe or effective in youth at high risk for developing BP who have not yet developed mania. In view of evidence for a sevenfold increase in AMPH prescriptions for children in the United States over the last decade[43] in parallel with a 40-fold increase in the diagnosis of childhood and adolescent BP in office-based medical settings,[44] there is an urgent need for additional research into potential iatrogenic effects of early psychostimulant treatment in high-risk populations.

EVIDENCE-BASED INTERVENTIONS
High Risk for Psychosis

In conjunction with the development of criteria for identifying individuals at high risk for psychosis, preliminary efforts have been made to develop interventions that are protective against the progression to psychosis in high-risk patients (**Table 1**). The first controlled prevention trial randomized a cohort of patients meeting high-risk criteria for psychosis to low-dose risperidone (mean dose, 1.3 mg/d; n = 31) combined with cognitive behavioral therapy or to need-based supportive psychotherapy (n = 28) for 6 months, after which patients were offered ongoing needs-based intervention for an additional 6 months.[45] By the end of the 6-month treatment phase, 10 (36%) of 28 patients who received needs-based supportive psychotherapy transitioned to psychosis compared with 3 (10%) of 31 patients receiving risperidone plus cognitive behavioral therapy (P = .03). During the 6-month follow-up phase, another three

Table 1
Intervention trials in patients at high risk for developing psychosis

Study	Design	Interventions/ Sample	Duration	Main Findings
McGorry et al,[45] 2002	Randomized Single blind	RSP, 1–2 mg/d + CBT (n = 31) NBI (n = 28)	6 mo	Transition rate: RSP + CBT: 36% vs NBI: 10% (P = .03) Positive symptoms: RSP + CBT = NBI Negative symptoms: RSP + CBT = NBI
McGlashan et al,[47] 2006	Randomized Double blind	OLZ, 5–15 mg/d (n = 31) PLB (n = 29)	12 mo	Transition rate: OLZ: 38% vs PLB: 16% (P = .08) Positive symptoms: OLZ > PLB Negative symptoms: OLZ = PLB
Yung et al,[46] 2011	Randomized Single blind	RSP, 0.5–2 mg/d + CT (n = 43) PLB + CT (n = 44) ST + PLB (n = 28)	6 mo	Transition rate: RSP + CT: 4.7% vs PLB + CT: 9.1% vs ST + PLB: 7.1% (P = .92) Positive symptoms: RSP + CT = PLB + CT = ST + PLB Negative symptoms: RSP + CT = PLB + CT = ST + PLB
Cornblatt et al,[34] 2007	Prospective Naturalistic	AD (n = 20) SGA antipsychotics (n = 28)	6 mo	Transition rate: AD: 0% vs SGA: 38% (P = .007) Positive symptoms: AD = SGA Negative symptoms: AD = SGA
Amminger et al,[48] 2010	Randomized Double blind	LCn-3 fatty acids (1.2 g/d) (n = 40) Placebo (n = 41)	12 wks	Transition rate: LCn-3: 4.9% vs PLB: 27.5% (P = .007) Positive symptoms: LCn-3 > PLB Negative symptoms: LCn-3 > PLB
Morrison et al,[49] 2004	Randomized Single blind	CT (n = 35) TAU (n = 23)	6 mo	Transition rate: CT: 6% vs TAU: 22% (P = .03) Positive symptoms: CT > TAU Negative symptoms: Not reported

Abbreviations: AD, antidepressants; CBT, cognitive behavioral therapy; CT, cognitive therapy; OLZ, olanzapine; NBI, needs-based intervention; PLB, placebo; RSP, risperidone; ST, supportive therapy; TAU, treatment as usual.

patients in the risperidone plus cognitive behavioral therapy group became psychotic and the original treatment group difference became nonsignificant. However, protection against transition was observed for patients that were adherent to risperidone therapy during the initial treatment phase. In a subsequent larger (n = 115) replication study, no differences were found in psychosis transition rates between high-risk participants who received 6 months of risperidone plus cognitive therapy compared with those who received placebo plus cognitive therapy.[46] In the latter study, a greater percentage of patients in the risperidone arm experienced weight gain (30%) compared with placebo (9.1%), although this difference was not statistically significant.

Another trial randomized patients at high risk for developing psychosis to olanzapine (5–15 mg/day; n = 31) or placebo (n = 29) for a 1-year double-blind treatment period followed by a 1-year no-treatment observational period.[47] During the treatment phase, 5 (16.1%) of 31 patients receiving olanzapine and 11 (37.9%) of 29 patients receiving placebo transitioned to psychosis, though this difference did not reach statistical significance (P = .08). The hazard ratio of conversion to psychosis for placebo-treated patients was 2.5 times greater than olanzapine-treated patients (P = .09). Prodromal-positive symptoms improved more in the olanzapine group than in the placebo group between Weeks 8 and 28 (P = .03). Olanzapine-treated patients gained significantly more weight than placebo-treated patients, and the rate of discontinuation was higher in the olanzapine (55%) than placebo (34%) arm. In the 1-year follow-up period, psychosis transition rates did not differ significantly between treatment groups.

A prospective naturalistic treatment study compared 48 adolescents at high risk for developing psychosis treated with antidepressant (n = 20) or SGA (n = 28) medications.[34] Of the 12 (25%) of 48 patients who transitioned to psychosis, all were prescribed SGAs, whereas none of the antidepressant-treated adolescents converted (P = .007). Importantly, 11 of the 12 converters were nonadherent to SGA treatment. Improvements in positive and negative symptoms were significant and similar in both treatment groups. It was concluded that that antidepressants may be advantageous over SGAs as a first-line treatment for patients at high risk for transitioning to psychosis, but interpretation was limited by nonrandom assignment and the widespread nonadherence to SGA treatment.

Nonpharmacologic interventions have also been evaluated in youth at high risk for developing psychosis. A double-blind trial randomized 81 patients at high risk for developing psychosis to 12-week treatment with 1.2 g/d of long chain omega-3 (LCn-3) fatty acids or placebo, followed by a 40-week observation period after treatment cessation (12 months total).[48] By the end of the 12-month study, 2 (4.9%) of 41 individuals in the LCn-3 fatty acid arm and 11 (27.5%) of 40 in the placebo arm transitioned to threshold psychosis (P = .007). During the 12-week treatment phase, LCn-3 fatty acids significantly reduced positive symptoms (P = .01), negative symptoms (P = .02), and general symptoms (P = .01) and improved functioning (P = .002) compared with placebo. The incidence of adverse effects did not differ between the treatment groups. It was concluded that LCn-3 fatty acids were safe and efficacious for preventing or delaying psychosis transitioning in high-risk patients. A controlled trial randomized 58 patients at high risk for developing psychosis to 6 months of cognitive therapy or treatment as usual, and all patients were monitored for a total of 12 months.[49] By the end of the 12-month study, 2 (6%) of 35 patients in the cognitive therapy arm and 5 (22%) of 23 in the treatment as usual arm had transitioned to threshold psychotic disorder (P = .028). The likelihood of being prescribed antipsychotic medications was also significantly reduced in the cognitive therapy arm compared with treatment as usual. These findings suggest the potential use of LCn-3 fatty acids or cognitive therapy as safe and efficacious first-line interventions for patients at high risk for SZ.

High Risk for BP

The potential negative effects of antidepressant and psychostimulant medications in youth at high risk for developing BP have prompted studies investigating the efficacy and safety of mood-stabilizer and antipsychotic medications for the treatment of prodromal mood symptoms in high-risk youth (**Table 2**). Lithium was evaluated for the treatment of MDD in 30 prepubertal children with a family history of BP (80%) or a multigenerational family history of MDD without BP (20%) in a 6-week double-blind placebo-controlled trial. In this study, lithium (mean serum level, 0.99 ± 0.16 mEq/L) was not more effective than placebo for treating prepubertal depression in these high-risk children.[50] A 12-week open-label study of divalproex for the treatment of 24 children and adolescents with at least one biologic parent with BP and at least one DSM-IV disorder (MDD, dysthymic disorder, cyclothymic disorder, or ADHD) and moderate affective symptoms found that 75% of patients were responders by primary outcome criteria ("very much improved" or "much improved" on the Clinical Global Impressions-Improvement scale).[51] However, a study of 56 youth ages 5 to 17 years with BP not otherwise specified or cyclothymia who also had at least one biologic parent with BP were randomly assigned to double-blind treatment with either divalproex or placebo for up to 5 years. The groups did not significantly differ in survival time for discontinuation for any reason ($P = .93$) or discontinuation because of a mood event ($P = .55$). Additionally, changes in mood symptom ratings and psychosocial functioning from baseline to study discontinuation did not differ between groups, suggesting that divalproex did not produce clinically meaningful improvements in this high-risk population.[52] Thus, it is unclear whether divalproex ultimately will have a role in treating this population acutely or for prophylaxis of mood disorder progression.

A 12-week single-blind study investigated quetiapine for the treatment of 20 adolescents with mood disorder diagnoses other than mania who had a first-degree relative with BP.[53] It was found that 87% of patients were responders as defined by an endpoint Clinical Global Impressions-Improvement scale score of "very much" or "much" improved. However, there was a statistically significant increase in body mass index, and more than half (55%) of the patients experienced somnolence during the course of the study.

All of these early intervention trials for youth at high risk for BP evaluated relatively acute outcomes, and were not long enough to assess prevention of the development of mania. Thus, to date, there have been no prospective prevention trials using pharmacologic interventions in children and adolescents at high risk for developing BP. However, Nadkarni and Fristad[54] found that multifamily psychoeducation groups exerted a protective effect on conversion to bipolar spectrum disorders among children with depressive spectrum disorders. Another 1-year open trial found that family-focused therapy with 13 children who had a parent with BP resulted in significant improvements in depression, hypomania, and psychosocial functioning scores.[55] In view of evidence for a protective effect of LCn-3 fatty acids in youth at high risk for developing psychosis,[48] it is relevant that preliminary prospective intervention trials have found that LCn-3 fatty acids administered as monotherapy or adjunctively significantly reduce depression or manic symptom severity in pediatric and adolescent patients with MDD[56] or BP.[57,58] These preliminary findings suggest that psychosocial therapy or LCn-3 fatty acids may represent candidate interventions for youth at high risk for developing BP, and warrant further evaluation in controlled trials.

Table 2
Intervention trials in patients at high risk for developing mania

Study	Design	Intervention	Target Dose	Duration	Findings
Geller et al,[50] 1998	Randomized Double blind	Lithium (n = 17) Placebo (n = 13)	Serum 0.9–1.3 mEq/L	6 wk	C–GAS: lithium = placebo
Chang et al,[51] 2003	Open–label	Divalproex (n = 24)	15–20 mg/kg/d	12 wk	↓ CGI–I, ↓ HAM-D, ↓ YMRS
Findling et al,[52] 2007	Randomized Double blind	Divalproex (n = 29) Placebo (n = 27)	10 mg/kg/d	<60 mo	CGAS: divalproex = placebo YMRS: divalproex = placebo CDRS–R: divalproex = placebo
DelBello et al,[53] 2007	Single blind	Quetiapine (n = 20)	300–600 mg/d	12 wk	CGI–I: quetiapine > placebo YMRS: quetiapine > placebo CDRS–R: quetiapine > placebo
Miklowitz et al,[55] 2011	Open	Family–focused therapy (n = 13)	3 Sessions/mo	4 mo	↓ CDRS–R, ↓ YMRS

Abbreviations: C–GAS, Children's Global Assessment Scale; CDRS–R, Children's Depression Rating Scale–Revised; CGI–I, Clinical Global Impressions–Improvement; HAM–D, Hamilton Rating Scale for Depression; YMRS, Young Mania Rating Scale.

CLINICAL VIGNETTE

"A.B." is a 16-year-old girl with a father with BP who presented with several months of depressed mood, hypersomnia, anhedonia, fatigue, anergia, episodes of spontaneous crying and feelings of guilt, and met DSM-IV-TR criteria for MDD. A.B. identified no precipitants for her depressive symptoms; denied significant anxiety symptoms or personal history of manic symptoms; and generally described good family relationships and fair (but recently declining) academic performance at a local, parochial school. There was no prior history of manic symptoms, anxiety, or ADHD. Additionally, there was no family history of antidepressant-induced manic symptoms in her mother or siblings. Citalopram was begun at a dose of 20 mg daily and after 5 weeks of treatment, A.B. had begun to improve but she still reported depressed mood and a moderate neurovegetative burden. To target her persistent depressed mood and neurovegetative symptoms, citalopram was increased to 30 mg daily. Three weeks after the increase in dose, A.B.'s mother reported concerns about her daughter's behavior, including her having been caught "sexting" several individuals with whom she had previously had superficial relationships and she had purchased several hundred dollars of clothing and lingerie at a local store. Additionally, A.B. required fewer than 4 hours of sleep per night, yet described her mood as "great" and reported racing thoughts, distractibility, and that her family and friends had noticed that she was talking "faster." At that time, her mental status examination was remarkable for the wearing of excessive make-up, a low-cut shirt, pressured speech, psychomotor agitation, elated mood, and expanded affective range. Further, A.B.'s thought processes were tangential and thought content was remarkable for grandiosity and sexual preoccupation. Citalopram was discontinued and quetiapine was begun at 100 mg daily and titrated to 300 mg daily with resolution of the manic symptoms within 1 week.

This case illustrates the potential risk of antidepressant-induced manic symptoms (AIMS) in adolescents with a family history of BP.[26] The emergence of manic symptoms occurred within several weeks of an increase in antidepressant dose and was not preceded by subsyndromal manic symptoms. Additionally, this patient's course raises the possibility that the use of a clinical staging model and alternative intervention (eg, psychotherapy or LCn-3 fatty acids) may have obviated the need for an antidepressant as the first-line intervention. Importantly, and of relevance to clinicians encountering treatment-emergent manic in high-risk youth who have been exposed to antidepressants, withdrawal of the selective serotonin reuptake inhibitor, and initiation of an SGA produced rapid, sustained improvement in manic symptoms. However, for less severe AIMS cases, it is possible that cessation of the antidepressant could be followed by close monitoring to see if manic symptoms abate naturally before antimanic medications are used. An alternate approach would have been to discuss the possibility of other medications with the family and patient, such as lamotrigine, quetiapine, or lithium. However, insufficient data exist to support the efficacy of these agents in depressed populations at high risk for BP, and future investigation should also include clinical and biologic predictors of AIMS in youth.

CONCLUSIONS AND FUTURE DIRECTIONS

Early research efforts have begun to develop and validate criteria to identify individuals at high risk for developing BP and SZ, and to evaluate pharmacologic and nonpharmacologic interventions for the treatment of prodromal symptoms in high-risk populations. Although there have been some promising findings from early intervention trials evaluating SGA medications, antidepressants, LCn-3 fatty acids, and cognitive-behavioral therapy in patients at high risk for developing psychosis, there is currently a dearth of prospective research in patients at high risk for developing mania. Indeed, the potential iatrogenic effects of antidepressant and psychostimulant medications, lack of efficacy of mood-stabilizer medications for prodromal mood symptoms, and adverse cardio-metabolic effects associated with SGA medications highlight the urgent need to identify and evaluate evidence-based treatments for youth at high risk for BP. These findings further emphasize the need to identify whether a patient is at high risk for developing mania or psychosis to exercise appropriate caution when prescribing standard of care medications. Preliminary evidence endorses the adoption of a clinical staging approach, and additional prospective research is warranted to evaluate the efficacy of candidate low-risk first-line interventions, including psychosocial or LCn-3 fatty acids, in youth at high risk for developing BP or SZ.

REFERENCES

1. Kessler RC, Merikangas KR, Wang PS. Prevalence, comorbidity, and service utilization for mood disorders in the United States at the beginning of the twenty-first century. Annu Rev Clin Psychol 2007;3:137–58.
2. Perlis RH, Dennehy EB, Miklowitz DJ, et al. Retrospective age at onset of bipolar disorder and outcome during two-year follow-up: results from the STEP-BD study. Bipolar Disord 2009;11:391–400.
3. Merikangas KR, Cui L, Kattan G, et al. Mania with and without depression in a community sample of US adolescents. Arch Gen Psychiatry 2012. [Epub ahead of print].
4. Smoller JW, Finn CT. Family, twin, and adoption studies of bipolar disorder. Am J Med Genet C Semin Med Genet 2003;123:48–58.
5. Berk M, Conus P, Lucas N, et al. Setting the stage: from prodrome to treatment resistance in bipolar disorder. Bipolar Disord 2007;9:671–8.
6. Conus P, Ward J, Hallam KT, et al. The proximal prodrome to first episode mania: a new target for early intervention. Bipolar Disord 2008;10:555–65.
7. Findling RL, Youngstrom EA, McNamara NK, et al. Early symptoms of mania and the role of parental risk. Bipolar Disord 2005;7:623–34.
8. McNamara RK, Nandagopal JJ, Strakowski SM, et al. Preventative strategies for early-onset bipolar disorder: towards a clinical staging model. CNS Drugs 2010; 24:983–96.
9. Strober M, Carlson G. Bipolar illness in adolescents with major depression: clinical, genetic, and psychopharmacologic predictors in a three- to four-year prospective follow-up investigation. Arch Gen Psychiatry 1982;39:549–55.
10. Birmaher B, Axelson D, Goldstein B, et al. Four-year longitudinal course of children and adolescents with bipolar spectrum disorders: the Course and Outcome of Bipolar Youth (COBY) study. Am J Psychiatry 2009;166:795–804.
11. Singh MK, DelBello MP, Kowatch RA, et al. Co-occurrence of bipolar and attention-deficit hyperactivity disorders in children. Bipolar Disord 2006;8:710–20.
12. Bechdolf A, Nelson B, Cotton SM, et al. A preliminary evaluation of the validity of at-risk criteria for bipolar disorders in help-seeking adolescents and young adults. J Affect Disord 2010;127:316–20.
13. Correll CU, Penzner JB, Lencz T, et al. Early identification and high-risk strategies for bipolar disorder. Bipolar Disord 2007;9:324–38.
14. Aleman A, Kahn RS, Selten JP. Sex differences in the risk of schizophrenia: evidence from meta-analysis. Arch Gen Psychiatry 2003;60:565–71.
15. Rosen JL, Miller TJ, D'Andrea JT, et al. Comorbid diagnoses in patients meeting criteria for the schizophrenia prodrome. Schizophr Res 2006;85:124–31.
16. Yung AR, Phillips LJ, Yuen HP, et al. Psychosis prediction: 12-month follow up of a high-risk ("prodromal") group. Schizophr Res 2003;60:21–32.

17. Fusar-Poli P, Bonoldi I, Yung AR, et al. Predicting psychosis: meta-analysis of transition outcomes in individuals at high clinical risk. Arch Gen Psychiatry 2012;69: 220–9.

18. Fusar-Poli P, Bechdolf A, Taylor MJ, et al. At risk for schizophrenic or affective psychoses? A meta-analysis of DSM/ICD diagnostic outcomes in individuals at high clinical risk. Schizophr Bull 2012. [Epub ahead of print].

19. Yung AR, Nelson B, Thompson AD, et al. Should a "Risk Syndrome for Psychosis" be included in the DSMV? Schizophr Res 2010;120:7–15.

20. Giedd JN, Lalonde FM, Celano MJ, et al. Anatomical brain magnetic resonance imaging of typically developing children and adolescents. J Am Acad Child Adolesc Psychiatry 2009;48:465–70.

21. LaRoche RB, Morgan RE. Adolescent fluoxetine exposure produces enduring, sex-specific alterations of visual discrimination and attention in rats. Neurotoxicol Teratol 2007;29:96–107.

22. McPherson CS, Lawrence AJ. Exposure to amphetamine in rats during periadolescence establishes behavioural and extrastriatal neural sensitization in adulthood. Int J Neuropsychopharmacol 2006;9:377–92.

23. Youngs RM, Chu MS, Meloni EG, et al. Lithium administration to preadolescent rats causes long-lasting increases in anxiety-like behavior and has molecular consequences. J Neurosci 2006;26:6031–9.

24. Correll CU, Manu P, Olshanskiy V, et al. Cardiometabolic risk of second-generation antipsychotic medications during first-time use in children and adolescents. JAMA 2009;302:1765–73.

25. McGorry PD, Hickie IB, Yung AR, et al. Clinical staging of psychiatric disorders: a heuristic framework for choosing earlier, safer and more effective interventions. Aust N Z J Psychiatry 2006;40:616–22.

26. Goldsmith M, Singh M, Chang K. Antidepressants and psychostimulants in pediatric populations. Is there an association with mania? Paediatr Drugs 2011;13: 225–39.

27. Martin A, Young C, Leckman JF, et al. Age effects on antidepressant-induced manic conversion. Arch Pediatr Adolesc Med 2004;158:773–80.

28. Cicero D, El-Mallakh RS, Holman J, et al. Antidepressant exposure in bipolar children. Psychiatry 2003;66:317–22.

29. Baumer FM, Howe M, Gallelli K, et al. A pilot study of antidepressant-induced mania in pediatric bipolar disorder: characteristics, risk factors, and the serotonin transporter gene. Biol Psychiatry 2006;60:1005–12.

30. Findling RL, Lingler J, Rowles BM, et al. A pilot pharmacotherapy trial for depressed youths at high genetic risk for bipolarity. J Child Adolesc Psychopharmacol 2008;18:615–21.

31. Post RM, Weiss SR. A speculative model of affective illness cyclicity based on patterns of drug tolerance observed in amygdala-kindled seizures. Mol Neurobiol 1996;13:33–60.

32. Joseph MF, Youngstrom EA, Soares JC. Antidepressant-coincident mania in children and adolescents treated with selective serotonin reuptake inhibitors. Future Neurol 2009;4:87–102.

33. Chang KD, Saxena K, Howe M, et al. Psychotropic medication exposure and age at onset of bipolar disorder in offspring of parents with bipolar disorder. J Child Adolesc Psychopharmacol 2010;20:25–32.

34. Cornblatt BA, Lencz T, Smith CW, et al. Can antidepressants be used to treat the schizophrenia prodrome? Results of a prospective, naturalistic treatment study of adolescents. J Clin Psychiatry 2007;68:546–57.

35. Fusar-Poli P, Valmaggia L, McGuire P. Can antidepressants prevent psychosis? Lancet 2007;370:1746–8.

36. Bell DS. The experimental reproduction of amphetamine psychosis. Arch Gen Psychiatry 1973;29:35–40.

37. Strakowski SM, Sax KW, Setters MJ, et al. Lack of enhanced response to repeated d-amphetamine challenge in first-episode psychosis: implications for a sensitization model of psychosis in humans. Biol Psychiatry 1997;42:749–55.

38. Laruelle M. The role of endogenous sensitization in the pathophysiology of schizophrenia: implications from recent brain imaging studies. Brain Res Brain Res Rev 2000;31:371–84.

39. DelBello MP, Soutullo CA, Hendricks W, et al. Prior stimulant treatment in adolescents with bipolar disorder: association with age at onset. Bipolar Disord 2001;3: 53–7.

40. Findling RL, Short EJ, McNamara NK, et al. Methylphenidate in the treatment of children and adolescents with bipolar disorder and attention-deficit/hyperactivity disorder. J Am Acad Child Adolesc Psychiatry 2007;46:1445–53.

41. Kowatch RA, Sethuraman G, Hume JH, et al. Combination pharmacotherapy in children and adolescents with bipolar disorder. Biol Psychiatry 2003;53:978–84.

42. Scheffer RE, Kowatch RA, Carmody T, et al. Randomized, placebo-controlled trial of mixed amphetamine salts for symptoms of comorbid ADHD in pediatric bipolar disorder after mood stabilization with divalproex sodium. Am J Psychiatry 2005; 162:58–64.

43. Mayes R, Bagwell C, Erkulwater J. ADHD and the rise in stimulant use among children. Harv Rev Psychiatry 2008;16:151–66.

44. Moreno C, Laje G, Blanco C, et al. National trends in the outpatient diagnosis and treatment of bipolar disorder in youth. Arch Gen Psychiatry 2007;64:1032–9.

45. McGorry PD, Yung AR, Phillips LJ, et al. Randomized controlled trial of interventions designed to reduce the risk of progression to first-episode psychosis in a clinical sample with subthreshold symptoms. Arch Gen Psychiatry 2002;59: 921–8.

46. Yung AR, Phillips LJ, Nelson B, et al. Randomized controlled trial of interventions for young people at ultra high risk for psychosis: 6-month analysis. J Clin Psychiatry 2011;72:430–40.

47. McGlashan TH, Zipursky RB, Perkins D, et al. Randomized, double-blind trial of olanzapine versus placebo in patients prodromally symptomatic for psychosis. Am J Psychiatry 2006;163:790–9.

48. Amminger GP, Schäfer MR, Papageorgiou K, et al. Long-chain omega-3 fatty acids for indicated prevention of psychotic disorders: a randomized, placebo-controlled trial. Arch Gen Psychiatry 2010;67:146–54.

49. Morrison AP, French P, Walford L, et al. Cognitive therapy for the prevention of psychosis in people at ultra-high risk: randomised controlled trial. Br J Psychiatry 2004;185:291–7.

50. Geller B, Cooper TB, Zimerman B, et al. Lithium for prepubertal depressed children with family history predictors of future bipolarity: a double-blind, placebo-controlled study. J Affect Disord 1998;51:165–75.

51. Chang KD, Dienes K, Blasey C, et al. Divalproex monotherapy in the treatment of bipolar offspring with mood and behavioral disorders and at least mild affective symptoms. Clin Psychiatry 2003;64:936–42.

52. Findling RL, Frazier TW, Youngstrom EA, et al. Double-blind, placebo-controlled trial of divalproex monotherapy in the treatment of symptomatic youth at high risk for developing bipolar disorder. J Clin Psychiatry 2007;68:781–8.

53. DelBello MP, Adler CM, Whitsel RM, et al. A 12-week single-blind trial of quetiapine for the treatment of mood symptoms in adolescents at high risk for developing bipolar I disorder. J Clin Psychiatry 2007;68:789–95.
54. Nadkarni RB, Fristad MA. Clinical course of children with a depressive spectrum disorder and transient manic symptoms. Bipolar Disord 2010;12:494–503.
55. Miklowitz DJ, Chang KD, Taylor DO, et al. Early psychosocial intervention for youth at risk for bipolar I or II disorder: a one-year treatment development trial. Bipolar Disord 2011;13:67–75.
56. Nemets H, Nemets B, Apter A, et al. Omega-3 treatment of childhood depression: a controlled, double-blind pilot study. Am J Psychiatry 2006;163:1098–100.
57. Clayton EH, Hanstock TL, Hirneth SJ, et al. Reduced mania and depression in juvenile bipolar disorder associated with long-chain omega-3 polyunsaturated fatty acid supplementation. Eur J Clin Nutr 2009;63:1037–40.
58. Wozniak J, Biederman J, Mick E, et al. Omega-3 fatty acid monotherapy for pediatric bipolar disorder: a prospective open-label trial. Eur Neuropsychopharmacol 2007;17:440–7.

The Neural Effects of Psychotropic Medications in Children and Adolescents

Manpreet K. Singh, MD, MS*, Kiki D. Chang, MD

KEYWORDS

- Medication • Neuroimaging • Pediatric • Psychopathology
- Magnetic resonance imaging

KEY POINTS

- Little is known about the neurobiological effects of psychotropic medications on the developing brain.
- An efficient way to elucidate neural mechanisms that underlie the effects of treatment is to use magnetic resonance imaging technology to assess in vivo brain differences in youth before and after an intervention has been made.
- Across disorders, the neurotropic effects of lithium on amygdala and hippocampal volumes appear to be normalizing and are correlated with symptom improvement, and there appears to be normalization of functional activations while performing a wide array of neurocognitive tasks after treatment with psychostimulants, antipsychotics, antidepressants, and mood stabilizers.
- Additional information is needed to better understand the critical periods of benefit from these interventions, and how they compare relative to one another.

INTRODUCTION

Children and adolescents are increasingly being diagnosed with psychopathology, with approximately 21% of youth in the United States ages 9 through 17 having a diagnosable mental illness with some degree of impairment.[1] An early onset of many psychiatric disorders in youth has been linked with a more severe course of illness, morbidities such as suicide attempts and substance abuse, as well as the presence of comorbidities and complications such as poor academic and job performance, interpersonal conflicts, or legal problems.[2–5] Despite vigorous efforts to find effective treatments for psychiatric conditions in youth, treatment challenges are frequent and illness carries high rates of complications, including mortality.[6]

Division of Child and Adolescent Psychiatry, Stanford University School of Medicine, 401 Quarry Road, Stanford, CA 94305-5719, USA
* Corresponding author.
E-mail address: mksingh@stanford.edu

Child Adolesc Psychiatric Clin N Am 21 (2012) 753–771
http://dx.doi.org/10.1016/j.chc.2012.07.010
1056-4993/12/$ – see front matter © 2012 Elsevier Inc. All rights reserved.

Comprehensive treatment plans are often required for youth with psychopathology to address a complex array of symptoms and associated morbidities. In general, a multimodal treatment approach combining pharmacologic agents and psychosocial interventions is suggested, with the goal of improving symptoms, providing psychoeducation about the mental illness, and promoting treatment adherence for relapse prevention and attenuation of long-term complications from the illness.[7,8] Clinicians are encouraged to advocate for prevention, early intervention, and biopsychosocial treatments that promote the healthy growth and development of all children affected by psychopathology, in any cultural context.[9] At this point, however, we know relatively little about the mechanisms that underlie treatment and presume that the effects of pharmacologic and nonpharmacologic interventions on the brain are multifactorial.

An efficient way to elucidate neural mechanisms that underlie the effects of treatment is to use magnetic resonance imaging (MRI) technology to assess in vivo brain differences in youth before and after an intervention has been made. For example, specific differences in brains exposed rather than unexposed to medications may suggest intrinsic biological pathways that may clarify the mechanisms by which such treatments are functioning to reduce symptom burden. In some instances, medications have been found to have either no effect or a normalizing effect on brain MRI findings compared with healthy controls.[10] Some neuroimaging studies have attempted to examine the effects of medications on structural and functional outcomes in the brain post hoc, and have found no direct influence of medication exposure on primary findings.[11,12] In other cases, researchers have tried to avoid the potential confounding effects of medications on brain MRI results by studying only unmedicated or medication-naïve youth.[13–16] Although there are some clear advantages to examining unmedicated youth with psychopathology, such individuals are difficult to find and may represent a subset of the population with relatively low symptom severity, thereby limiting generalizability of the results to the overall population.

This article evaluates studies in which medications were not treated as a confounder, but rather as a variable of interest on neural outcome. Structural, functional, neurochemical, and other neuroimaging modalities used to study the neurophysiologic alterations associated with psychotropic medication exposure in youth are reviewed. In addition, the authors review neuroimaging studies examining the effects of psychotherapeutic interventions, in an effort to explore the potential effects of nonpharmacologic treatment in selected disorders. After reviewing each modality as it applies to youth with various psychiatric diagnoses, the article concludes by illustrating how taken together, these studies suggest that therapeutic interventions during childhood do indeed affect brain structure and function in a detectable manner. Finally, areas of future study that will further explain the biological correlates of treating psychopathology are proposed.

METHODS

A literature search using PubMed was conducted to identify peer-reviewed neuroimaging studies of children and adolescents for the period 1966 to June 2012. The following terms were included in the search: "medication" or "psychotropic" or "psychotherapy" or "treatment" with "psychiatric" or diagnostic categories, and "adolescents," "children," "youth," "juvenile," or "pediatric," followed by "neuroimaging," "magnetic resonance imaging (MRI)," "diffusion tensor imaging (DTI)," "functional MRI (fMRI)," or "spectroscopy (MRS)." References from identified articles were also reviewed to ensure that all relevant articles were included.

RESULTS

Data were reviewed from more than 50 studies published from 1966 to 2012 that reported on neuroimaging applications in selected child psychiatric diagnoses. Available data were examined from structural MRI, diffusion tensor imaging (DTI), functional MRI (fMRI), and magnetic resonance spectroscopy (MRS) studies in youth with selected psychiatric disorders including anorexia nervosa (AN), attention deficit with hyperactivity disorder (ADHD), autism, bipolar disorder (BD), depressive disorders, obsessive-compulsive disorder (OCD), and schizophrenia.

Anorexia Nervosa

In youth with eating disorders such as AN, some studies have demonstrated that the cognitive effects of this disorder may be ameliorated by intervention in general. Although weight recovery is the main treatment end point for youth with this disorder, an understanding of the interaction between specific mechanisms by which weight recovery is achieved and neurocognitive outcomes is still under development. For example, 9 patients with AN were assessed by neuroimaging before and after 7 months of inpatient multidisciplinary treatment, involving a combination of biological management (eg, with selective serotonin reuptake inhibitors [SSRIs]), nutritional rehabilitation, a behavioral program standardized to improve eating patterns and weight, individual and group cognitive treatment, and parent counseling, all aimed at weight recovery.[17] Before treatment, the AN group showed significantly higher activation than controls in temporal and parietal areas, and especially in the temporal superior gyrus, during performance of a working memory task. A negative correlation was found between brain activation and body mass index and a positive correlation was found between activation and depressive symptomatology. At follow-up after weight recovery, AN patients showed a decrease in brain activation in these areas and did not present differences relative to controls, suggesting that differences with respect to controls disappeared after weight recovery. These investigators also showed that posterior gray matter structural deficits assessed by serial voxel-based morphometry (VBM)[18] and prefrontal N-acetyl aspartate (NAA), and other neurochemical deficits assessed by MRS,[19] are also reversible by nutritional recovery. The multimodal approach used by these researchers provides them with the opportunity to develop important theoretical models of how treatment of AN can influence all levels of brain function. Future studies would benefit from teasing apart the specific neural effects of the various interventions (biological and psychosocial) presented to this population.

Attention Deficit with Hyperactivity

In youth with ADHD, a few studies have examined the neural effects of psychostimulant medications. One study showed that total frontal, prefrontal, and caudate volumes were larger for children and adolescents with ADHD compared with controls, and that youth with ADHD without a treatment history had smaller right anterior cingulate cortex (ACC) volumes than those of ADHD youth with a treatment history.[20] Although the treatment group and the nontreatment group were comparable in terms of ADHD symptom severity assessed by parents, this study did not explicitly evaluate or control for symptom severity, which may have biased their results such that those who received treatment had more severe illness warranting pharmacologic intervention in comparison with those who did not receive treatment.

Structural MRI for ADHD

Because ADHD persists into adulthood in 50% to 70% of cases, a recent meta-analysis aiming to identify MRI-based structural differences between adults and children with ADHD discovered significant positive effects of treatment.[21] Specifically, volumetric reductions in basal ganglia regions (eg, right globus pallidus, right putamen, and caudate), as well as alterations in limbic regions (ACC and amygdala), were more pronounced in nontreated populations and appeared to diminish over time from childhood to adulthood. Treatment also appeared to have a normalizing effect on brain structure such that a higher percentage of treated participants showed fewer structural anomalies than those who were untreated. Consistent with this study, another meta-analysis of structural imaging data also found abnormalities in the basal ganglia associated with ADHD.[22] This analysis evaluated the effects of age and treatment in these studies, and found that patients with ADHD may catch up on disorder-related developmental delay with the use of stimulant medication, which was associated with normalization of structural abnormalities in the lentiform nucleus extending into the caudate nucleus. Both of these meta-analyses demonstrate the need for within-subject prospective studies to confirm the impact of psychostimulants on brain structure in youth with ADHD.

Functional MRI for ADHD

fMRI studies in this area used longitudinal designs by performing prestimulant and poststimulant exposure fMRI scans. In an fMRI study of 18 youths with ADHD, researchers used a Sternberg working memory task in a randomized, double-blind, placebo-controlled design. Results demonstrated that a clinically effective dose of a psychostimulant led to the recruitment of additional brain regions that were not engaged in the networks when participants were on placebo.[23] In addition, psychostimulant therapy strengthened connectivity between frontoparietal networks that were engaged during working memory, with many connectivity changes being directly related to improved working memory reaction time. This study showed strong evidence for regional functional connectivity changes following medication in structures previously implicated as abnormal in ADHD, such as anterior cingulate, ventrolateral prefrontal cortex, and precuneus, suggesting a mechanism underlying the beneficial effects of medication on working memory performance.

In another fMRI study designed to assess the effects of single-dose methylphenidate on error-processing regions of the brain during a stop task, 12 medication-naïve boys with ADHD were scanned twice, under either a single clinical dose of methylphenidate or placebo, in a randomized, double-blind design.[24] Brain activation was compared within patients under either drug condition, and to test for the potential normalization effects of methylphenidate, brain activation in ADHD patients under either drug condition was compared with that of 13 healthy age-matched boys. This study found that during failed inhibition, boys with ADHD taking placebo showed reduced brain activation relative to control subjects in performance-monitoring areas of dorsomedial and left ventrolateral prefrontal cortices, thalamus, cingulate, and parietal regions. Methylphenidate, in comparison with placebo, upregulated activation in these brain regions within patients and normalized all activation differences between patients and control subjects. During successful inhibition, methylphenidate normalized reduced activation observed in patients taking placebo compared with control subjects in parietotemporal and cerebellar regions. This study demonstrated that a single dose of a psychostimulant normalizes levels of brain activity in attentional brain networks in youth with ADHD.

Functional near-infrared spectroscopy for ADHD

Similar to ADHD, olfactory sensitivity, discrimination, and identification are mediated by dopamine metabolism. Twenty-seven youths with ADHD and a history of chronic methylphenidate exposure were washed out from their medication and assessed along with healthy controls for olfactory function by functional near-infrared spectros-copy (fNIRS) during presentation of 2-phenylethanol.[25] Results from this study showed that cessation of methylphenidate led to significant increases in olfactory discrimination, but decreased inferior frontal and temporal brain activation in youth with ADHD. Of interest, this activation pattern associated with olfaction normalized with the reintroduction of medication to the ADHD group, providing in vivo evidence that psychostimulants modulate related dopaminergic systems.

Magnetic resonance spectroscopy for ADHD

Data demonstrating macroscopic structural and functional brain changes in youth with ADHD suggest underlying cellular and molecular changes that may be due to treat-ment. MRS is a noninvasive neuroimaging method that yields molecular-level bio-chemical data to quantitatively examine neuronal function. Several studies in youth with ADHD have demonstrated in vivo neurochemical changes in response to different medication treatments. In a case series of 2 children showing symptom improvement with methylphenidate and 2 children treated with atomoxetine, a decrease in the gluta-mate/creatine ratio (mean change 56.1%) was observed in the striatum between 14 and 18 weeks of therapy in all 4 children with ADHD.[26] In the prefrontal cortex, how-ever, changes in the glutamate/creatine ratio were noted only in subjects receiving atomoxetine.[26] In another study by the same group, MRS data were collected from the prefrontal cortex and striatum in 14 children with ADHD, before and after treatment with psychostimulants or atomoxetine.[27] The glutamate/glutamine/γ-aminobutyric acid-to-creatine/phosphocreatine ratio decreased significantly in the striatum, sug-gesting that striatal glutamate may be involved in treatment response in ADHD.

Treatment of the prefrontal region for ADHD

Hammerness and colleagues[28] recently found that glutamatergic abnormalities may also be ameliorated with treatment in a prefrontal region of youth with ADHD. In an open-label design, adolescents with ADHD were scanned by MRS in the ACC before and after administration of extended-release methylphenidate. Untreated youth with ADHD showed higher metabolite ratios (glutamate/myoinositol, glutamine/myoino-sitol, glutamate + glutamine/myoinositol) in the ACC compared with controls and treated ADHD youth, but these group differences did not reach statistical significance. Although these preliminary findings suggest possible glutamatergic abnormalities in adolescents with ADHD, which may normalize with methylphenidate treatment, a larger sample and controlled study design are needed to confirm these results.

Another study using a pretest and posttest design examined the effect on prefrontal neurometabolites of 12 weeks of treatment with long-acting methylphenidate, 20 mg per day, in 21 medication-naïve children with ADHD.[29] These youths had increases in NAA/creatine ratios and decreases in glutamate/creatine, choline/creatine, and myoinositol/creatine ratios in the right and left prefrontal cortices after stimulant treat-ment. The investigators speculated that the significant neurochemical changes may reflect medication-related functional improvement and improved neuroplasticity in the prefrontal cortices of children with ADHD.

Behavioral treatment for ADHD

Behavioral treatment of ADHD symptoms appears to also have an effect on brain func-tioning. In a recent study of youth attending summer camp training for treatment of ADHD, fMRI with a Go/No-Go paradigm was performed twice in 12 children with ADHD before and after a response cost and token (RCT) program, and in 12 healthy control children, to investigate the influence of RCT training on attention and impul-sivity.[30] The No-Go condition revealed weak activation in the dorsal part of the

ACC, parietal cortex, and dorsolateral prefrontal cortex (DLPFC) before the training in children with ADHD compared with healthy children, which was significantly more pronounced after the training. This increase in hemodynamic response was not attributed merely to repetition of the measurement, because the effect was not observed in healthy children. The increase in hemodynamic response in the ACC and right DLPFC was significantly associated with a reduction in response-time variability and clinical symptoms in ADHD patients. This study showed that after the RCT training, youth with ADHD showed more pronounced activation of cortical structures that function in response monitoring and self-control.

Combination treatments for ADHD
Collectively these studies suggest significant effects of pharmacologic and behavioral interventions on brain structure and function in youth with ADHD. Additional controlled studies and longer-term follow-up would aid in determining the long-term benefits of these interventions in ameliorating brain dysfunction associated with ADHD.

Autism

Despite a wealth of preclinical investigation, there are surprisingly few human studies in youth with autism that directly examine the effects of intervention on brain functioning. One study examined functional connectivity during a phonological decision-making task in adolescents with autism-spectrum disorders.[31] This study found that in youth taking propranolol, there was increased functional connectivity in regions including the left inferior frontal cortex, left fusiform gyrus, left parietal cortex, and left middle temporal gyrus.

A few other studies in youth with autism have evaluated the effects of medication directly on receptor and transporter functioning in the brain. For example, a positron emission tomography (PET) study showed that a high value of dopamine D2 receptor binding in the caudate and putamen decreased by about 10% toward the normal level after treating 6 children between 3 and 5 years of age with infantile autism for 3 months with enzymatic cofactor 6R-L-erythro-5,6,7,8-tetrahydrobiopterin.[32] Another study aimed to correlate striatal dopamine transporter (DAT) binding and cerebrospinal fluid insulin-like growth factor 1 (CSF IGF-1) with clinical response in autistic children (n = 13, age 5–16 years) after 6 months of fluoxetine treatment.[33] Good clinical responders (n = 6) had a decrease ($P = .031$) in DAT binding as assessed using single-photon emission computed tomography with [^{123}I]nor-β-CIT (2β-carbomethoxy-3β-(4-iodo-phenyl)nortropane), whereas poor responders had a trend toward an increase. This study showed that fluoxetine decreases DAT binding, which may also have a neuroprotective effect against dopamine-induced neurotoxicity in autistic children.

Medications do not appear to have any direct effects on white matter microstructure, as described in youth and young adults with high-functioning autism.[34] However, long-term cognitive and behavioral therapies beginning in adolescence have been shown to improve structural integrity in the uncinate fasciculus in low-functioning young adults with autism.[35] These few studies in youth with autism point to specific mechanisms by which interventions may reduce symptom severity, but additional studies are needed to specifically evaluate how these interventions work to provide neural protection.

Bipolar Disorder

There are several emerging pharmacologic neuroimaging studies in youth with BD. Bipolar symptoms are severe in youth and create a significant level of impairment, such that it is challenging to find youth unmedicated for this disorder when they enroll in a neuroimaging study. Moreover, sometimes youth with BD do not show significant departures from normal development in brain structure and function, possibly because of the normalizing effects of medication. Researchers have attempted to evaluate the contribution of medication to neural effects insofar as examining subsamples of youth with and without medication exposure, or to compare neuroimaging outcome measures among youth with specific medication exposures. For example, a recent study showed that youth with BD who were exposed to lithium had larger hippocampal volumes than those who were not exposed to lithium.[36] Other studies have found that youth with BD who had past exposure to mood stabilizers (either lithium or divalproex) had significantly greater posterior subgenual ACC and amygdalar volumes compared with BD youth without mood-stabilizer exposure and controls.[37,38] The effects on white matter microstructure have been less studied, with one post hoc analysis finding no effects of medication exposure on DTI findings in youth with BD.[39]

Functional MRI for bipolar disorder
Recently, a few researchers have begun to directly examine the effects of pharmaco-logic intervention in fMRI activation in youth with BD. In an open-label study, Chang and colleagues[40] examined the neural effects of lamotrigine in adolescents with bipolar depression and found that BD youth treated with lamotrigine for 8 weeks demonstrated less amygdala activation when viewing negative stimuli as depressive symptoms improved; whether the changes in fMRI activation were due to lamotrigine exposure or improvements in depressive symptoms (as a consequence of lamotrigine treatment) could not be determined. Another study examined 17 youths with BD after 14 weeks of treatment with a second-generation antipsychotic (SGA) followed by adjunctive lamotrigine monotherapy, and compared fMRI activation with that of healthy subjects while performing an affective color-matching task.[41] The investiga-tors observed treatment-related decreases in the ventromedial prefrontal cortex (VMPFC) and the DLPFC in the BD subjects, showing that pharmacotherapy resulted in differential brain activation patterns within the BD group, with persistently increased activity in the affective regions and decreased activity in the cognitive regions relative to a healthy comparison group. This same group showed that treatment with an SGA followed by lamotrigine monotherapy enhanced ventrolateral prefrontal cortical (VLPFC) and temporal lobe activity during a response-inhibition task, demonstrating reversal of disorder-relevant neural circuitry dysfunction in patients with adolescent BD.[42] Behavioral performance was not slowed down in patients on this treatment regimen. Finally, an affective working memory task was presented before and after sequential treatment for 8 weeks with an SGA followed by 6 weeks of lamotrigine to previously unmedicated youth with BD, showing that pharmacotherapy resulted in normalization of symptoms and higher prefrontal cortical and cognitive regional acti-vation in youth with BD versus healthy subjects, but did not normalize amygdala over-activation.[43] Improvement on Young Mania Rating Scale (YMRS) score significantly correlated with decreased activity in the VMPFC within the patient group, suggesting a normalizing effect of treatment on fMRI activation, which may be due to either direct medication effects or improvement in symptoms.

Other studies have looked more broadly at the effects of pharmacotherapy on neu-rocognitive systems in pediatric BD. Wegbreit and colleagues[44] aimed to determine functional connectivity differences in youth with BD who were responders (n = 22) versus nonresponders (n = 12) to 1 of 3 mood-stabilizing medications (divalproex, ris-peridone, or lamotrigine) and compared with healthy controls (n = 14). Participants performed a color-matching task during fMRI whereby they had to match the color of positive, negative, or neutral words with colored dots. A frontolimbic network was identified that showed impaired functional integration in youth with BD relative to healthy controls when participants viewed negatively valenced words. Medication responders in the BD group showed greater connectivity of the amygdala into the network before and after treatment compared with nonresponders, with responders showing a pattern more similar to healthy controls than to nonresponders. The degree of amygdala functional connectivity predicted medication response as well as the improvement in YMRS scores across responders and nonresponders regardless of medication type. From these results the investigators inferred that increased functional integration of the amygdala within the frontolimbic network might be a biomarker of broad responsivity to mood stabilizers in BD.

Differential neural effects of medications for bipolar disorder

Differential neural effects between two medications have also been demonstrated. Pavuluri and colleagues[45–47] recently investigated the relative effects of risperidone and divalproex on 3 different cognitive functions in unmedicated manic patients randomized to either treatment or healthy control. In the first task, participants matched the color of a positive, negative, or neutral word with one of two colored circles. After treatment and relative to healthy controls, the risperidone-treated group showed increased activation in the right pregenual and subgenual ACC, and decreased activation in the bilateral middle frontal gyrus, left inferior, medial, and right middle frontal gyri, left inferior parietal lobe, and right striatum. In the divalproex-treated group, relative to healthy controls, increased activations were found in the right superior temporal gyrus, left medial frontal gyrus, and right precuneus. The differential effects of medication were also evaluated in this sample while subjects performed a response inhibition task whereby a motor response, already "on the way" to execution, had to be voluntarily inhibited in trials where a stop signal was presented.[46] Youth taking risperidone and divalproex differentially engaged an evaluative affective circuit (EAC: bilateral inferior frontal gyrus, middle frontal gyrus, ACC, middle temporal gyrus, insulae, caudate, and putamen) during task performance. Within the EAC, posttreatment and relative to healthy controls, greater engagement was seen in left insula in the risperidone group and left subgenual ACC in the divalproex group. Finally, during a working memory task under emotional duress, divalproex enhanced activation in a frontotemporal circuit whereas risperidone increased activation in the dopamine (D2) receptor-rich ventral striatum.[47] Thus, risperidone and divalproex yield differential patterns of neural activity during emotion processing, response inhibition, and working memory tasks in youth with BD. These studies illustrate that psychotropic medication effects on the brain may be task dependent as well as specific for different types of medications.

Multimodal neuroimaging for bipolar disorder

In a multimodal neuroimaging study, Chang and colleagues[48] examined the effect of divalproex on brain structure, chemistry, and function in symptomatic youth at high risk for BD. Although there were no detectable effects on brain structure or neurochemistry after 12 weeks of treatment with divalproex, decreases in prefrontal brain activation correlated with decreases in depressive symptom severity.[48] Thus, this change in brain activation may have been due to symptom improvement rather than direct effects of the medication. A placebo arm may help to differentiate medication effects from changes resulting from symptomatic change.

Magnetic resonance spectroscopy for bipolar disorder

Other studies have used MRS in youth with BD, primarily using proton (^{1}H-MRS) acquisitions focused on key prefrontal cortical regions. For example, studies of youth with BD have shown altered medial and dorsolateral prefrontal concentrations of NAA and phosphocreatine/creatine, healthy nerve cell markers putatively involved in maintaining energy production and myelin formation in the brain.[49] In addition, higher prefrontal myoinositol levels, a marker for cellular metabolism and second-messenger signaling pathways, have also been found in youth with[50] or at familial risk[51] for BD. These levels appear to be sensitive to lithium treatment in that children with BD exposed to lithium have relative decreases in prefrontal myoinositol.[52] Some, but not all, prior studies have demonstrated that alterations in neurometabolite concentrations may explain the pathophysiology of BD[53] and may be sensitive to the effects of psychotropic medications in this population.

Lithium treatment for bipolar disorder

Both NAA and myoinositol concentrations have changed in response to lithium treatment in pediatric populations.[52,54] Specifically, Davanzo and colleagues[52] found that after 1 week of acute lithium treatment, baseline elevated levels of myoinositol/creatine ratios in the ACC in 11 youths with BD decreased, and this decrement was higher for lithium responders than for nonresponders. However, Patel and colleagues[55] observed that in 12- to 18-year-old youth with bipolar depression, lithium did not have any acute (1 week) or chronic (42 days) effects on myoinositol levels in the medial and lateral prefrontal cortices. In a different study, Patel and colleagues[54] did find that after 42 days of lithium administration, a sample of 12- to 18-year-old youth with BD demonstrated reductions in NAA concentration in the ventral but not the lateral prefrontal cortex. In this study, there was a time-by-remission-status interaction of NAA concentrations in the right ventrolateral prefrontal cortex, such that youth who remitted developed decreased mean NAA concentration from day 7 to day 42 whereas nonremitters showed an increase in mean NAA concentration during that same time period. The investigators speculated that higher lithium levels earlier in the treatment course might have resulted in lithium-induced increases in prefrontal metabolism.[54] However, in adults, chronic lithium exposure has been shown to nonselectively increase NAA concentrations in prefrontal, temporal, parietal, and occipital regions,[56] thereby perhaps increasing neuronal viability and function. Some of these findings suggest that by modulating neurometabolites involved in neuronal cell fluid balance and the second-messenger–related neurometabolite myoinositol, lithium exerts its action either by fluid shifts or through intracellular calcium signaling pathways. These studies provide clues about the mechanisms by which lithium and other mood stabilizers exert their therapeutic effect,[57] and are consistent with the aforementioned effects of lithium on brain regional volume.

Prefrontal neurometabolite concentrations in bipolar disorder

Prefrontal neurometabolite levels in youth have also been examined after treatment with divalproex[48] and the atypical antipsychotic olanzapine.[58] In a cohort of youth at high risk for developing BD, there were no statistically changes in pre-divalproex to post-divalproex NAA/creatine ratios, but there was a large effect size (d = 0.94) for a decrease in right dorsolateral prefrontal NAA/creatine after treatment with divalproex. Hospitalized adolescents with bipolar I disorder, experiencing a manic or mixed episode, who achieved remission with olanzapine demonstrated increases in ventral prefrontal NAA compared with nonremitting patients, who showed decreases in prefrontal NAA concentrations. Thus it is unclear as to exactly what these increases or decreases in NAA/creatine ratios mean, but given the potential neurogenic effects of these medications in rat brains[59] and neural stem cells,[60] additional studies examining in vivo effects of these medications in individuals with BD would help clarify their role in reversing the pathophysiologic effects of this disorder.

Another prefrontal neurometabolite measurable by ¹H-MRS that may be associated with abnormal mood regulation is the excitatory neurotransmitter glutamate, its precursor and storage form glutamine, or a combined contribution of glutamate and glutamine (Glx). Moore and colleagues[61] used ¹H-MRS and found decreased levels of glutamine in the ACC in unmedicated youth with BD in comparison with healthy controls and medicated youth on a variety of different agents for BD. This group also found that unmedicated children with BD exhibiting manic symptoms severe enough to warrant treatment had lower Glx to creatine ratios in the ACC than children with BD who were stably treated with risperidone.[62] Mania severity correlated negatively with ACC Glx/creatine levels.

Medications outcomes in bipolar disorder

Taken together, these studies suggest that medications appear to consistently have a normalizing effect on brain function and on some brain volumes in youth with BD. This notion is also consistent with findings from studies in adults with BD.[63] Larger controlled studies in individuals who were previously medication naïve would aid in understanding the specific effects of medication exposure on neural activation in BD.

Depressive Disorders

Youth with depressive disorders demonstrate abnormalities in brain structure and function.[64] However, although effective treatments are available, the impact of treatment of depression on the brain in youth is understudied. In the only fMRI study examining changes in brain activity with treatment in pediatric depression, Tao and colleagues[65] showed that after 8 weeks of open-label fluoxetine treatment, 19 depressed youths with baseline overactivation in prefrontal and temporal regions showed normalization of brain activation in these areas. Further region-of-interest analyses of the areas involved in emotion processing indicated that before treatment, depressed youth had significantly greater activations of fearful relative to neutral facial expressions than did healthy comparison subjects in the amygdala, orbitofrontal cortex, and subgenual ACC bilaterally. Fluoxetine treatment appeared to decrease activations in all 3 regions. This study is limited by the lack of depressed youth exposed to a placebo to substantiate that fluoxetine was truly normalizing activations in these regions.

A smaller open-label study evaluated the potential neurochemical benefit of supplementing fluoxetine with creatine for 8 weeks in 5 adolescent females who had been stabilized on fluoxetine but continued to have persistent depressive symptoms.[66] This study used phosphorus MRS and found that compared with healthy controls, creatine-treated adolescents demonstrated a significant increase in brain phosphocreatine concentration ($P = .02$) on follow-up MRS brain scans. This study warrants replication because of its small sample size and lack of a placebo control group. Moreover, additional neuroimaging studies are needed to investigate the neural effects of widely accepted pharmacologic and psychotherapeutic treatments for pediatric depression.

Obsessive-Compulsive Disorder

A single case report describes the pharmacologic effect of paroxetine on neurochemistry in an 8-year-old with OCD.[67] In this report, OCD symptoms improved markedly in an 8-year-old girl treated for 14 months with the SSRI paroxetine (titrated from 10 to 40 mg/d). Paroxetine dose was then decreased in 10-mg decrements and discontinued without symptom recurrence. Serial ¹H-MRS examinations were acquired before and after 12 weeks of paroxetine treatment (40 mg/d) and 3 months after discontinuation of medication. A striking decrease in caudate Glx was observed after 12 weeks of treatment, which persisted after discontinuation of medication. These data provide support for a reversible glutamatergically mediated dysfunction of the caudate nucleus in OCD that may serve as a marker for pathophysiology and treatment response. It is clear that more investigation in this area would advance our understanding of brain-based disease and treatment correlates.

Schizophrenia

Children and adolescents with schizophrenia share a similar pattern of phenomeno-logic, genetic, and cognitive abnormalities with adults with this disorder. However, early-onset schizophrenia (before age 18 years) is associated with a higher frequency of developmental delays and schizophrenia-spectrum disorders in family members along with a worse long-term outcome. Neurobiologically, schizophrenia in childhood is associated with a high frequency of cytogenetic abnormalities such as de novo chromosomal aberrations, and brain-imaging research in adolescents with schizo-phrenia has revealed a progressive loss of cortical gray matter after onset of psychosis and subtle abnormalities in white matter microstructure.[68] Although more likely to be treatment-refractory than adults with schizophrenia, there are some data supporting that youth with schizophrenia are particularly responsive to clozapine.

Caudate volume in schizophrenia treated with clozapine

The neural effects of this medication were demonstrated in a study of 8 adolescents with early-onset psychosis who were scanned along with matched controls at base-line before starting clozapine, and a rescanned after 2 years of treatment with cloza-pine.[69] Caudate volume was found to be higher than normal in the patients at the initial scanning, showing a slope of declining volume between scans, and did not differ significantly between the patients and the healthy control subjects at the second scan-ning. This study suggested a potential beneficial role of atypical antipsychotics in normalizing striatal volumes after a period of maintenance treatment.

Cortical thickness in schizophrenia treated with clozapine and olanzapine

Another study compared the effects of clozapine and its nearest related drug, olanza-pine, on brain cortical thickness in youth with schizophrenia, contrasted with gray matter trajectories of matched healthy controls.[70] There were no significant differ-ences in the trajectories of cortical thickness between clozapine-treated and olanza-pine-treated groups, except in a small area in the right prefrontal cortex where olanzapine-treated youth had a thicker cortex. Both treatment groups showed relative cortical thinning over time compared with healthy controls. The fact that olanzapine showed a generally comparable neural trajectory to clozapine provides clinicians with additional information during their discussion with patients about choice of medication for long-term use in this population, particularly in treatment-refractory states.[71]

Cortical thickness and remission status in schizophrenia

Remission status also appears to affect cortical thickness. One study aimed to ex-amine cortical thickness in 56 youths with childhood-onset schizophrenia between the time of hospital admission and discharge, on average 3 months later.[72] This study found that compared with patients with continued symptoms, the patients who were remitted at discharge (n = 16 [29%]) had thicker regional cortex in left orbitofrontal, left superior, and middle temporal gyri, and bilateral postcentral and angular gyri ($P \leq .008$). Although a specific medication was not evaluated, this study still provides some neuroanatomic correlates of clinical remission in schizophrenia as well as preliminary evidence that response to treatment may be mediated by these cortical brain regions.

Structural brain changes in schizophrenia

Because schizophrenia is characterized by a chronic course, structural brain changes seen over time in some patients may relate to poor outcome, whereas other changes may be predictive of recovery.[73] There are data about the safety and efficacy of multimodal interventions for childhood-onset schizophrenia starting even in the prodromal phases of illness. However, just as for depression, there are few studies that have examined the neural processes that might underlie their benefit. It is certainly possible that intervention may not directly influence the neural processes studied at all. For example, in one study examining prefrontal neurochemical levels in children with symptoms of schizophrenia-spectrum disorders (n = 16; mean age 11 years) and a healthy comparison group (n = 12; mean age 10.8 years), mean ratios of NAA/creatine were significantly lower in schizophrenia-spectrum subjects than in the comparison group (1.67 vs 1.92; $P<.05$), but medication status did not affect results in schizophrenia-spectrum subjects.[74] However, post hoc analyses searching for medication effects are often underpowered to detect significant or specific differences in medicated and unmedicated subsamples. Taken together, the preliminary findings in youth with schizophrenia suggest that atypical antipsychotics in this population tend to normalize brain structure, although perhaps not completely. Antipsychotic effects on brain function, connectivity, and white matter of youth with schizophrenia-spectrum disorders are not known.

CLINICAL VIGNETTE

Although neuroimaging cannot currently be used to diagnose youth with psychopathology,[75] one can imagine that this tool will become more accessible and, it is hoped, lead to more targeted treatments for youth with psychiatric illnesses. In some young individuals, treatments directed to more specific brain structures such as repetitive transcranial magnetic stimulation have shown some promise for tolerability and efficacy.[76] For the great majority of youth, however, pharmacologic and psychosocial interventions will likely remain the mainstay of treatment. A hypothetical example is given here to illustrate how information from neuroimaging studies might advance our treatments for youth with severe psychiatric illness.

A 16-year-old girl presents to the clinic after a week of euphoria, decreased need for sleep, increased goal-directed activities, racing thoughts, grandiosity, distractibility, increased motor activity, and hypersexuality, preceded by a 2-week period of depressed mood, suicidal ideation, irritability, lethargy, and hypersomnia. These symptoms are above and beyond what would be expected of a typical adolescent, and she meets criteria for bipolar I disorder. Currently unmedicated, she and her family elect to first undergo multimodal neuroimaging. Her structural MRI scan shows that she has reduced volumes in the subgenual anterior cingulate cortex, amygdala, and hippocampus. Her fMRI scan shows amygdalar overactivation and impaired functional integration of limbic structures with prefrontal areas during emotional tasks. Her MRS scan shows increased prefrontal myoinositol, decreased NAA, and decreased glutamine levels. With hope that lithium might restore her structural and neurochemical aberrances, the clinician begins a trial of lithium for 12 weeks. The patient achieves remission of her manic symptoms and receives a follow-up MRI scan, which reveals normalization of subgenual ACC, amygdalar, and hippocampal volumes, restoration of typical neurometabolite levels, and normalization of activation patterns and improved functional integration between limbic structures and the prefrontal cortex. Three months later, she experiences another depressive episode and is rescanned. Amygdalar and VLPFC activation is high during an fMRI emotion task, and prefrontal glutamate levels are increased. After 8 weeks of adjunctive lamotrigine she is rescanned, with normalization of activation in these areas. With additional family and individual therapy, the patient remains in remission for the next 2 years.

SUMMARY

Neuroimaging studies have shown great promise in advancing our understanding of potential mechanisms of action of effective treatments for a range of psychiatric disorders. The good news is that, taken together, intervention appears to have a normalizing effect on brain structure and function in youth suffering from psychopathology. Across disorders, the neurotropic effects of lithium on amygdala and hippocampal volumes appear to be normalizing and are correlated with symptom improvement, and there appears to be normalization of functional activations while performing a wide array of neurocognitive tasks after treatment with psychostimulants, antipsychotics, antidepressants, and mood stabilizers (**Fig. 1**). Additional information is needed to better understand the critical periods of benefit from these interventions, and how they compare relative to one another. These kinds of investigations will enrich the field of child psychiatry and substantiate the importance of early identification and intervention in youth. Longitudinal studies tracking youth well into adulthood will also provide important supporting evidence for the long-term beneficial effects or deleterious consequences of treatment.

It is also clear from this review that using neuroimaging tools to probe intervention effects in psychiatry may be associated with unique methodological considerations. Such factors include the psychometric effects of repeated scans, how to assess potential relations between the effects of an intervention on symptoms and on specific structural, neurochemical, or brain activation patterns, and how to best make causal inferences about intervention effects on brain function.[77] For example, it is often unclear from the studies described whether neural differences observed after treatment are due to the intervention or due to the symptom improvement that resulted from the intervention (ie, we do not know if we are observing a medication effect or a brain-improvement effect with changing symptoms). Future studies should be designed with placebo arms to distinguish these related but separate effects on brain structure and function.

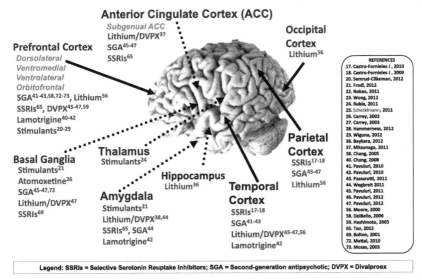

Fig. 1. Selected brain regions affected by medication exposure in youth versus healthy volunteers. Superscript numbers indicate appropriate references listed on the right. DVPX, divalproex; SGA, second-generation antipsychotic; SSRIs, selective serotonin reuptake inhibitors.

In addition, the study of treatment effects in disorders that manifest in childhood presents additional unique challenges related to brain maturation, analysis methods, and the potential for motion artifacts. Methodological advancements to minimize confounders associated with artifact and optimize analytical techniques to enable predictive inferences will be important steps in advancing this field. It is also true that the interventions examined in the literature reviewed were studied in youth who need them rather than experimentally exposing these interventions to typically developing healthy youth, which proves to be ethically challenging. For example, whereas it may be the case that lithium restores brain structure and function in youth with BD, it is less clear whether it has the same effect in healthy youth. This aspect limits our interpretation of the results, as there may be an interaction between certain neural characteristics and medications that produce a unique effect, one that may not be generalizable to all humans.

There are many justifiable concerns about the adverse effects of psychotropic medication on the developing body and brain. All of the studies in this review reported either null effect or benefit of treatment, but our knowledge of the long-term risks of the various interventions is very limited. However, we do know from prospective observations about the short-term risks of untreated depression, BD, schizophrenia, and other psychiatric disorders in which the levels of morbidity and mortality are very high if left untreated. Therefore, while there are adverse effects that may arise in both the body and the brain, the potential beneficial effects on the brain require further understanding. This kind of investigation is certain to substantiate why behavioral and functional improvements are observed at the clinical level. Nevertheless, adverse brain effects should also be studied with neuroimaging. It would be important to determine if there are predictors of response as well as predictors of adverse effects that are detectable. For example, is it possible that neuroimaging could help us determine which depressed adolescents will respond well to SSRIs and which would have a high likelihood of developing antidepressant-induced mania?[78]

When we learn more about the effects of treatment on brain structure and function, and if there is a particular window during development when they are optimal (or most problematic), we can begin to develop more targeted and thoughtful approaches to treatment. The possibility remains that acute intervention with proper medications at a critical point in time will allow for shorter duration of treatment needed, and perhaps neuroprotection or neuroplastic change that will then eliminate the need for a lifetime of medications. This dream is one shared by all practitioners caring for youth with psychopathology, who wish that these youth achieve full and permanent remission of all symptoms and are able to eventually be taking as few medications as possible, and ideally be medication free, before reaching adulthood.

REFERENCES

1. Opler M, Sodhi D, Zaveri D, et al. Primary psychiatric prevention in children and adolescents. Ann Clin Psychiatry 2010;22(4):220–34.
2. Carlson GA, Kotov R, Chang SW, et al. Early determinants of four-year clinical outcomes in bipolar disorder with psychosis. Bipolar Disord 2012;14(1):19–30.
3. Olino TM, Seeley JR, Lewinsohn PM. Conduct disorder and psychosocial outcomes at age 30: early adult psychopathology as a potential mediator. J Abnorm Child Psychol 2010;38(8):1139–49.
4. Birmaher B, Axelson D. Course and outcome of bipolar spectrum disorder in children and adolescents: a review of the existing literature. Dev Psychopathol 2006; 18(4):1023–35.

5. Klein DN, Shankman SA, Rose S. Dysthymic disorder and double depression: prediction of 10-year course trajectories and outcomes. J Psychiatr Res 2008; 42(5):408–15.

6. Brezo J, Paris J, Barker ED, et al. Natural history of suicidal behaviors in a population-based sample of young adults. Psychol Med 2007;37(11):1563–74.

7. Birmaher B, Brent D, Bernet W, et al. Practice parameter for the assessment and treatment of children and adolescents with depressive disorders. J Am Acad Child Adolesc Psychiatry 2007;46(11):1503–26.

8. Pliszka S. Practice parameter for the assessment and treatment of children and adolescents with attention-deficit/hyperactivity disorder. J Am Acad Child Adolesc Psychiatry 2007;46(7):894–921.

9. McClellan J, Kowatch R, Findling RL. Practice parameter for the assessment and treatment of children and adolescents with bipolar disorder. J Am Acad Child Adolesc Psychiatry 2007;46(1):107–25.

10. Phillips ML, Travis MJ, Fagiolini A, et al. Medication effects in neuroimaging studies of bipolar disorder. Am J Psychiatry 2008;165(3):313–20.

11. Singh MK, Chang KD, Mazaika P, et al. Neural correlates of response inhibition in pediatric bipolar disorder. J Child Adolesc Psychopharmacol 2010;20(1):15–24.

12. Singh M, Spielman D, Adleman N, et al. Brain glutamatergic characteristics of pediatric offspring of parents with bipolar disorder. Psychiatry Res 2010;182(2): 165–71.

13. Guyer AE, Choate VR, Detloff A, et al. Striatal functional alteration during incentive anticipation in pediatric anxiety disorders. Am J Psychiatry 2012;169(2): 205–12.

14. Chantiluke K, Halari R, Simic M, et al. Fronto-striato-cerebellar dysregulation in adolescents with depression during motivated attention. Biol Psychiatry 2012; 71(1):59–67.

15. Freitag CM, Luders E, Hulst HE, et al. Total brain volume and corpus callosum size in medication-naïve adolescents and young adults with autism spectrum disorder. Biol Psychiatry 2009;66(4):316–9.

16. Dickstein DP, van der Veen JW, Knopf L, et al. Proton magnetic resonance spectroscopy in youth with severe mood dysregulation. Psychiatry Res 2008;163(1):30–9.

17. Castro-Fornieles J, Caldú X, Andrés-Perpiñá S, et al. A cross-sectional and follow-up functional MRI study with a working memory task in adolescent anorexia nervosa. Neuropsychologia 2010;48(14):4111–6.

18. Castro-Fornieles J, Bargalló N, Lázaro L, et al. A cross-sectional and follow-up voxel-based morphometric MRI study in adolescent anorexia nervosa. J Psychiatr Res 2009;43(3):331–40.

19. Castro-Fornieles J, Bargalló N, Lázaro L, et al. Adolescent anorexia nervosa: cross-sectional and follow-up frontal gray matter disturbances detected with proton magnetic resonance spectroscopy. J Psychiatr Res 2007;41(11):952–8.

20. Semrud-Clikeman M, Pliszka SR, Bledsoe J, et al. Volumetric MRI differences in treatment naive and chronically treated adolescents with ADHD-combined type. J Atten Disord 2012. Available at: http://www.ncbi.nlm.nih.gov/pubmed/22653807. Accessed June 30, 2012.

21. Frodl T, Skokauskas N. Meta-analysis of structural MRI studies in children and adults with attention deficit hyperactivity disorder indicates treatment effects. Acta Psychiatr Scand 2012;125(2):114–26.

22. Nakao T, Radua J, Rubia K, et al. Gray matter volume abnormalities in ADHD: voxel-based meta-analysis exploring the effects of age and stimulant medication. Am J Psychiatry 2011;168(11):1154–63.

23. Wong CG, Stevens MC. The effects of stimulant medication on working memory functional connectivity in attention-deficit/hyperactivity disorder. Biol Psychiatry 2012;71(5):458–66.

24. Rubia K, Halari R, Mohammad AM, et al. Methylphenidate normalizes frontocingulate underactivation during error processing in attention-deficit/hyperactivity disorder. Biol Psychiatry 2011;70(3):255–62.

25. Schecklmann M, Schaldecker M, Aucktor S, et al. Effects of methylphenidate on olfaction and frontal and temporal brain oxygenation in children with ADHD. J Psychiatr Res 2011;45(11):1463–70.

26. Carrey N, MacMaster FP, Sparkes SJ, et al. Glutamatergic changes with treatment in attention deficit hyperactivity disorder: a preliminary case series. J Child Adolesc Psychopharmacol 2002;12(4):331–6.

27. Carrey N, MacMaster FP, Fogel J, et al. Metabolite changes resulting from treatment in children with ADHD: a 1H-MRS study. Clin Neuropharmacol 2003;26(4): 218–21.

28. Hammerness P, Biederman J, Petty C, et al. Brain biochemical effects of methylphenidate treatment using proton magnetic spectroscopy in youth with attention-deficit hyperactivity disorder: a controlled pilot study. CNS Neurosci Ther 2012; 18(1):34–40.

29. Wiguna T, Guerrero AP, Wibisono S, et al. Effect of 12-week administration of 20-mg long-acting methylphenidate on Glu/Cr, NAA/Cr, Cho/Cr, and mI/Cr ratios in the prefrontal cortices of school-age children in Indonesia: a study using ^{1}H magnetic resonance spectroscopy (MRS). Clin Neuropharmacol 2012;35(2): 81–5.

30. Siniatchkin M, Glatthaar N, von Müller GG, et al. Behavioural treatment increases activity in the cognitive neuronal networks in children with attention deficit/hyperactivity disorder. Brain Topogr 2012;25(3):332–44.

31. Narayanan A, White CA, Saklayen S, et al. Effect of propranolol on functional connectivity in autism spectrum disorder—a pilot study. Brain Imaging Behav 2010;4(2):189–97.

32. Fernell E, Watanabe Y, Adolfsson I, et al. Possible effects of tetrahydrobiopterin treatment in six children with autism—clinical and positron emission tomography data: a pilot study. Dev Med Child Neurol 1997;39(5):313–8.

33. Makkonen I, Kokki H, Kuikka J, et al. Effects of fluoxetine treatment on striatal dopamine transporter binding and cerebrospinal fluid insulin-like growth factor-1 in children with autism. Neuropediatrics 2011;42(5):207–9.

34. Lange N, Dubray MB, Lee JE, et al. Atypical diffusion tensor hemispheric asymmetry in autism. Autism Res 2010;3(6):350–8.

35. Pardini M, Elia M, Garaci FG, et al. Long-term cognitive and behavioral therapies, combined with augmentative communication, are related to uncinate fasciculus integrity in autism. J Autism Dev Disord 2012;42(4):585–92.

36. Baykara B, Inal-Emiroglu N, Karabay N, et al. Increased hippocampal volumes in lithium treated adolescents with bipolar disorders: a structural MRI study. J Affect Disord 2012;138(3):433–9.

37. Mitsunaga MM, Garrett A, Howe M, et al. Increased subgenual cingulate cortex volume in pediatric bipolar disorder associated with mood stabilizer exposure. J Child Adolesc Psychopharmacol 2011;21(2):149–55.

38. Chang K, Karchemskiy A, Barnea-Goraly N, et al. Reduced amygdalar gray matter volume in familial pediatric bipolar disorder. J Am Acad Child Adolesc Psychiatry 2005;44(6):565–73.

39. Barnea-Goraly N, Chang KD, Karchemskiy A, et al. Limbic and corpus callosum aberrations in adolescents with bipolar disorder: a tract-based spatial statistics analysis. Biol Psychiatry 2009;66(3):238–44.
40. Chang KD, Wagner C, Garrett A, et al. A preliminary functional magnetic resonance imaging study of prefrontal-amygdalar activation changes in adolescents with bipolar depression treated with lamotrigine. Bipolar Disord 2008;10(3): 426–31.
41. Pavuluri MN, Passarotti AM, Parnes SA, et al. A pharmacological functional magnetic resonance imaging study probing the interface of cognitive and emotional brain systems in pediatric bipolar disorder. J Child Adolesc Psychopharmacol 2010;20(5):395–406.
42. Pavuluri MN, Passarotti AM, Harral EM, et al. Enhanced prefrontal function with pharmacotherapy on a response inhibition task in adolescent bipolar disorder. J Clin Psychiatry 2010;71(11):1526–34.
43. Passarotti AM, Sweeney JA, Pavuluri MN. Fronto-limbic dysfunction in mania pretreatment and persistent amygdala over-activity post-treatment in pediatric bipolar disorder. Psychopharmacology (Berl) 2011;216(4):485–99.
44. Wegbreit E, Ellis JA, Nandam A, et al. Amygdala functional connectivity predicts pharmacotherapy outcome in pediatric bipolar disorder. Brain Connect 2011; 1(5):411–22.
45. Pavuluri MN, Passarotti AM, Lu LH, et al. Double-blind randomized trial of risperidone versus divalproex in pediatric bipolar disorder: fMRI outcomes. Psychiatry Res 2011;193(1):28–37.
46. Pavuluri MN, Ellis JA, Wegbreit E, et al. Pharmacotherapy impacts functional connectivity among affective circuits during response inhibition in pediatric mania. Behav Brain Res 2012;226(2):493–503.
47. Pavuluri MN, Passarotti AM, Fitzgerald JM, et al. Risperidone and divalproex differentially engage the fronto-striato-temporal circuitry in pediatric mania: a pharmacological functional magnetic resonance imaging study. J Am Acad Child Adolesc Psychiatry 2012;51(2):157–170.e5.
48. Chang K, Karchemskiy A, Kelley R, et al. Effect of divalproex on brain morphometry, chemistry, and function in youth at high-risk for bipolar disorder: a pilot study. J Child Adolesc Psychopharmacol 2009;19(1):51–9.
49. Chang K, Adleman N, Dienes K, et al. Decreased N-acetylaspartate in children with familial bipolar disorder. Biol Psychiatry 2003;53(11):1059–65.
50. Patel NC, Cecil KM, Strakowski SM, et al. Neurochemical alterations in adolescent bipolar depression: a proton magnetic resonance spectroscopy pilot study of the prefrontal cortex. J Child Adolesc Psychopharmacol 2008;18(6): 623–7.
51. Cecil KM, DelBello MP, Sellars MC, et al. Proton magnetic resonance spectroscopy of the frontal lobe and cerebellar vermis in children with a mood disorder and a familial risk for bipolar disorders. J Child Adolesc Psychopharmacol 2003;13(4):545–55.
52. Davanzo P, Thomas MA, Yue K, et al. Decreased anterior cingulate myo-inositol/creatine spectroscopy resonance with lithium treatment in children with bipolar disorder. Neuropsychopharmacology 2001;24(4):359–69.
53. Yildiz-Yesiloglu A, Ankerst DP. Neurochemical alterations of the brain in bipolar disorder and their implications for pathophysiology: a systematic review of the in vivo proton magnetic resonance spectroscopy findings. Prog Neuropsychopharmacol Biol Psychiatry 2006;30(6):969–95.

54. Patel NC, DelBello MP, Cecil KM, et al. Temporal change in N-acetyl-aspartate concentrations in adolescents with bipolar depression treated with lithium. J Child Adolesc Psychopharmacol 2008;18(2):132–9.

55. Patel NC, DelBello MP, Cecil KM, et al. Lithium treatment effects on Myo-inositol in adolescents with bipolar depression. Biol Psychiatry 2006;60(9):998–1004.

56. Moore GJ, Bebchuk JM, Hasanat K, et al. Lithium increases N-acetyl-aspartate in the human brain: in vivo evidence in support of bcl-2's neurotrophic effects? Biol Psychiatry 2000;48(1):1–8.

57. Glitz DA, Manji HK, Moore GJ. Mood disorders: treatment-induced changes in brain neurochemistry and structure. Semin Clin Neuropsychiatry 2002;7(4): 269–80.

58. DelBello MP, Cecil KM, Adler CM, et al. Neurochemical effects of olanzapine in first-hospitalization manic adolescents: a proton magnetic resonance spectroscopy study. Neuropsychopharmacology 2006;31(6):1264–73.

59. Hashimoto R, Fujimaki K, Jeong MR, et al. Neuroprotective actions of lithium. Seishin Shinkeigaku Zasshi 2003;105(1):81–6 [in Japanese].

60. Laeng P, Pitts RL, Lemire AL, et al. The mood stabilizer valproic acid stimulates GABA neurogenesis from rat forebrain stem cells. J Neurochem 2004;91(1): 238–51.

61. Moore CM, Frazier JA, Glod CA, et al. Glutamine and glutamate levels in children and adolescents with bipolar disorder: a 4.0-T proton magnetic resonance spectroscopy study of the anterior cingulate cortex. J Am Acad Child Adolesc Psychiatry 2007;46(4):524–34.

62. Moore CM, Biederman J, Wozniak J, et al. Mania, glutamate/glutamine and risperidone in pediatric bipolar disorder: a proton magnetic resonance spectroscopy study of the anterior cingulate cortex. J Affect Disord 2007;99(1–3):19–25.

63. Hafeman DM, Chang KD, Garrett AS, et al. Effects of medication on neuroimaging findings in bipolar disorder: an updated review. Bipolar Disord 2012;14(4): 375–410.

64. Hulvershorn LA, Cullen K, Anand A. Toward dysfunctional connectivity: a review of neuroimaging findings in pediatric major depressive disorder. Brain Imaging Behav 2011;5(4):307–28.

65. Tao R, Calley CS, Hart J, et al. Brain activity in adolescent major depressive disorder before and after fluoxetine treatment. Am J Psychiatry 2012;169(4): 381–8.

66. Kondo DG, Sung YH, Hellem TL, et al. Open-label adjunctive creatine for female adolescents with SSRI-resistant major depressive disorder: a 31-phosphorus magnetic resonance spectroscopy study. J Affect Disord 2011;135(1–3):354–61.

67. Bolton J, Moore GJ, MacMillan S, et al. Case study: caudate glutamatergic changes with paroxetine persist after medication discontinuation in pediatric OCD. J Am Acad Child Adolesc Psychiatry 2001;40(8):903–6.

68. Kumra S, Asarnow R, Grace A, et al. From bench to bedside: translating new research from genetics and neuroimaging into treatment development for early-onset schizophrenia. Early Interv Psychiatry 2009;3(4):243–58.

69. Frazier JA, Giedd JN, Kaysen D, et al. Childhood-onset schizophrenia: brain MRI rescan after 2 years of clozapine maintenance treatment. Am J Psychiatry 1996; 153(4):564–6.

70. Mattai A, Chavez A, Greenstein D, et al. Effects of clozapine and olanzapine on cortical thickness in childhood-onset schizophrenia. Schizophr Res 2010;116(1): 44–8.

71. Mozes T, Greenberg Y, Spivak B, et al. Olanzapine treatment in chronic drug-resistant childhood-onset schizophrenia: an open-label study. J Child Adolesc Psychopharmacol 2003;13(3):311–7.
72. Greenstein DK, Wolfe S, Gochman P, et al. Remission status and cortical thickness in childhood-onset schizophrenia. J Am Acad Child Adolesc Psychiatry 2008;47(10):1133–40.
73. DeLisi LE, Sakuma M, Ge S, et al. Association of brain structural change with the heterogeneous course of schizophrenia from early childhood through five years subsequent to a first hospitalization. Psychiatry Res 1998;84(2–3):75–88.
74. Brooks WM, Hodde-Vargas J, Vargas LA, et al. Frontal lobe of children with schizophrenia spectrum disorders: a proton magnetic resonance spectroscopic study. Biol Psychiatry 1998;43(4):263–9.
75. Chang K, Adleman N, Wagner C, et al. Will neuroimaging ever be used to diagnose pediatric bipolar disorder? Dev Psychopathol 2006;18(4):1133–46.
76. Mattai A, Miller R, Weisinger B, et al. Tolerability of transcranial direct current stimulation in childhood-onset schizophrenia. Brain Stimul 2011;4(4):275–80.
77. Dichter GS, Sikich L, Song A, et al. Functional neuroimaging of treatment effects in psychiatry: methodological challenges and recommendations. Int J Neurosci 2012. Available at: http://www.ncbi.nlm.nih.gov/pubmed/22471393. Accessed July 5, 2012.
78. Goldsmith M, Singh M, Chang K. Antidepressants and psychostimulants in pediatric populations: is there an association with mania? Paediatr Drugs 2011;13(4):225–43.

Psychiatric Pharmacogenomics in Pediatric Psychopharmacology

Christopher A. Wall, MD*, Paul E. Croarkin, DO,
Cosima Swintak, MD, Brett A. Koplin, MD

KEYWORDS

- Pharmacogenomics • Psychopharmacology • Pediatric • Metabolism • Dopamine
- Serotonin • Transporter • Receptor

KEY POINTS

- Psychiatric pharmacogenomics is the study of how gene variations influence the response of an individual to treatment with psychotropic medications.
- Metabolic enzymes, frequently referred to as cytochrome P-450 enzymes, are the most commonly tested genes in pharmacogenomic practice and assist in understanding the pharmacokinetics of drug metabolism.
- More recently, neuron function genes are being studied to assist in understanding the pharmacodynamic qualities of an individual's medication response.
- Literature regarding pharmacogenomics is expanding rapidly and can be quite challenging to practicing physicians.
- Most psychiatric pharmacogenomic studies have focused on the adult population, with relatively few studies in youth.
- The interpretation of psychiatric pharmacogenomic testing is an emerging clinical tool designed to guide prescribers to choose medications that cause fewer adverse drug effects and improve chances of having a therapeutic response.

OVERVIEW OF PSYCHIATRIC PHARMACOGENOMICS

Stimulants, antidepressants, and antipsychotics are some of the most frequently prescribed medications in youth in the United States.[1] A recent multiyear survey by Comer and colleagues[2] reported psychotropic medications being prescribed to youth (ages 6–17) at roughly 9% of all office visits to a US physician. Furthermore, the rate for multiclass psychotropic prescribing in youth has approached 20% over the same period.

When a psychotropic medication is necessary, families, children, and their prescribing clinicians naturally are motivated to identify the "right medication" from the very first prescription. Unfortunately, the initial psychopharmacologic agents in the child and adolescent population are usually chosen based on empiric response.

Division of Child and Adolescent Psychiatry, Department of Psychiatry and Psychology, Mayo Clinic, 200 1st Street South West, Rochester, MN 55905, USA
* Corresponding author.
E-mail address: wall.chris@mayo.edu

Child Adolesc Psychiatric Clin N Am 21 (2012) 773–788
http://dx.doi.org/10.1016/j.chc.2012.07.001

Nearly all prescribing decisions are based on information about the patient's illness process, target symptoms, and family medication experiences within the context of the experience of the clinician, subspecialty practice guidelines, and results delivered from pharmaceutical trials.[3] Although this approach is effective for many patients, there remains a significant number of less fortunate youth that struggle with treatment-resistant symptoms and medication-related side effects. In an editorial from 2011, Emslie noted, "there are no radically new treatments on the horizon for the treatment of depression, and so we have to do better with the treatments we have available."[4] To date, much of the available literature on pharmacogenomic testing in the pediatric population has focused on the spectrum of efficacy related to cancer treatments.[5–10] Impressive results in leukemia remission rates have been described as partly caused by advancements in pharmacogenomically derived individualized prescribing practices. Cheok and colleagues[10] highlighted the progress made in the treatment of acute lymphoblastic leukemia in children noting the disease as being lethal four decades ago to current cure rates exceeding 80%. Similar to Emslie's comments, progress in the treatment of acute lymphoblastic leukemia is largely caused by the optimization of existing treatment modalities rather than the discovery of new antileukemic agents. Furthermore, as Pickar[11] suggested, there is no specialty where the need for pharmacogenetics seems more compelling than for psychiatry.

By definition, psychiatric pharmacogenomics (PGx) is the study of how gene variations influence the responses of a patient to treatment with psychotropic medications.[12] When discussing pharmacogenomic studies, it is important to have an understanding of the targeted genes and their function. For ease of understanding and navigation of the ever-expanding literature, currently available PGx testing (**Table 1**) can be divided into two primary categories: metabolic enzymes (ie, the cytochrome P-450 [CYP] enzyme system also referred to as "pharmacokinetics"); and genes that effect neuronal function (ie, the dopamine transporter and receptor genes frequently referred to as "pharmacodynamics").

Many of these PGx target genes have also been studied in relation to their influence on disease vulnerability; however, this research is beyond the scope of this article. It should also be noted that hundreds of discrete PGx candidate genes and pathways have been discussed in several thousands of published articles that comprise the

Table 1 Currently testable genotypes	
Complete Name	**Abbreviation**
Cytochrome P-450 2D6 gene	CYP2D6
Cytochrome P-450 2C19 gene	CYP2C19
Cytochrome P-450 2C9 gene	CYP2C9
Cytochrome P-450 1A2 gene	CYP1A2
Catecholamine O-methyltransferase gene	COMT
Norepinephrine transporter gene	SLC6A2
Dopamine transporter gene	SLC6A3
Serotonin transporter gene	SLC6A4
Serotonin 1A receptor gene	HTR1A
Serotonin 2A receptor gene	HTR2A
Serotonin 2C receptor gene	HTR2C
D_2 dopamine receptor gene	DRD2
D_3 dopamine receptor gene	DRD3
D_4 dopamine receptor gene	DRD4

extant literature.[13] Because this is a clinically focused article, an exhaustive review of each candidate gene is clearly beyond the scope of this discussion.

Although the use of pharmacogenomics is only just emerging in routine clinical practice, evidence has demonstrated specific patients with either limited metabolic capacity or neuron function gene polymorphisms in target genes that place them at well-documented increased risk of experiencing medication-related side effects and ineffective medication trials. Over the past decade, PGx testing has become far more cost-effective and with this decreased cost it has been predicted that pharmacogenomic testing will routinely be ordered to guide the selection and dosing of psychotropic medications.[14] This article provides an overview of where PGx testing stands as an emerging clinical tool in modern psychotropic prescribing practice, specifically in the pediatric population. This practical discussion is organized around the state of PGx research when choosing psychopharmacologic interventions in the most commonly encountered mental illnesses in youth.

ATTENTION-DEFICIT/HYPERACTIVITY DISORDER

The most frequent reason for pediatric psychotropic office visits is for attention-deficit/hyperactivity disorder (ADHD) and associated disruptive behavior disorders, which accounted for nearly half of all reported visits.[2] The foundation of modern psychopharmacology in the treatment of ADHD remains the stimulant class.[15] It is estimated that approximately 75% of children and adolescents prescribed stimulants ultimately are clinical responders. Despite this success, there remains a significant amount of variability in treatment response, optimal dosage needed, and tolerability. Genetic factors have increasingly been demonstrated to play a role in this variability.[16]

Pharmacogenomic Mechanism and Target in ADHD

Generally, stimulants are believed to work by dopaminergic and noradrenergic activity enhancement. Pharmacogenomic association studies have therefore frequently targeted variations in the dopamine transporter gene (SLC6A3) and dopamine receptor gene (DRD4). More recently, genes systematically studied are the α_{2A}-adrenergic receptor (ADRA2A) and the norepinephrine transporter (SLC6A2).

Dopamine transporter gene

The most frequently studied pharmacogenomic target in ADHD is the dopamine transporter genes, more specifically the SLC6A3 gene. To date, there has been some suggestion of a reduced effect of methylphenidate (MPH) being associated with the 10-repeat polymorphism in specific ancestral populations. However, the overall assessment of the pharmacogenomic literature has been inconclusive regarding the role of SLC6A3 in associations with clinical response.[17–31] Therefore, it has been suggested that other gene regions be studied in future ADHD pharmacogenomic research.[16]

Dopamine receptor gene

The second-most frequently studied gene region in ADHD pharmacogenomics is DRD4. Contradictory results regarding DRD4 and clinically meaningful response to MPH, and emergence of side effects have been reported thus far.[17,25,26,28,31–37] The role for DRD4 as an individually meaningful gene target in ADHD pharmacogenomics also remains an open question.

Adrenergic receptor gene

Several studies have suggested that there is a positive association between variation in ADRA2A as having a positive association between MPH and clinical response.[38–40] Given the hypothesized role of ADRA2A in attentional ability, specifically in the prefrontal cortex, this remains an intriguing PGx target of interest. However, a report by Contini and colleagues[41] did not confirm a relationship between ADRA2A and response to MPH in adult patients with ADHD.

Drug Metabolism

At the level of drug metabolism, CYP has been suggested as relevant to the clinical response to atomoxetine. Specifically, CYP2D6 is a highly polymorphic enzyme that influences metabolism and subsequently influences atomoxetine treatment response and adverse effects. Michelson and colleagues[42] reviewed response to atomoxetine in children and adolescents using data from multiple studies and found a greater improvement in poor metabolizers versus extensive (normal) metabolizers. However, the poor metabolizers group also showed a tendency for increased treatment-related adverse events including increased heart rate and blood pressure.

Clinical Results of Pharmacogenomics for ADHD

In summary, over the past two decades, considerable efforts have been made to identify genes involved in clinical and etiologic features of ADHD. The result has been a large and conflicting literature of candidate gene associations.[43] Future studies will likely use the new technology of genome-wide association studies. Early findings from this approach have begun to implicate more complex processes, such as neuronal migration and cell adhesion and cell division, as potentially important in the cause of ADHD.[44] However, from a clinical standpoint, the results from ADHD pharmacogenomic studies have not yet been translatable to clinically relevant practice enhancement at the level of the individual prescription.

DEPRESSION AND ANXIETY

Selective serotonin reuptake inhibitors (SSRIs) have been carefully studied and reported as effective in the treatment of adolescent major depression and anxiety disorders.[45–50] Unfortunately, between one-third and one-half of those with anxiety and depression fail to respond to appropriate treatment with an SSRI.[51] Pharmacogenomic factors are hypothesized to play a role in the variability of medication response and adverse drug effects. Several pharmacogenomic targets have been explored thus far ranging from metabolic enzymes to the serotonin transporter and receptor polymorphisms. Very few pharmacogenomic trials of antidepressants in the pediatric population have been performed to date.[52–54] However, a recent, high-quality review of pharmacogenomic studies of antidepressant response has indicated several candidate genes involved in the pharmacokinetics and pharmacodynamics of these drugs.[55]

Pharmacogenomic Mechanism and Target in Depression and Anxiety

The serotonin transporter (SLC6A4) is the main target of SSRIs and a target for tricyclic antidepressants and selective norepinephrine reuptake inhibitors. SLC6A4 has been the most often studied gene in antidepressant pharmacogenomics. Polymorphisms in the SLC6A4 gene seem to consistently influence response to SSRIs but not other types of antidepressants or placebo.[56] Although several polymorphisms of this gene exist, the most frequently studied area of the gene is in the promoter region, also known as 5-HTTLPR. Three studies have investigated the association of 5-HTTLPR and remission in response to citalopram in the 4041 patient STAR*D sample.[57–59] The studies report different results ranging from no evidence of association in an ancestrally homogenous large sample with treatment remission to improved response rates in those subjects who identified themselves as white non-Hispanics.

Serotonin transporter polymorphisms have been implicated in emergence of antidepressant-induced mania in youth.[53] Several studies have also investigated the association between antidepressant-induced mania in adults and candidate genetic variants focusing on 5-HTTLPR.[60–64] However, a recent review and meta-analysis by Biernacka and colleagues[65] suggest that insufficient published data exist to confirm an association between 5HTTLPR and antidepressant-induced mania.

Another frequently studied gene in the pharmacogenomics of antidepressants is the postsynaptic serotonin receptor 2A (5HTR2A) gene. Evidence suggests that genetic variability of the 5HTR2A gene could be of value in predicting antidepressant response.[66–81] However, because several variants of the gene exist, a consensus of which variants or combinations are the most predictive has not emerged.[55]

Drug Metabolism

Metabolic enzymes are some of the most frequently tested genes in PGx practice. The importance of these enzymes is derived from the fundamental concerns inherent in drug–drug interactions and dosing decisions. Of all the metabolic genes, CYP2D6 has the highest variability, is the most frequently tested, and is arguably the most clinically relevant in the practice of PGx. CYP2D6 polymorphisms have been implicated as playing a role in issues ranging from poor medication response to an increased risk of adverse events, such as analgesic toxicity in infants and children, and have recently been postulated to play a role in suicide completion.[12,82–93] It is estimated that 15% to 25% of the population are either poor or ultrarapid metabolizers at CYP2D6.[3] Ethnic variations in CYP2D6 expression have also been reported.[13,88,94–96] For example, Northern European populations are more likely to carry the *4 polymorphism (inactive), whereas North African populations have a higher rate of expressing the *2A polymorphism (ultrarapid). Because most antidepressant and antipsychotic agents are metabolized to some degree by this pathway, knowledge of an individual's genotype may be of considerable importance when making prescribing decisions. Similarly, although to a lesser degree, other clinically testable CYP enzymes, such as CYP2C9, CYP2C19, and CYP1A2, play an important role in the metabolism of various antidepressants (**Table 2**).[3,97]

Recently, a specific marker within the promoter region of the catechol O-methyltransferase gene, which catalyzes the O-methylation of catecholamine neurotransmitters, has been hypothesized to influence response to SSRI therapy of patients with major depressive disorder (MDD).[98] Although this has not been studied in the pediatric population, this remains an interesting and testable PGx target.

PSYCHOTIC, MANIC, AND AUTISM SPECTRUM DISORDERS

Although psychosis, mania, and autism spectrum disorders are distinct in presentation and heritability, they share a common psychopharmacologic approach, namely the use of symptom-improving mood stabilizers and antipsychotic agents.

Pharmacogenomic Mechanism and Target in Psychotic, Manic, and Spectrum Disorders

Several mood stabilizers and antipsychotics have been studied from the perspective of treatment response and adverse effects using PGx techniques and a host of candidate gene targets (**Table 3**)[3,53,65,99–122]:

- ~40% of antipsychotics are major substrates of CYP2D6 enzymes
- 23% are major substrates of CYP3A4
- 18% are major substrates of CYP1A2

Table 2
Antidepressant metabolism by CYP enzyme

CYP Enzyme	Primarily Metabolized	Substantially Metabolized	Minimally Metabolized
2D6	Amitriptyline Desipramine Doxepin Fluoxetine Nortriptyline Paroxetine Venlafaxine	Buproprion Duloxetine Imipramine Trazodone	Citalopram Escitalopram Fluvoxamine Mirtazapine Sertraline
2C19	Amitriptyline Citalopram Clomipramine Escitalopram	Doxepin Imipramine Moclobemide Nortriptyline Sertraline	Venlafaxine Trazodone
1A2	Fluvoxamine	Clomipramine Duloxetine Imipramine	Amitriptyline Mirtazapine Trazodone
2C9	None	Amitriptyline Fluoxetine	Sertraline Venlafaxine
3A4	Mirtazapine Reboxetine Trazodone Vilazodone	Citalopram Desvenlafaxine	Sertraline Venlafaxine

Therefore, a focus on the metabolic genes for antipsychotics and mood stabilizing agents is a rational place to start when considering PGx in the pediatric population.

Drug Metabolism

It is reasonable to conclude that if an individual is discovered to be a poor metabolizer at CYP2D6 or CYP1A2, the choice in antipsychotic should be guided by this knowledge.

Table 3
Antipsychotic metabolism by CYP enzyme

CYP Enzyme	Primarily Metabolized	Substantially Metabolized	Minimally Metabolized
2D6	Chlorpromazine Haloperidol Perphenazine Risperidone Thioridazine	Aripiprazole Olanzapine	Clozapine Quetiapine Ziprasidone
2C19	None	Clozapine	Thioridazine
1A2	Clozapine Olanzapine Thioridazine	Chlorpromazine	Haloperidol Thioridazine
3A4	Haloperidol Quetiapine Ziprasidone	Olanzapine	Clozapine Risperidone

Early work examined the role of 5-HT2A receptor polymorphisms in clozapine response. Studies have shown associations between the 102 C allele and 452Tyr allele and response. However, these have not been replicated consistently and are thought to contribute to only a modest influence on treatment response. Case control and meta-analytic studies have also suggested that 5-HT$_{2C}$ receptor polymorphisms play a role in clozapine response, but this has not been definitively demonstrated.[123]

Associations of Polymorphisms on Antipsychotic Efficacy and Adverse Effects

Recently, Correia and colleagues[112] examined putative candidate genes related to efficacy and adverse effects in 45 subjects with autism (mean age, 8.67; standard deviation, 4.3) treated with risperidone. This study found associations with HTR2A, DRD3, HTR2C, and ABCB1 polymorphisms were predictors of clinical improvement with risperidone therapy. Furthermore, several polymorphisms seemed to influence prolactin elevation, whereas HTR2C and some CYP2D6 polymorphisms were associated with risperidone-induced increases in body mass index or waist circumference. Interestingly, the CYP2D6 ultrarapid metabolizer phenotype conferred a lower increase in body mass index and waist circumference compared with extensive metabolizers. Regarding HTR2C variants, the C/C genotype in females and the C genotype in males had smaller increases in body mass index and waist circumference compared with the GG phenotype.[112] These findings have not been uniformly reported. However, this line of research serves to demonstrate the potential future clinical use of pharmacogenomic testing in children and adolescents who will be treated with atypical antipsychotics.

One final, compelling example involves carbamazepine. Stevens-Johnson syndrome and toxic epidermal necrolysis are two rare, but life-threatening dermatologic conditions that involve the separation of epidermis from dermis as a result of cell death. These are associated with certain medications including antibiotics and mood stabilizers, such as carbamazepine. In 2004, Chung and colleagues[124] demonstrated a strong association between the HLA-B*1502 allele in Han Chinese patients and Stevens-Johnson syndrome from carbamazepine treatment. In 2007, this culminated in a US Food and Drug Administration label change that recommended genetic testing for Asian patients before initiating carbamazepine. In cases in which Asian patients have the HLA-B*1502 allele, alternative treatments should be considered unless the potential benefit of treatment with carbamazepine greatly exceeds the potential for Stevens-Johnson syndrome or toxic epidermal necrolysis.[125] With the availability of genetic testing for this polymorphism, this recommendation is hard for clinicians to ignore.

CLINICAL VIGNETTE: FEMALE ADOLESCENT GENOTYPED FOR ANTIDEPRESSANTS

A hospitalized 16-year-old white girl became increasingly nonfunctional in the setting of worsening depressive symptoms and reported medication side effects. Her functioning had regressed to the point of minimal to no independent activities of daily living and her parents reporting feeling overwhelmed with the struggle to find "something" that could help their daughter. Her admission medications included sertraline, 250 mg daily (2C19, 2D6, 2C9, 3A4); mirtazapine, 60 mg nightly (2D6, 1A2, 3A4); and trazodone, 400 mg nightly (3A4, 2D6, 2C19, 1A2). Cytochrome P-450 genotyping revealed her to be a CYP2D6 poor metabolizer and a CYP2C19 intermediate metabolizer. Over the course of 11 days, her medications were tapered and she eventually reported significant improvement in her mood. Because sleep remained a concern, ramelteon, 8 mg nightly (1A2), was initiated with excellent response and no reported side effects. At the time of dismissal, she denied any depressive symptoms, became vigorously involved in hospital and family activities, and acknowledged enthusiasm to return home to get her driver's license.

CONCLUSIONS AND FUTURE DIRECTIONS

Currently available pharmacogenomic technology offers patients and prescribers an opportunity to move closer to the ultimate goal of truly individualized prescriptions, a goal that is especially critical in the youth that present with serious psychiatric illnesses. Relatively few studies of pharmacogenomic factors in the pediatric population have been performed to date; however, the results from adult trials and clinical extrapolation provide some guidance. A clear role in drug toxicity and efficacy has been established for some gene–drug combinations.[126] Therefore, when an individual is discovered to possess a poor or ultrarapid metabolizer status for a drug that relies heavily on that pathway for metabolism, it is imprudent to ignore the objective evidence and continue prescribing "as usual."

Once informed with PGx data, one should discuss limitations of testing, and the emerging potential to reduce side effect burden and the ability to choose a more appropriate medication through a rational decision-making process. Although the promise of pharmacogenomics is still developing, the era of widespread use and clinically meaningful application of testing results is rapidly evolving.

Although several studies have been reported here showing significant progress in the understanding of pharmacogenomics in youth, such as in the treatment of ADHD and illnesses requiring an antidepressant, clinical adoption of PGx testing lags behind the emerging evidence. However, when pharmacogenomically avoidable events are reported, such as the death of a child exposed to fluoxetine, with CYP2D6 poor metabolism,[127] it is important that clinicians act on the available evidence. As reported, some populations of patients may also be more pharmacogenomically vulnerable to serious adverse effects, such as the Stevens-Johnson syndrome reported in Asians with an allelic variant that are treated with carbamazepine.[124]

Cost and Availability of PGx Testing

A frequent concern regarding PGx testing is cost and availability. Although the costs of this testing are not insignificant, they are improving and will continue to decrease, subsequently posing less of a barrier in the future.[126,128] When weighed against the expense and suffering associated with adverse drug effects and nontherapeutic medication trials, the use of PGx to protect patients will become a more common practice for an increasingly large number of gene–drug combinations. Regarding concerns related to access and availability, several commercially available companies provide pharmacogenomic testing services in the form of mailable "kits." However, the interpretation and reporting of the testing is variable. Some companies choose to simply provide "genotyping" data, requiring clinical interpretation by the ordering physician, whereas others use an algorithm that suggests clinical interpretation related to specific medications for that individual. For practicing clinicians, interpretive reports must be comprehensible to be used.

When to do PGx Testing

At this time, based on the available scientific and clinical evidence, the authors suggest PGx testing when a patient or their family is reporting minimal response to "typically" therapeutic doses when medication compliance is confirmed. Although one failed medication trial may be enough evidence of concern for some clinicians, two or more unsuccessful medication trials should compel the clinician to objectively assess pharmacogenomic variables that may be impacting medication response. Furthermore, if there is a clear report of significant side effects, such as an unusual increase in irritability, lethargy, activation, or other unexpected physiologic signs (ie, marked changes in blood pressure, pulse), PGx testing should be strongly considered. Finally, as with all medications, it is crucial to carefully investigate and monitor symptoms that patients report in association with medication initiation and titration. Clearly, individual responses to medications exist and our field is beginning to understand some of the genetic factors associated with observed variability. As clinicians become increasingly comfortable with the application and verbiage associated with PGx, and as pharmaceutical trials include PGx testing as a part of drug development and analysis, many future children and adolescents will be afforded truly individualized prescriptions.

REFERENCES

1. Paulose-Ram R, Safran MA, Jonas BS, et al. Trends in psychotropic medication use among U.S. adults. Pharmacoepidemiol Drug Saf 2007;16(5):560–70.
2. Comer JS, Olfson M, Mojtabai R. National trends in child and adolescent psychotropic polypharmacy in office-based practice, 1996–2007. J Am Acad Child Adolesc Psychiatry 2010;49(10):1001–10.
3. Wall CA, Oldenkamp C, Swintak C. Safety and efficacy pharmacogenomics in pediatric psychopharmacology. Prim Psychiatr 2010;17(5):53–8.
4. Emslie GJ. The psychopharmacology of adolescent depression. J Child Adolesc Psychopharmacol 2012;22(1):2–4.
5. Brenner TL, Pui CH, Evans WE. Pharmacogenomics of childhood acute lymphoblastic leukemia. Curr Opin Mol Ther 2001;3(6):567–78.
6. Cheok MH, Evans WE. Acute lymphoblastic leukaemia: a model for the pharmacogenomics of cancer therapy. Nat Rev Cancer 2006;6(2):117–29.
7. Ansari M, Krajinovic M. Pharmacogenomics of acute leukemia. Pharmacogenomics 2007;8(7):817–34.
8. Ansari M, Krajinovic M. Pharmacogenomics in cancer treatment defining genetic bases for inter-individual differences in responses to chemotherapy. Curr Opin Pediatr 2007;19(1):15–22.
9. Pottier N, Cheok M, Kager L. Antileukemic drug effects in childhood acute lymphoblastic leukemia. Expert Rev Clin Pharmacol 2008;1(3):401–13.
10. Cheok MH, Pottier N, Kager L, et al. Pharmacogenetics in acute lymphoblastic leukemia. Semin Hematol 2009;46(1):39–51.
11. Pickar D. Pharmacogenomics of psychiatric drug treatment. Psychiatr Clin North Am 2003;26(2):303–21.
12. Mrazek DA. Psychiatric pharmacogenomics. 1st edition. In: David Mrazek, editor. Oxford University Press; Apr 2010. ISBN13: 9780195367294, ISBN10: 0195367294 Hardback, 280 pages. 2010.
13. Scott SA. Personalizing medicine with clinical pharmacogenetics. Genet Med 2011;13(12):987–95.
14. Mrazek DA. Psychiatric pharmacogenomic testing in clinical practice. Dialogues Clin Neurosci 2010;12(1):66–73.
15. Pliszka S, AACAP Work Group on Quality Issues. Practice parameter for the assessment and treatment of children and adolescents with attention-deficit/hyperactivity disorder. J Am Acad Child Adolesc Psychiatry 2007;46(7):894–921.
16. Kieling C, Genro JP, Hutz MH, et al. A current update on ADHD pharmacogenomics. Pharmacogenomics 2010;11(3):407–19.
17. Winsberg BG, Comings DE. Association of the dopamine transporter gene (DAT1) with poor methylphenidate response. J Am Acad Child Adolesc Psychiatry 1999;38(12):1474–7.

18. Roman T, Szobot C, Martins S, et al. Dopamine transporter gene and response to methylphenidate in attention-deficit/hyperactivity disorder. Pharmacogenetics 2002;12(6):497–9.
19. Kirley A, Lowe N, Hawi Z, et al. Association of the 480 bp DAT1 allele with methylphenidate response in a sample of Irish children with ADHD. Am J Med Genet B Neuropsychiatr Genet 2003;121(1):50–4.
20. Stein MA, Waldman ID, Sarampote CS, et al. Dopamine transporter genotype and methylphenidate dose response in children with ADHD. Neuropsychopharmacology 2005;30(7):1374–82.
21. van der Meulen EM, Bakker SC, Pauls DL, et al. High sibling correlation on methylphenidate response but no association with DAT1-10R homozygosity in Dutch sibpairs with ADHD. J Child Psychol Psychiatry 2005;46(10):1074–80.
22. Langley K, Turic D, Peirce TR, et al. No support for association between the dopamine transporter (DAT1) gene and ADHD. Am J Med Genet B Neuropsychiatr Genet 2005;139(1):7–10.
23. Cheon KA, Ryu YH, Kim JW, et al. The homozygosity for 10-repeat allele at dopamine transporter gene and dopamine transporter density in Korean children with attention deficit hyperactivity disorder: relating to treatment response to methylphenidate. Eur Neuropsychopharmacol 2005;15(1):95–101.
24. Mick E, Biederman J, Spencer T, et al. Absence of association with DAT1 polymorphism and response to methylphenidate in a sample of adults with ADHD. Am J Med Genet B Neuropsychiatr Genet 2006;141(8):890–4.
25. McGough J, McCracken J, Swanson J, et al. Pharmacogenetics of methylphenidate response in preschoolers with ADHD. J Am Acad Child Adolesc Psychiatry 2006; 45(11):1314–22.
26. Zeni CP, Guimaräes AP, Polanczyk GV, et al. No significant association between response to methylphenidate and genes of the dopaminergic and serotonergic systems in a sample of Brazilian children with attention-deficit/hyperactivity disorder. Am J Med Genet B Neuropsychiatr Genet 2007;144(3):391–4.
27. Joober R, Grizenko N, Sengupta S, et al. Dopamine transporter 3Ä≤-UTR VNTR genotype and ADHD: a pharmaco-behavioural genetic study with methylphenidate. Neuropsychopharmacology 2007;32(6):1370–6.
28. Tharoor H, Lobos EA, Todd RD, et al. Association of dopamine, serotonin, and nicotinic gene polymorphisms with methylphenidate response in ADHD. Am J Med Genet B Neuropsychiatr Genet 2008;147(4):527–30.
29. Purper-Ouakil D, Wohl M, Orejarena S, et al. Pharmacogenetics of methylphenidate response in attention deficit/hyperactivity disorder: association with the dopamine transporter gene (SLC6A3). Am J Med Genet B Neuropsychiatr Genet 2008;147(8):1425–30.
30. Kooij JS, Boonstra AM, Vermeulen SH, et al. Response to methylphenidate in adults with ADHD is associated with a polymorphism in SLC6A3 (DAT1). Am J Med Genet B Neuropsychiatr Genet 2008;147(2):201–8.
31. Kereszturi E, Tarnok Z, Bognar E, et al. Catechol-O-methyltransferase Val158-Met polymorphism is associated with methylphenidate response in ADHD children. Am J Med Genet B Neuropsychiatr Genet 2008;147(8):1431–5.
32. Tahir E, Yazgan Y, Cirakoglu B, et al. Association and linkage of DRD4 and DRD5 with attention deficit hyperactivity disorder (ADHD) in a sample of Turkish children. Mol Psychiatry 2000;5(4):396–404.
33. Seeger G, Schloss P, Schmidt MH. Marker gene polymorphisms in hyperkinetic disorder: predictors of clinical response to treatment with methylphenidate? Neurosci Lett 2001;313(1–2):45–8.

34. Hamarman S, Fossella J, Ulger C, et al. Dopamine receptor 4 (DRD4) 7-repeat allele predicts methylphenidate dose response in children with attention deficit hyperactivity disorder: a pharmacogenetic study. J Child Adolesc Psychopharmacol 2005;14(4):564–74.
35. Cheon KA, Kim BN, Cho SC. Association of 4-repeat allele of the dopamine D4 receptor gene exon III polymorphism and response to methylphenidate treatment in Korean ADHD children. Neuropsychopharmacology 2007;32(6):1377–83.
36. McGough JJ, McCracken JT, Loo SK, et al. A candidate gene analysis of methylphenidate response in attention-deficit/hyperactivity disorder. J Am Acad Child Adolesc Psychiatry 2009;48(12):1155–64.
37. Mrazek DA. Pharmacogenomics of methylphenidate response: making progress. J Am Acad Child Adolesc Psychiatry 2009;48(12):1140–2.
38. Polanczyk G, Zeni C, Genro JP, et al. Association of the adrenergic Œ±2A receptor gene with methylphenidate improvement of inattentive symptoms in children and adolescents with attention-deficit/hyperactivity disorder. Arch Gen Psychiatry 2007;64(2):218–24.
39. da Silva TL, Pianca TG, Roman T, et al. Adrenergic alpha2A receptor gene and response to methylphenidate in attention-deficit/hyperactivity disorder-predominantly inattentive type. J Neural Transm 2008;115(2):341–5.
40. Cheon KA, Cho DY, Koo MS, et al. Association between homozygosity of a G Allele of the alpha-2a-adrenergic receptor gene and methylphenidate response in Korean children and adolescents with attention-deficit/hyperactivity disorder. Biol Psychiatry 2009;65(7):564–70.
41. Contini V, Victor MM, Cerqueira CCS, et al. Adrenergic alpha2A receptor gene is not associated with methylphenidate response in adults with ADHD. Eur Arch Psychiatry Clin Neurosci 2011;261(3):205–11.
42. Michelson D, Read HA, Ruff DD, et al. CYP2D6 and clinical response to atomoxetine in children and adolescents with ADHD. J Am Acad Child Adolesc Psychiatry 2007;46(2):242–51.
43. Gizer IR, Ficks C, Waldman ID. Candidate gene studies of ADHD: a meta-analytic review. Hum Genet 2009;126(1):51–90.
44. Banaschewski T, Becker K, Scherag S, et al. Molecular genetics of attention-deficit/hyperactivity disorder: an overview. Eur Child Adolesc Psychiatry 2010;19(3):237–57.
45. Emslie GJ, John Rush A, Weinberg WA, et al. A double-blind, randomized, placebo-controlled trial of fluoxetine in children and adolescents with depression. Arch Gen Psychiatry 1997;54(11):1031–7.
46. Birmaher B, Axelson DA, Monk K, et al. Fluoxetine for the treatment of childhood anxiety disorders. J Am Acad Child Adolesc Psychiatry 2003;42(4):415–23.
47. Williams TP, Miller BD. Pharmacologic management of anxiety disorders in children and adolescents. Curr Opin Pediatr 2003;15(5):483–90.
48. Geller DA, Wagner KD, Emslie G, et al. Paroxetine treatment in children and adolescents with obsessive-compulsive disorder: a randomized, multicenter, double-blind, placebo-controlled trial. J Am Acad Child Adolesc Psychiatry 2004;43(11):1387–96.
49. Wagner KD, Berard R, Stein MB, et al. A multicenter, randomized, double-blind, placebo-controlled trial of paroxetine in children and adolescents with social anxiety disorder. Arch Gen Psychiatry 2004;61(11):1153–62.
50. Emslie GJ, Ryan ND, Wagner KD. Major depressive disorder in children and adolescents: clinical trial design and antidepressant efficacy. J Clin Psychiatry 2005;66(Suppl 7):14–20.

51. Thase ME, Haight BR, Richard N, et al. Remission rates following antidepressant therapy with bupropion or selective serotonin reuptake inhibitors: a meta-analysis of original data from 7 randomized controlled trials. J Clin Psychiatry 2005;66(8):974–81.

52. Joyce PR, Mulder RT, Luty SE, et al. Age-dependent antidepressant pharmacogenomics: polymorphisms of the serotonin transporter and G protein beta3 subunit as predictors of response to fluoxetine and nortriptyline. Int J Neuropsychopharmacol 2003;6(4):339–46.

53. Baumer FM, Howe M, Gallelli K, et al. A pilot study of antidepressant-induced mania in pediatric bipolar disorder: characteristics, risk factors, and the serotonin transporter gene. Biol Psychiatry 2006;60(9):1005–12.

54. Kronenberg S, Apter A, Brent D, et al. Serotonin transporter polymorphism (5-HTTLPR) and citalopram effectiveness and side effects in children with depression and/or anxiety disorders. J Child Adolesc Psychopharmacol 2007;17(6):741–50.

55. Horstmann S, Binder EB. Pharmacogenomics of antidepressant drugs. Pharmacol Ther 2009;124(1):57–73.

56. Durham LK, Webb SM, Milos PM, et al. The serotonin transporter polymorphism, 5HTTLPR, is associated with a faster response time to sertraline in an elderly population with major depressive disorder. Psychopharmacology 2004;174(4):525–9.

57. Kraft JB, Peters EJ, Slager SL, et al. Analysis of association between the serotonin transporter and antidepressant response in a large clinical sample. Biol Psychiatry 2007;61(6):734–42.

58. Hu XZ, Rush AJ, Charney D, et al. Association between a functional serotonin transporter promoter polymorphism and citalopram treatment in adult outpatients with major depression. Arch Gen Psychiatry 2007;64(7):783–92.

59. Mrazek DA, Rush AJ, Biernacka JM, et al. SLC6A4 variation and citalopram response. Am J Med Genet B Neuropsychiatr Genet 2009;150(3):341–51.

60. Mundo E, Walker M, Cate T, et al. The role of serotonin transporter protein gene in antidepressant-induced mania in bipolar disorder: preliminary findings. Arch Gen Psychiatry 2001;58(6):539–44.

61. Rousseva A, Henry C, van den Bulke D, et al. Antidepressant-induced mania, rapid cycling and the serotonin transporter gene polymorphism. Pharmacogenomics J 2003;3(2):101–4.

62. Serretti A, Artioli P, Zanardi R, et al. Genetic features of antidepressant induced mania and hypo-mania in bipolar disorder. Psychopharmacology 2004;174(4):504–11.

63. Masoliver E, Menoyo A, Pérez V, et al. Serotonin transporter linked promoter (polymorphism) in the serotonin transporter gene may be associated with antidepressant-induced mania in bipolar disorder. Psychiatr Genet 2006;16(1):25–9.

64. Ferreira AD, Neves FS, da Rocha FF, et al. The role of 5-HTTLPR polymorphism in antidepressant-associated mania in bipolar disorder. J Affect Disord 2009;112(1–3):267–72.

65. Biernacka JM, McElroy SL, Crow S, et al. Pharmacogenomics of antidepressant induced mania: a review and meta-analysis of the serotonin transporter gene (5HTTLPR) association. J Affect Disord 2012;136(1–2):e21–9.

66. Minov C, Baghai TC, Schüle C, et al. Serotonin-2A-receptor and -transporter polymorphisms: Lack of association in patients with major depression. Neurosci Lett 2001;303(2):119–22.

67. Cusin C, Serretti A, Zanardi R, et al. Influence of monoamine oxidase A and serotonin receptor 2A polymorphisms in SSRI antidepressant activity. Int J Neuropsychopharmacol 2002;5(1):27–35.
68. Sato K, Yoshida K, Takahashi H, et al. Association between -1438 G/A promoter polymorphism in the 5-HT(2A) receptor gene and fluvoxamine response in Japanese patients with major depressive disorder. Neuropsychobiology 2002; 46(3):136–40.
69. Peters EJ, Slager SL, McGrath PJ, et al. Investigation of serotonin-related genes in antidepressant response. Mol Psychiatry 2004;9(9):879–89.
70. Choi MJ, Kang RH, Ham BJ, et al. Serotonin receptor 2A gene polymorphism (-1438A/G) and short-term treatment response to citalopram. Neuropsychobiology 2005;52(3):155–62.
71. McMahon FJ, Buervenich S, Charney D, et al. Variation in the gene encoding the serotonin 2A receptor is associated with outcome of antidepressant treatment. Am J Hum Genet 2006;78(5):804–14.
72. Kato M, Fukuda T, Wakeno M, et al. Effects of the serotonin type 2A, 3A and 3B receptor and the serotonin transporter genes on paroxetine and fluvoxamine efficacy and adverse drug reactions in depressed Japanese patients. Neuropsychobiology 2006;53(4):186–95.
73. Hong CJ, Chen TJ, Yu YWY, et al. Response to fluoxetine and serotonin 1A receptor (C-1019 G) polymorphism in Taiwan Chinese major depressive disorder. Pharmacogenomics J 2006;6(1):27–33.
74. Kang RH, Choi MJ, Paik JW, et al. Effect of serotonin receptor 2A gene polymorphism on mirtazapine response in major depression. Int J Psychiatry Med 2007; 37(3):315–29.
75. Horstmann S, Lucae S, Menke A, et al. Association of GRIK4 and HTR2A genes with antidepressant treatment in the MARS cohort of depressed inpatients. Eur Neuropsychopharmacol 2008;18:S214–5.
76. Perlis RH, Fijal B, Adams DH, et al. Variation in catechol-O-methyltransferase is associated with duloxetine response in a clinical trial for major depressive disorder. Biol Psychiatry 2009;65(9):785–91.
77. Uher R, Huezo-Diaz P, Perroud N, et al. Genetic predictors of response to antidepressants in the GENDEP project. Pharmacogenomics J 2009;9(4):225–33.
78. Lucae S, Ising M, Horstmann S, et al. HTR2A gene variation is involved in antidepressant treatment response. Eur Neuropsychopharmacol 2010;20(1):65–8.
79. Kato M, Serretti A. Review and meta-analysis of antidepressant pharmacogenetic findings in major depressive disorder. Mol Psychiatry 2010;15(5): 473–500.
80. Lohoff FW, Aquino TD, Narasimhan S, et al. Serotonin receptor 2A (HTR2A) gene polymorphism predicts treatment response to venlafaxine XR in generalized anxiety disorder. Pharmacogenomics J 2011. http://dx.doi.org/10.1038/tpj.2011.47.
81. Lee MS. Pharmacogenetics in the treatment of depression in Asia. Asia Pac Psychiatry 2011;3(3):107–8.
82. Bertilsson L, Aberg-Wistedt A, Gustafsson LL, et al. Extremely rapid hydroxylation of debrisoquine: a case report with implication for treatment with nortriptyline and other tricyclic antidepressants. Ther Drug Monit 1985;7(4): 478–80.
83. Yu A, Haining RL. Comparative contribution to dextromethorphan metabolism by cytochrome P450 isoforms in vitro: can dextromethorphan be used as a dual probe for both CYP2D6 and CYP3A activities? Drug Metab Dispos 2001;29(11):1514–20.

84. Kirchheiner J, Brøsen K, Dahl ML, et al. CYP2D6 and CYP2C19 genotype-based dose recommendations for antidepressants: a first step towards subpopulation-specific dosages. Acta Psychiatr Scand 2001;104(3):173–92.

85. Bertilsson L, Dahl ML, Dalén P, et al. Molecular genetics of CYP2D6: Clinical relevance with focus on psychotropic drugs. Br J Clin Pharmacol 2002;53(2):111–22.

86. Ingelman-Sundberg M. Genetic polymorphisms of cytochrome P450 2D6 (CYP2D6): clinical consequences, evolutionary aspects and functional diversity. Pharmacogenomics J 2005;5(1):6–13.

87. Koren G, Cairns J, Chitayat D, et al. Pharmacogenetics of morphine poisoning in a breastfed neonate of a codeine-prescribed mother. Lancet 2006;368(9536):704.

88. Bertilsson L. Metabolism of antidepressant and neuroleptic drugs by cytochrome P450s: clinical and interethnic aspects. Clin Pharmacol Ther 2007;82(5):606–9.

89. Zhou SF. Polymorphism of human cytochrome p450 2D6 and its clinical significance: part I. Clin Pharm 2009;48(11):689–723.

90. Zhou SF. Polymorphism of human cytochrome P450 2D6 and its clinical significance: part II. Clin Pharm 2009;48(12):761–804.

91. Bertilsson L. CYP2D6, serotonin, and suicideal relationship? Clin Pharmacol Ther 2010;88(3):304–5.

92. Zackrisson AL, Lindblom B, Ahlner J. High frequency of occurrence of CYP2D6 gene duplication/multiduplication indicating ultrarapid metabolism among suicide cases. Clin Pharmacol Ther 2010;88(3):354–9.

93. Piatkov I, Jones T, Van Vuuren RJ. Suicide cases and venlafaxine. Acta Neuropsychiatr 2011;23(4):156–60.

94. Tan CH, Shinfuku N, Sim K. Psychotropic prescription practices in east Asia: looking back and peering ahead. Curr Opin Psychiatry 2008;21(6):645–50.

95. Guilherme SK. Ethnic differences in drug therapy: a pharmacogenomics perspective. Expert Rev Clin Pharmacol 2008;1(3):337–9.

96. McGraw J, Waller D. Cytochrome P450 variations in different ethnic populations. Expert Opin Drug Meta Toxicol 2012;8(3):371–82.

97. Black Iii JL, O'Kane DJ, Mrazek DA. The impact of CYP allelic variation on antidepressant metabolism: a review. Expert Opin Drug Meta Toxicol 2007;3(1):21–31.

98. Ji Y, Biernacka J, Snyder K, et al. Catechol O-methyltransferase pharmacogenomics and selective serotonin reuptake inhibitor response. Pharmacogenomics J 2012;12(1):78–85.

99. Brudnak MA. Application of genomeceuticals to the molecular and immunological aspects of autism. Med Hypotheses 2001;57(2):186–91.

100. Arranz MJ, Kerwin RW. Pharmacogenetic and pharmacogenomic research for the prediction of response to antipsychotics in schizophrenia. Drug Dev Res 2003;60(2):104–10.

101. Leeder JS. Developmental and pediatric pharmacogenomics. Pharmacogenomics 2003;4(3):331–41.

102. Ogden CA, Rich ME, Schork NJ, et al. Candidate genes, pathways and mechanisms for bipolar (manic-depressive) and related disorders: an expanded convergent functional genomics approach. Mol Psychiatry 2004;9(11):1007–29.

103. Ackenheil M, Weber K. Differing response to antipsychotic therapy in schizophrenia: pharmacogenomic aspects. Dialogues Clin Neurosci 2004;6(1):71–7.

104. Kirchheiner J, Nickchen K, Bauer M, et al. Pharmacogenetics of antidepressants and antipsychotics: the contribution of allelic variations to the phenotype of drug response. Mol Psychiatry 2004;9(5):442–73.

105. Muller DJ, Muglia P, Fortune T, et al. Pharmacogenetics of antipsychotic-induced weight gain. Pharm Res 2004;49(4):309–29.
106. Reynolds GP, Templeman LA, Zhang ZJ. The role of 5-HT2C receptor polymorphisms in the pharmacogenetics of antipsychotic drug treatment. Prog Neuropsychopharmacol Biol Psychiatry 2005;29(6):1021–8.
107. Escamilla M. Variation in the malic enzyme 2 gene: implications for the pharmacogenomics of psychotic disorders. Pharmacogenomics 2007;8(7):691–5.
108. Arranz MJ, De Leon J. Pharmacogenetics and pharmacogenomics of schizophrenia: a review of last decade of research. Mol Psychiatry 2007;12(8):707–47.
109. Rege S. Antipsychotic induced weight gain in schizophrenia: mechanisms and management. Aust N Z J Psychiatry 2008;42(5):369–81.
110. Fijal BA, Kinon BJ, Kapur S, et al. Candidate-gene association analysis of response to risperidone in African-American and white patients with schizophrenia. Pharmacogenomics J 2009;9(5):311–8.
111. Bishop JR, Bishop DL. Iloperidone for the treatment of schizophrenia. Drugs Today (Barc) 2010;46(8):567–79.
112. Correia CT, Almeida JP, Santos PE, et al. Pharmacogenetics of risperidone therapy in autism: association analysis of eight candidate genes with drug efficacy and adverse drug reactions. Pharmacogenomics J 2010;10(5):418–30.
113. Zandi PP, Judy JT. The promise and reality of pharmacogenetics in psychiatry. Clin Lab Med 2010;30(4):931–74.
114. Luykx JJ, Boks MPM, Terwindt APR, et al. The involvement of GSK3Œ≤ in bipolar disorder: integrating evidence from multiple types of genetic studies. Eur Neuropsychopharmacol 2010;20(6):357–68.
115. Liu BC, Zhang J, Wang L, et al. HTR2C promoter polymorphisms are associated with risperidone efficacy in Chinese female patients. Pharmacogenomics 2010;11(5):685–92.
116. McCarthy MJ, Leckband SG, Kelsoe JR. Pharmacogenetics of lithium response in bipolar disorder. Pharmacogenomics 2010;11(10):1439–65.
117. Squassina A, Manchia M, Manolopoulos VG, et al. Realities and expectations of pharmacogenomics and personalized medicine: impact of translating genetic knowledge into clinical practice. Pharmacogenomics 2010;11(8):1149–67.
118. Squassina A, Manchia M, Del Zompo M. Pharmacogenomics of mood stabilizers in the treatment of bipolar disorder. Hum Genomics Proteomics 2010;2010:159761.
119. Arranz MJ, Rivera M, Munro JC. Pharmacogenetics of response to antipsychotics in patients with schizophrenia. CNS Drugs 2011;25(11):933–9.
120. Houston J, Dharia S, Bishop JR, et al. Association of DRD2 and ANKK1 polymorphisms with prolactin increase in olanzapine-treated women. Psychiatry Res 2011;187(1–2):74–9.
121. Cacabelos R, Hashimoto R, Takeda M. Pharmacogenomics of antipsychotics efficacy for schizophrenia. Psychiatry Clin Neurosci 2011;65(1):3–19.
122. Fleeman N, Dundar Y, Dickson R, et al. Cytochrome P450 testing for prescribing antipsychotics in adults with schizophrenia: systematic review and meta-analyses. Pharmacogenomics J 2011;11(1):1–14.
123. Veenstra-VanderWeele J, Anderson GM, Cook EH Jr. Pharmacogenetics and the serotonin system: initial studies and future directions. Eur J Pharmacol 2000;410(2–3):165–81.
124. Chung WH, Hung SI, Hong HS, et al. A marker for Stevens-Johnson syndrome. Nature 2004;428(6982):486.

125. Ferrell PB Jr, McLeod HL. Carbamazepine, HLA-B*1502 and risk of Stevens-Johnson syndrome and toxic epidermal necrolysis: US FDA recommendations. Pharmacogenomics 2008;9(10):1543–6.

126. Mrazek DA, Lerman C. Facilitating clinical implementation of pharmacogenomics. JAMA 2011;306(3):304–5.

127. Sallee FR, DeVane CL, Ferrell RE. Fluoxetine-related death in a child with cytochrome P-450 2D6 genetic deficiency. J Child Adolesc Psychopharmacol 2000; 10(1):27–34.

128. Williams MS. Insurance coverage for pharmacogenomic testing in the USA. Personalized Medicine 2007;4(4):479–87.

Psychopharmacologic Treatment for Pediatric Anxiety Disorders

Todd E. Peters, MD[a],*, Sucheta Connolly, MD[b]

KEYWORDS

• Children • Anxiety • Psychopharmacology • SSRI • Review

KEY POINTS

- Strong empiric evidence supports the use of psychotherapy as a first-line agent for anxiety disorders of mild to moderate severity in children and adolescents.
- Solid, empirically based data support the use of combination therapy (cognitive-behavioral therapy + antidepressants) in youth diagnosed with obsessive-compulsive disorder, generalized anxiety disorder, social anxiety disorder, and social phobia when symptoms become more severely impairing.
- Comorbid disorders often warrant antidepressant use earlier in the treatment course.
- A relative lack of data supports pharmacologic treatment of several prominent anxiety disorders in children, including posttraumatic disorder and panic disorder.
- No current data are available on long-term effects of antidepressant use on the developing brain in youth, especially on potential side effects and theoretical risk for increased suicidality.
- Untreated anxiety disorders in youth can lead to significant impairments in school performance, family functioning, and potential disability/further impairment in adulthood.

OVERVIEW

Experiencing anxiety or fear is a normal part of life. It functions as an automatic response to dangerous situations, either perceived or real. From a developmental standpoint, different types of anxiety symptoms are present throughout life, from stranger anxiety as an infant and separation anxiety as a toddler, to worries about potential physical harm in early childhood, and later social concerns and existential worry in adolescence. However, these normative worries can worsen, causing

[a] Department of Psychiatry, Division of Child and Adolescent Psychiatry, Vanderbilt University School of Medicine, Vanderbilt Psychiatric Hospital, 1601 23rd Avenue South, Nashville, TN 37212-8645, USA; [b] Institute for Juvenile Research (MC 747), Department of Psychiatry, Pediatric Stress and Anxiety Disorders Clinic, University of Illinois at Chicago, 1747 West Roosevelt Road, Room 155, Chicago, IL 60608, USA
* Corresponding author. Vanderbilt Psychiatric Hospital, 1601 23rd Avenue South, Nashville, TN 37212-8645.
E-mail address: todd.peters@vanderbilt.edu

Child Adolesc Psychiatric Clin N Am 21 (2012) 789–806
http://dx.doi.org/10.1016/j.chc.2012.07.007
1056-4993/12/$ – see front matter © 2012 Elsevier Inc. All rights reserved.
childpsych.theclinics.com

prominent distress and impairment in multiple spheres of life, leading to anxiety disorders.[1] Anxiety disorders in childhood are common, with 12-month prevalence rates of 10% to 20%.[2–6] Anxiety disorders are often very impairing and evolve during childhood, which can lead to other psychological disorders in adolescence and adulthood. Anxiety disorders in early childhood predict other mental health issues in adolescents, including conduct disorder, attention-deficit/hyperactivity disorder, depression, and, most commonly, other anxiety disorders,[7,8] and can lead to incapacitating symptoms into adulthood.

Several general principles apply to treatment of all anxiety disorders in youth. Psychotherapy, primarily cognitive-behavioral therapy (CBT), is considered the first-line treatment for anxiety disorders of mild severity. Psychotherapeutic treatment is outside of the scope of this article, but other extensive review articles address these treatment modalities.[9–11] As anxiety worsens to a moderate or severe level, strong data support the use of pharmacologic agents, especially selective serotonin reuptake inhibitors (SSRIs), in combination with psychotherapy for most anxiety disorders.[12,13] Despite this evidence, the U.S. Food and Drug Administration (FDA) has only approved SSRI use for obsessive-compulsive disorder (OCD) in children (fluoxetine, sertraline, and fluvoxamine, along with clomipramine). However, SSRIs are commonly used off-label in the treatment of anxiety in childhood and adolescence and are considered the first-line pharmacologic agents for anxiety disorders in youth.[14,15] **Table 1** provides details on randomized controlled trials of antidepressant agents.

This article reviews the literature on psychopharmacological management of 7 of the 8 anxiety disorders in youth as stated in the *Diagnostic and Statistical Manual of Mental Disorders* (Fourth Edition, Text Revision) (DSM-IV-TR):

1. Separation anxiety disorder (SAD)
2. Specific phobia
3. Generalized anxiety disorder (GAD)
4. Panic disorder
5. Social phobia (SoP)/anxiety (including discussion of selective mutism)
6. OCD
7. Posttraumatic stress disorder (PTSD)

Specific phobia, an anxiety disorder commonly seen in childhood, is mainly treated with exposure-focused CBT. However, for severe impairment, medications such as SSRIs[16] and short-term use of benzodiazepines and β-blockers can be considered to reduce anxiety severity and increase participation in exposures.

This article reviews the empiric data surrounding psychopharmacologic treatment of these disorders, focusing primarily on randomized placebo-controlled trials and providing updated data from the previous installation of this topic in this journal.[17] The potential side effects, complications, and safety concerns associated with SSRI use for treating children with anxiety disorders are discussed, including in very young children (ages 0–6 years). Treatment of the most prevalent comorbid conditions and how these impact the treatment of anxiety disorders are addressed.

PHARMACOLOGIC MANAGEMENT OF GAD, SAD, AND SOCIAL PHOBIA

GAD, SAD, and SoP (also known as *social anxiety disorder*) are common anxiety disorders diagnosed in childhood that often cause significant impairment that impacts the child and family. These diagnoses are often clustered together for research purposes because of a high level of co-occurrence and overlap between symptom constellations. These disorders are linked to 2 additional conditions or symptom complexes seen in anxious youth: school refusal behavior andelective mutism.

Table 1
Placebo-controlled pharmacologic treatment studies for anxiety disorders in youth

Disorder	Medication Class	Author	Treatment	Demographics	Diagnoses	Results
SoP, GAD, SAD	SSRI	Black & Uhde,[19] 1994	Fluoxetine (12–27 mg/d)	N = 15; age: 6–11 y	SM plus SoP or AD	Fluoxetine > PLC
		RUPP,[26] 2001	Fluvoxamine (50–250 mg/d child, max 300 mg/d adolescent)	N = 128; age: 6–17 y	SoP, SAD, GAD	Fluvoxamine > PLC
		Rynn et al,[27] 2001	Sertraline (50 mg/d)	N = 22; age: 5–17 y	GAD	Sertraline > PLC
		Birmaher et al,[28] 2003	Fluoxetine (20 mg/d)	N = 74; age: 7–17 y	GAD, SoP, SAD	Fluoxetine > PLC, Fluoxetine > PLC, Fluoxetine = PLC
		Wagner et al,[29] 2004	Paroxetine (10–50 mg/d)	N = 322; age: 8–17 y	SoP	Paroxetine > PLC
	TCA	Gittleman-Klein & Klein,[35] 1971	Imipramine (100–200 mg/d)	N = 35; age: 6–14 y	School phobia with anxiety disorders	Imipramine > PLC
		Berney et al,[36] 1981	Clomipramine (40–75 mg/d)	N = 51; age: 9–14 y	School refusal	Clomipramine = PLC
		Klein et al,[37] 1992	Imipramine (75–275 mg/d)	N = 21; age: 6–15 y	SAD with or without school phobia	Imipramine = PLC
	SNRI	March et al,[33] 2007	Venlafaxine ER (37.5–225 mg/d)	N = 293; age: 8–17 y	SoP	Venlafaxine > PLC
		Rynn et al,[34] 2007	Venlafaxine ER (37.5–225 mg/d)	N = 220; age: 6–17 y	GAD	Venlafaxine > PLC
	Benzodiazepines	Bernstein et al,[41] 1990	Alprazolam (0.75–4.0 mg/d) vs imipramine (50–175 mg/d)	N = 24; age: 7–18 y	School refusal, SAD	Alprazolam = Imipramine = PLC
		Simeon et al,[42] 1992	Alprazolam (0.5–3.5 mg/d)	N = 30; age: 8–17 y	OAD, AD	Alprazolam = PLC
		Graae et al,[43] 1994	Clonazepam (0.5–2.0 mg/d)	N = 15; age: 7–13 y	SAD	Clonazepam = PLC
OCD	SSRI	March et al,[61] 1998	Sertraline (max 200 mg/d)	N = 187; age: 6–17 y	OCD	Sertraline > PLC
		Riddle et al,[65] 2001	Fluvoxamine (50–200 mg/d)	N = 120; age: 8–17 y	OCD	Fluvoxamine > PLC
		Geller et al,[63] 2001	Fluoxetine (max 60 mg/d)	N = 103; age: 7–17 y	OCD	Fluoxetine > PLC
		Geller et al,[66] 2004	Paroxetine (10–50 mg/d)	N = 207; age: 7–17 y	OCD	Paroxetine > PLC
		March et al, 2004	Sertraline (25–200 mg/d) only vs CBT only vs combination	N = 112; age: 7–17 y	OCD	Combination > CBT = Sertraline > PLC
	TCA	Flament et al, 1985	Clomipramine (max 200 mg/d)	N = 60; age: 10–17 y	OCD	Clomipramine > PLC
PTSD	SSRI	Cohen et al,[79] 2007	TF-CBT + sertraline or TF-CBT + placebo	N = 24; age 10–17 y (female only)	PTSD	TF-CBT + sertraline > TF-CBT + placebo
		Robb et al, 2008	Sertraline (50–200 mg/d)	N = 131; age: 6–17 y	PTSD	Sertraline = PLC

Abbreviations: AD, avoidant disorder; ER, extended release; GAD, generalized anxiety disorder; max, maximum; OAD, overanxious disorder; PLC, placebo; PTSD, posttraumatic stress disorder; RUPP, Research Unit on Pediatric Psychopharmacology; SAD, separation anxiety disorder; SM, selective mutism; SNRI, serotonin-norepinephrine reuptake inhibitor; SoP, social phobia; TCA, tricyclic antidepressant; TF-CBT, trauma-focused cognitive behavioral therapy.

Many investigators argue that selective mutism is an anxiety disorder variant, and particularly associated with SoP.[18] Studies have shown that up to 68% to 97% of children with a diagnosis of selective mutism meet criteria for SoP or avoidant behavior.[19,20] Thirteen placebo-controlled pharmacologic trials support the use of antidepressant medications in youth with anxiety disorders, with most supporting SSRIs as the first choice for treatment of more severe symptoms (see **Table 1**).

SSRIs

Several studies in the 1990s, including chart reviews,[21,22] open-label trials,[23–25] and one smaller randomized, placebo-controlled trial for children with selective mutism and SoP,[19] showed promising results that SSRIs were likely effective in the treatment of pediatric anxiety disorders. During this time (1996), the National Institute of Mental Health established the Research Unit on Pediatric Psychopharmacology (RUPP) networks to systematically and safely investigate pharmacologic treatment for psychiatric disorders in childhood. One such branch, entitled the RUPP Anxiety Disorders Study Group, recruited 128 children diagnosed with SoP, SAD, or GAD, for whom a 3-week, lead-in psychosocial intervention failed, into an 8-week, double-blind study with either fluvoxamine or placebo. Overall, this study showed a profound improvement of clinical status in the fluvoxamine group, with a 76% acute response versus a 29% response in the placebo group, with a poorer outcome seen in those with severe illness and a diagnosis of SoP.[26]

This hallmark study paved the way for additional medication-based randomized controlled trials that used other SSRIs in the 2000s.

One small study (N = 22) investigated the efficacy of low-dose sertraline (50 mg/d) versus placebo for 9 weeks in children diagnosed with GAD. The results showed clear clinical improvement in the sertraline group (90%) versus the placebo group (10%); however, only 2 of 11 patients in the sertraline group had a marked improvement, with a remission rate of 18%.[27]

A larger (N = 74) study followed, comparing fluoxetine fixed-dosing (20 mg) versus placebo over a 12-week period in youth diagnosed with GAD, SAD, and SoP. Fluoxetine showed a significant improvement over placebo (response rates: 61% vs 35%), with specific improvement in global functional status. However, children with SoP and GAD showed a more marked improvement than those diagnosed with SAD.[28]

In 2004, a large (N = 322) multisite study was published evaluating the safety and effectiveness of paroxetine use in youth with SoP.[29] This study showed a clear, favorable short-term response rate for paroxetine compared with placebo (78% vs 39%). However, a plethora of adverse effects were present in those taking paroxetine, including increased insomnia, nausea/vomiting, and decreased appetite, along with worsened nervousness, hostility, and signs of potential activation in younger children.

Since this study, paroxetine has fallen out of favor for use in youth because of its short half-life and associated side effects, and is commonly not considered a first-line agent for youth with anxiety disorders.

More recently, 2 randomized controlled trials investigated the use of SSRIs versus therapeutic interventions.

The first study compared the efficacy of social effectiveness therapy (SET-C) versus fluoxetine monotherapy (with a placebo/control arm) in youth with SoP.[30] Low to moderate dosing of fluoxetine (10–40 mg) during the 12-week treatment course was more efficacious than placebo overall. SET-C and fluoxetine were both effective in diminishing behavioral avoidance and social distress, but SET-C was superior to fluoxetine through the enhancement of social skills, showing continued improvement throughout the entire 12-week treatment course.[31]

Another study, entitled the Child-Adolescent Anxiety Multimodal Study (CAMS), was the first study to compare monotherapy with combined treatment for SAD, GAD, and SoP. CAMS was a large (N = 488) 12-week multisite trial with 3 treatment arms (sertraline up to 200mg; CBT; and combination of sertraline and CBT) and a placebo control arm.[31]

The results showed that all treatment arms had superior clinical improvement compared with placebo, as rated very much or much improved on the Clinician Global Impression-Improvement scale. However, maximum benefit was achieved with combination therapy, with 80.7% for combination, 59.7% for CBT only, 54.9% for sertraline only, and 23.7% for placebo. The strongest predictors for overall remission were[32]

- Lack of other internalizing disorders
- Lower baseline anxiety levels
- Younger age
- Lack of SoP
- Nonminority status

Based on these results, the authors recommended that all 3 treatments be considered for youth with non-OCD anxiety disorders, with consideration of individual and family preferences along with availability of high-quality CBT providers in the patient's respective community.

The American Academy of Child and Adolescent Psychiatry (AACAP) practice parameters for anxiety disorders in youth designated SSRI use as "clinical guidelines," in which this treatment should be considered in most if not all patients (apply approximately 75% of the time).[12]

Serotonin-Norepinephrine Reuptake Inhibitors and Tricyclic Antidepressants

Three large randomized controlled trials have investigated the use of venlafaxine extended-release (ER) tablets in children with SoP and GAD.

A 16-week, placebo-controlled study investigating use of venlafaxine ER in SoP showed statistically significant improvement in those treated with up to 225 mg of venlafaxine ER compared with placebo (56% vs 37% treatment response on the Clinical Global Impression Improvement [CGI-I] scale, respectively).[33]

Rynn and colleagues[34] included data from 2 randomized controlled trials (N = 320) on venlafaxine ER as a treatment for GAD.

The first study showed a clear response to venlafaxine ER compared with placebo, whereas the second study showed some improvement of secondary measures, but this was not clinically significant compared with placebo. The combined response rates between studies showed a statistically significant improvement with venlafaxine ER compared with placebo (69% vs 48%). Based on these preliminary studies, venlafaxine may be considered for treatment of GAD and SoP, but only after failure of several SSRIs, with close monitoring for potential side effects or adverse effects (see later section on potential side effects).[8]

Several small randomized controlled trials examining tricyclic antidepressants (TCAs) as a potential treatment option for youth with SoP, GAD, and SAD have yielded disparate results.

The first study, published in 1971, investigated imipramine as a potential treatment option for "school phobia," in which most children would meet criteria for SAD based on study parameters. Imipramine was found to be superior to placebo in this limited study.[35]

Two subsequent studies examining school phobia/refusal could not replicate the outcomes of the 1971 study; no statistically significant differences were seen between the placebo and TCA treatment group (both clomipramine and imipramine were studied).[36,37]

In 2000, Bernstein and others[38] examined 47 school-refusing youth with comorbid anxiety and major depressive disorders, offering double-blind combination therapy for all participants with imipramine + CBT versus placebo + CBT. Imipramine + CBT was found to be superior to placebo + CBT in this study. A naturalistic follow-up study of these patients after 1 year found that for those with comorbid disorders and severe impairment, symptoms persisted over time, requiring more long-term maintenance treatment (both psychotherapy and pharmacologic) to maintain gains.[39,40]

Despite these mixed positive results, TCAs should be used with great caution in children because of the negative side-effect profile, including cardiac conduction issues and the greater risk for lethality in overdose.

Benzodiazepines and Other Agents

Several trials in the early 1990s investigated the use of benzodiazepines in children with anxiety disorders,[41–43] including alprazolam and clonazepam. Despite multiple trials, benzodiazepines have not been shown to be efficacious as a single agent for the treatment of anxiety disorders in youth.[15] However, benzodiazepines can be considered as an augmenting agent to target acute anxiety symptoms during progressive titration of antidepressant agents, which can take up to 4 to 6 weeks to reach maximal effect and may initially cause rebound anxiety symptoms. Benzodiazepines can also be considered for children who are having difficulty engaging in exposure-based CBT because of severe or extreme anxiety symptoms.[44] Caution must be exercised with the use of benzodiazepines in children, and these agents should be avoided with comorbid substance abuse disorders; see later section on side effects of treatment for additional data.

Buspirone has been suggested as an alternate agent or adjuvant agent to consider with failure of SSRI- or serotonin-norepinephrine reuptake inhibitor (SNRI)–based treatment.[8,12] Buspirone has proven efficacious for some adults with GAD; however, no randomized controlled trials have investigated the use of buspirone in children or adolescents. An open trial with buspirone in children with mixed anxiety disorders showed significant improvement without prominent side effects.[45] Another study showed that children may benefit from lower doses of buspirone (5–7.5 mg twice daily), and older adolescents may require higher doses for similar response without significant side effects (5–30 mg twice daily).[46] The most prominent side effects seen in this study were lightheadedness (68%), headache (48%), and dyspepsia (20%).

PHARMACOLOGIC MANAGEMENT OF PANIC DISORDER

Despite an extensive history of treatment trials for panic disorder in the adult literature, no randomized controlled trials exist in youth for this disorder. This lack of studies has been attributed to a limited understanding of the developmental course of panic disorder in children and adolescents. Many children experience panic attacks that are impairing with a range of anxiety disorders but do not meet full criteria for having a panic disorder as currently defined in DSM-IV-TR.

A small open-label pilot study looking at the use of SSRIs in adolescents with panic disorder and associated comorbid disorders showed much or very much improvement in up to 75% of patients with several SSRIs—fluoxetine, sertraline, and paroxetine—when used as single-treatment agents or in combination with benzodiazepines (clonazepam or lorazepam) for more severe symptoms.[44]

An open treatment study of mixed anxiety disorders in youth determined that fluoxetine treatment was helpful in alleviating several anxiety symptoms, including panic, in children (mean dose = 24 mg) and adolescents (mean dose = 40 mg).[24]

Paroxetine also showed significant clinical improvement of panic symptoms in children with panic disorder along with comorbid disorders in a small (N = 18) retrospective chart review in 2001.[47] However, despite this medication being well tolerated in this study, paroxetine has fallen out of favor with some child and adolescent psychiatrists because of its negative side-effect profile (including significant discontinuation syndrome) and perceived lack of efficacy in treating major depressive disorder in youths.

In December 2004, the European Medicines Agency's Committee for Medicinal Products for Human Use recommended that paroxetine should not be prescribed to children.[48] Providers should exercise caution in using paroxetine in children based on the black box warning for potential increased suicidal thoughts in adolescents and young adults associated with all SSRI agents.

PHARMACOLOGIC MANAGEMENT OF OCD

OCD in children and adolescents is highly prevalent (1%–2% of the population) and often undetected and untreated in the general population. The diagnosis of OCD follows a strong familial link, with a risk of OCD diagnosis in up to 12% of first-degree relatives.[49] Environmental influences significantly impact the manifestation of the disorder.[50] Additionally, a small subset of OCD cases have been associated with a potential underlying immunologic response to group A β-hemolytic streptococcal infection that causes inflammation of the basal ganglia, leading to a syndrome of OCD, symptoms of hyperactivity, and tic-like behavior or Tourette syndrome, entitled *pediatric autoimmune neuropsychiatric disorders associated with streptococcus* (PANDAS),[51–53] although controversy exists regarding this diagnosis.[54,55]

No controversy exists, however, in examining the evidence for OCD treatment in children and adolescents. After thorough assessment and subsequent diagnosis of OCD, CBT is strongly recommended as the first-line treatment for mild to moderate severity of symptoms, with antidepressant medication recommended as an adjunctive treatment for more moderate to severe cases. Rigorous clinical data support this recommendation for combination therapy; the AACAP considers this the "clinical standard" of treatment.[50] OCD is the only FDA-approved indication for serotonin reuptake inhibitor (SRI) use in children and adolescents with anxiety, with fluoxetine, sertraline, fluvoxamine, and clomipramine the approved agents. Aside from severity scales, the main clinical question is often when to initiate pharmacologic treatment in combination with CBT. Pharmacotherapy may be considered earlier if comorbid diagnoses are present, especially associated mood and anxiety disorders that commonly respond well to SSRI-based treatment. These comorbid disorders can impact the child's ability to participate in exposure-based treatments. Earlier initiation of medications can be prompted by familial factors, such as[56]

- Poor insight into the disease
- Limited follow-up or practice of treatment strategies outside of the session
- Continued accommodations of behavior or a child's resistance to treatment

Additionally, the shortage of clinicians who can provide exposure-based CBT in the community directly impacts the availability of care. However, a recent study shows that, for youth with OCD who are initially treated with SSRIs and have a partial response, augmentation with OCD-specific brief (12-week) CBT can provide superior clinical response (68.6%) compared with continued medication treatment alone (30.0%) or continued medication management plus instructions in CBT strategies (34.0%).[57]

SRIs, Including Clomipramine

Agents with high serotonergic effects have shown the most promise in the treatment of OCD in both youth and adults. The first placebo-controlled trials for the treatment of OCD in children and adolescents studied clomipramine,[58,59] which gained FDA approval in 1989. In subsequent studies, clomipramine has been shown to be superior to less serotonergic TCAs, such as desipramine.[60]

These initial studies, along with the effectiveness with highly serotonergic agents in adult OCD research, led to several industry-sponsored, placebo-controlled, randomized trials that showed the effectiveness of sertraline,[61] fluoxetine,[62–64] fluvoxamine,[65] and paroxetine[66] over placebo for children with OCD. A meta-analysis performed in 2003 examining all randomized controlled trials of medications targeting youth with OCD determined a clear statistical significance between SRI use and placebo (number needed to treat was approximately 4–6).[67] In this same study, no one SSRI clearly distinguished itself. However, some evidence suggested that clomipramine may have higher efficacy than SSRIs for the treatment of pediatric OCD. Despite this evidence, SSRIs are routinely used as first-line agents for youth with OCD in clinical practice because of a more favorable side-effect profile and less cardiac risk associated with general use and after overdose attempts.

Pediatric OCD treatment study

The nearly universal recommendation for a combination of psychotherapy, mainly exposure-based CBT, and SSRI treatment for youth with moderate to severe anxiety disorders was clearly exemplified in the Pediatric OCD Treatment Study (POTS) sponsored by the National Institute of Mental Health.[68,69] POTS was created as the first randomized placebo-controlled trial in the pediatric OCD population comparing monotherapy, including exposure and response prevention-based CBT and sertraline, versus a combination of the treatments. This study included 3 clinical sites and involved 112 youth with moderate to severe OCD symptoms, as shown by a score of 16 or higher on the Children's Yale-Brown Obsessive-Compulsive Scale (CY-BOCS). The results showed that combination therapy was clearly more efficacious in symptom reduction than either sertraline or CBT alone (clinical remission was 53.6% for combined treatment, 39.3% for CBT alone, 21.4% for sertraline alone, and 3.6% for placebo). All active treatment arms also independently showed superior efficacy in symptom reduction compared with the placebo control group. However, in terms of symptom reduction for the separate monotherapies, the CBT and sertraline groups did not differentiate from each other in a statistically significant fashion. The authors also reviewed clinical remission, which was specified as a CY-BOCS score of less than 10, and determined that the combination and CBT groups had superior results to the placebo group. However, the sertraline group did not show superior results over placebo in terms of remission, and no statistically significant difference was seen between combination therapy and CBT monotherapy in terms of overall remission rate. Some center-specific differences were seen regarding the efficacy of monotherapy, with one center showing more favorable results with CBT compared with sertraline alone, and the other site showing more favorable results with medication monotherapy compared with CBT alone. All sites determined that combination therapy was superior to all other treatments. This study determined an overall effect size of 0.66 for sertraline therapy in the studied population.[69]

Augmentation Strategies for Partial Response or SRI Treatment Resistance

Based on the recent AACAP practice parameters, treatment resistance in pediatric OCD is supported after failure of response to 2 SRIs (either 2 SSRIs or 1 SSRI and clomipramine) after at least 10 weeks of treatment at maximum tolerated dosing, along with adequate CBT-based treatment.[50] In these situations, clinicians have shown some benefit with cautiously combining lower doses of an SSRI, especially fluvoxamine, with clomipramine, monitoring closely for signs of serotonin overload or serotonin syndrome. Changing from an SRI to SNRI-based therapy, such as venlafaxine and duloxetine, has also been helpful in some refractory patients.[50]

Other medications have been shown to be beneficial as an add-on therapy to SRIs in clinical practice. Several randomized controlled trials have used atypical antipsychotics as augmentation agents in adult OCD; these results have been extrapolated to pediatric OCD treatment, especially for those with severe obsessive/compulsive symptoms, associated tic disorders, pervasive developmental disorders, or struggles with mood instability.[50] Clonazepam has also been combined with SRI use in several smaller trials in pediatric OCD.[70] However, benzodiazepines should be used cautiously in younger children because of a higher risk of adverse effects (see later section on adverse effects). Other treatment strategies, such as recent use of the glutamate antagonists memantine and riluzole, have been trialed but currently do not have enough data to support their regular use in the pediatric OCD population.[50]

PHARMACOLOGIC MANAGEMENT OF PTSD

Trauma in childhood continues to be a prevalent cause of anxiety in children and adolescents; greater than 1 in 4 children will experience a significant traumatic event before adulthood.[71] To meet diagnostic criteria for PTSD, children must be able to describe a traumatic event and associated symptoms in relation to this event.[72] Reports have shown a high lifetime prevalence of PTSD of up to 9.2% in the general population,[73] with many other children likely experiencing subthreshold symptomatology or not meeting full criteria for the disorder. However, those with subthreshold symptoms are often as functionally impaired as those who meet criteria for PTSD.[74]

Trauma-focused psychotherapy is considered the first-line treatment for youth with PTSD. Trauma-focused CBT (TF-CBT) has the strongest empiric support for treatment in youth, but individual psychodynamic strategies and trauma-focused family therapy have also shown benefit in children and adolescents. In contrast, pharmacotherapy with SSRIs for PTSD in youth has less empiric support compared with other anxiety disorders. In the latest PTSD practice parameters from the AACAP, SSRIs are considered an "option" for treatment, which is defined as an acceptable form of treatment based on some empiric evidence or expert opinion, but lacking strong evidence or consensus among child and adolescent psychiatrists.[72] These results are in stark comparison to the adult literature for PTSD, which shows sound efficacy for multiple antidepressant agents. This divide shows the inherent difficulty in applying the adult literature carte blanche for the pediatric population, proving once again that children are not just "little adults."

SSRIs

Initial open studies investigating SSRIs in pediatric PTSD showed some clinical improvement.[75-77] However, 2 recent randomized controlled trials have attempted to determine the efficacy of SSRI use in this population with disappointing results.

The first study of 67 youth with PTSD comparing sertraline versus placebo showed clinical improvement in both groups (with a strong placebo effect) but did not determine sertraline to be superior to placebo.[78]

The second study explored the use of combination therapy with TF-CBT + sertraline versus TF-CBT + placebo in 24 youth with PTSD caused by a history of sexual abuse. This study again showed improvement in both groups without statistically significant differences between groups.[79]

Because of the limited effect of SSRIs in these studies, the general opinion regarding treatment of pediatric PTSD does not support the use of SSRI as the only treatment strategy; instead, the most common treatment strategy is to start with trauma-focused psychotherapy and augment with an SSRI only in the presence of very severe initial symptoms or limited clinical response from psychotherapy alone. However, for children with comorbid psychiatric disorders with a strong efficacy for SSRI-based treatment, such as major depressive disorder or other anxiety disorders (such as OCD or GAD), initiation of an SSRI may be considered earlier in the treatment course.[72]

Other Medication Strategies for PTSD

Additional treatment strategies are based on the underlying evidence of neurochemical changes evident in youth experiencing PTSD. Evidence in the pediatric population with PTSD shows heightened adrenergic tone, resulting in hyperresponsiveness of these associated pathways. In turn, α- and β-adrenergic blockers are frequently used with some benefit in children, with several open trials supporting use of both clonidine[80–82] and propranolol.[83] Research has also shown increased dopamine levels in adults and youth with PTSD, supporting the heightened fear response seen in patients with trauma-based anxiety disorders. In an effort to target excessive dopamine levels, neuroleptic agents such as atypical antipsychotics are frequently used in youth with prominent PTSD symptoms. One open study of risperidone use in this population showed high rates of remission (13 of 18 children with severe PTSD symptoms), but these children also had high levels of comorbid disorders, such as bipolar disorder, which, when effectively treated with risperidone, may have contributed to these promising results.[84] In clinical practice, atypical antipsychotics are often used to target prominent symptoms of dissociation or active auditory/visual hallucinations that are more likely attributable to PTSD than to a primary psychotic process. It is recommended that, as children progress in the treatment process for PTSD, the need for continued antipsychotic medications be reassessed to reduce the risk for metabolic syndrome associated with long-term antipsychotic use.

CLINICAL CONSIDERATIONS AND POTENTIAL ADVERSE EFFECTS FROM PHARMACOLOGIC TREATMENT

Pharmacotherapy, especially SSRI-based treatment, is usually well tolerated in children and adolescents with anxiety disorders. The frequency of adverse effects in youth often correlates with that seen in research on adult anxiety disorders. However, certain treatments for anxiety disorders may be linked to certain adverse effects, which should be closely monitored.

SSRI Adverse Effects

Based on the data from prior treatment studies for non-OCD anxiety disorders, children who were treated with SSRIs experienced increased rates of gastrointestinal issues and hyperkinetic behavior compared with the placebo group.[15,26]

Less common, but potentially more serious or impairing, are concerns of behavioral activation and disinhibition. In the initial treatment course, care must be taken to review whether a child is simply showing improved mood from early benefits of medication use versus activation or disinhibition from SSRI use, which may increase the risk for further elevation of mood and potential medication-induced mania. Furthermore, as anxiety improves, children may display normal oppositionality and assertiveness versus overcompliance related to anxiety. This issue must be discussed with the family and not mislabeled as disinhibition.

Even less commonly, SSRIs can cause issues with tremors, tics, enuresis, sedation, affective blunting, profound apathy, or akathisia. Many of these symptoms may improve or resolve after lowering the dose of the current medication or transitioning to another SSRI[15]; however, intolerance may be class-related or from an underlying undiagnosed bipolar disorder. These symptoms, along with sexual side effects, may contribute to compliance issues in this population, warranting close assessment for these underlying symptoms.[8,85]

The black box criteria for increased risk of suicidal thoughts must be reviewed with all patients and families before antidepressant therapy is initiated. However, this risk is likely diminished for those taking SSRIs for anxiety disorders, especially OCD, for which it is negligible (number needed to harm = 200).[86]

SSRI Age-Related Adverse Effects

Several potential age-related adverse effects within the pediatric population must be considered when treating anxiety disorders.

- Nausea/vomiting and activation are more common in younger children than in adolescents.
- Age-specific peak plasma concentrations have been seen with some SSRIs, including fluvoxamine, which may relate to the potential for increased side effects in younger populations.[87]
- In very young children (age 0–6 years), trying psychotherapy for at least 12 weeks is recommended before considering antidepressant use because of the relative lack of empiric data. If a lack of response or limited partial response is seen, initiation of a very low dose of fluoxetine (1–5 mg/d) may be considered to target severe anxiety symptoms. If this treatment is ineffective, transitioning to another SSRI may be warranted.[8,88]
- Benzodiazepines should not be used routinely in very young children and be used sparingly in older children because of concerns regarding excessive sedation, impact on short-term memory and learning, potential physiologic dependence or withdrawal symptoms, or a paradoxic reaction, including activation, disinhibition, irritability, or oppositional behavior.[43,89–92]

Long-Term Effects of Antidepressant Use in Youth

No studies have been completed assessing long-term antidepressant use in youth with anxiety disorders. This lack of data should be discussed with families before initiation of antidepressants and weighed against the risk of negative effects of untreated anxiety symptoms on normal brain development. After the patient experiences a period of relative stability on an antidepressant medication (12 months), clinicians should consider a slow taper and eventual discontinuation during a period of low stress (often summer vacation or holidays) if tolerated. If symptoms relapse, the dose can be retitrated or restarted to target these worsening symptoms.[15,93]

CLINICAL VIGNETTE

A 10-year-old boy presented for initial psychiatric treatment after becoming increasingly anxious over the previous 6 months. He became significantly preoccupied with his morning routine during this time, which caused him to be late to school each day and caused frequent arguments and conflict with his parents. Before leaving home for school, he must watch his goldfish swim "up, then down and to the left...or something bad will happen." He endorses fear that his family will die if he does not perform this activity "or we will have to move out of our home because it will fall apart." Although he normally receives stellar grades in school, his performance has declined despite extra time spent on homework. He realizes that his thoughts are excessive; however, he feels that he cannot stop for fear of harming others. He also endorsed worsening neurovegetative symptoms during this time, noting difficulty initiating sleep, anhedonia, decreased energy, and limited appetite. He also developed a fear of eating certain foods aside from crackers, pretzels, and cereal, concerned that he may choke or asphyxiate while eating. His decreased parenteral intake caused significant weight loss and borderline bradycardia.

He was admitted to a partial hospital program for medical workup (which was unremarkable) and ongoing psychiatric care. After admission, a fear hierarchy was created to target obsessive/compulsive symptoms. He met with a nutritionist who, through the help of the primary team, developed a plan for reintroducing avoided foods over time to meet caloric goals. He was started on sertraline shortly after admission, progressively titrating the dose from 12.5 mg to 75 mg daily by the time of discharge. Because of ongoing profound obsessive/compulsive symptoms, which severely impacted his ability to function, he was started on low-dose risperidone (0.5 mg/d) as brief augmentation until reaching therapeutic effects from sertraline dosing. Through a combination of cognitive-behavioral strategies and pharmacologic treatment, he was able to increase and vary his food intake. He was also able to gradually expose himself to several anxiety provoking situations, "riding the wave of anxiety." The authors' team also focused on working with his parents to help them avoid accommodating his OCD symptoms, modeling strategies for combating anxious thoughts and leading exposures at home. These treatments eventually attenuated the duration and severity of anxiety symptoms overall and allowed the patient to successfully return to school with continued outpatient supports.

SUMMARY/FUTURE DIRECTIONS

Over the past 10 to 20 years, several major placebo-controlled trials have investigated psychopharmacologic treatment for anxiety disorders in youth. Strong empiric evidence supports the use of psychotherapy, especially exposure-based CBT strategies, as a first-line agent for anxiety disorders of mild to moderate severity in children and adolescents. When anxiety symptoms become more severely impairing, solid empirically based data support the use of combination therapy (CBT + antidepressants) in youth diagnosed with OCD (SSRIs and clomipramine), GAD, SAD, and SoP (SSRIs). Comorbid disorders, such as underlying depressive disorders or additional anxiety disorders, often warrant antidepressant use earlier in the treatment course to target these confounding symptoms.

Despite these advances, many areas for future study remain in the field of psychopharmacology for childhood anxiety disorders. Few studies compare psychopharmacologic treatment with psychotherapy and other psychosocial interventions, although this gap has closed substantially over the past decade.[31,32,69] A relative lack of data supports pharmacologic treatment of several prominent anxiety disorders in children, including PTSD and panic disorder. Many other treatment strategies for augmentation, such as benzodiazepine and atypical antipsychotic use, are extrapolated from the adult anxiety treatment data and are not supported by rigorous medication trials in children. Most importantly, no current data exist regarding the long-term effects of antidepressant use on the developing brain in this population, which hampers the ability to use this medication more judiciously in this population, especially given the concerns of potential side effects and theoretical risk for increased suicidality.

Additionally, there is a general shortage of child and adolescent mental health providers throughout the nation and world who are trained in CBT approaches for treating anxious children. In turn, a strong need exists to have primary care providers screen all youth for anxiety disorders and triage accordingly for treatment. Because of this lack of providers and screening, many children with anxiety disorders will remain underdiagnosed and undertreated. Untreated anxiety disorders in youth can lead to significant impairments in school performance and family functioning, and potential disability/further impairment in adulthood. It is essential for future research to focus on the early identification of anxiety disorders, thereby enabling training of a wider range of health providers regarding CBT and medications, and development of evidence-based treatment strategies to make it feasible for community providers to address these prevalent disorders in youth.

REFERENCES

1. Krain AL, Ghaffari M, Freeman J, et al. Anxiety disorders. In: Martin A, Volkmar FR, editors. Lewis's child and adolescent psychiatry. Philadelphia: Lippincott, Williams & Wilkins; 2007. p. 538–47.
2. Achenbach TM, Howell CT, McConaughy SH, et al. Six-year predictors of problems in a national sample of children and youth: I. Cross-informant syndromes. J Am Acad Child Adolesc Psychiatry 1995;34:336–47.
3. Gurley D, Cohen P, Pine DS, et al. Discriminating depression and anxiety in youth: a role for diagnostic criteria. J Affect Disord 1996;39:191–200.
4. Costello EJ, Mustillo S, Erkanli A, et al. Prevalence and development of psychiatric disorders in childhood and adolescence. Arch Gen Psychiatry 2003;60:837–44.
5. Costello EJ, Egger HL, Angold A. Developmental epidemiology of anxiety disorders. In: Ollendick TH, March JS, editors. Phobic and anxiety disorders in children and adolescents. New York: Oxford University Press; 2004. p. 334–80.
6. Marmorstein NR. Generalized versus performance-focused social phobia: patterns of comorbidity among male and female youth. J Anxiety Disord 2006; 20:778–93.
7. Bitner A, Egger HL, Erkanli A, et al. What do childhood anxiety disorders predict? J Child Psychol Psychiatry 2007;48:1174–83.
8. Connolly SD, Suarez L, Sylvester C. Assessment and treatment of anxiety disorders in children and adolescents. Curr Psychiatry Rep 2011;13:99–110.
9. Seligman LD, Ollendick TH. Cognitive-behavioral therapy for anxiety disorders in youth. Child Adolesc Psychiatr Clin N Am 2011;20:217–38.
10. Kircanski K, Peris TS, Piancentini JC. Cognitive-behavioral therapy for obsessive-compulsive disorder in children and adolescents. Child Adolesc Psychiatr Clin N Am 2011;20:239–54.
11. Dorsey S, Briggs EC, Woods BA. Cognitive-behavioral treatment for posttraumatic stress disorder in children and adolescents. Child Adolesc Psychiatr Clin N Am 2011;20:255–70.
12. American Academy of Child and Adolescent Psychiatry. Practice parameter for the assessment and treatment of children and adolescents with anxiety disorders. J Am Acad Child Adolesc Psychiatry 2003;46:267–83.
13. Walkup JT, Albano AM, Piancentini J, et al. Cognitive behavioral therapy, sertraline, or a combination in childhood anxiety. N Engl J Med 2008;359:2753–66.

14. Seidel L, Walkup JT. Selective serotonin reuptake inhibitor use in the treatment of pediatric non-obsessive-compulsive disorder anxiety disorders. J Child Adolesc Psychopharmacol 2006;16:171–9.

15. Reinblatt SP, Riddle MA. The pharmacological management of childhood anxiety disorders: a review. Psychopharmacology 2007;191:67–86.

16. Ginsburg GS, Walkup JT. Specific phobia. In: Ollendick TH, March JS, editors. Phobic and anxiety disorders in children and adolescents. New York: Oxford University Press; 2004. p. 175–97.

17. Waslick B. Psychopharmacology interventions for pediatric anxiety disorders: a research update. Child Adolesc Psychiatr Clin N Am 2006;15:51–71.

18. Viana AG, Beidel DC, Rabian B. Selective mutism: a review and integration of the last 15 years. Clin Psychol Rev 2009;29:57–67.

19. Black B, Uhde TW. Treatment of elective mutism with fluoxetine: a double-blind, placebo-controlled study. J Am Acad Child Adolesc Psychiatry 1994;33:1000–6.

20. Kristensen H. Selective mutism and comorbidity with developmental disorder/delay, anxiety disorder, and elimination disorder. J Am Acad Child Adolesc Psychiatry 2000;39:249–56.

21. Lepola U, Leinonen E, Koponen H. Citalopram in the treatment of early-onset panic disorder and school phobia. Pharmacopsychiatry 1996;29:30–2.

22. Mancini C, Van Ameringen M, Oakman JM, et al. Serotonergic agents in the treatment of social phobia in children and adolescents: a case series. Depress Anxiety 1999;10:33–9.

23. Birmaher B, Waterman GS, Ryan N, et al. Fluoxetine for childhood anxiety disorders. J Am Acad Child Adolesc Psychiatry 1994;33:993–9.

24. Fairbanks JM, Pine DS, Tancer NK, et al. Open fluoxetine treatment of mixed anxiety disorders in children and adolescents. J Child Adolesc Psychopharmacol 1997;7:17–29.

25. Compton SN, Grant PJ, Chrisman AK, et al. Sertraline in children and adolescents with social anxiety disorder: an open trial. J Am Acad Child Adolesc Psychiatry 2001;40:564–71.

26. Research Unit on Pediatric Psychopharmacology Anxiety Disorders Study Group. Fluvoxamine for the treatment of anxiety disorders in children and adolescents. The Research Unit on Pediatric Psychopharmacology Anxiety Study Group. N Engl J Med 2001;344:1279–85.

27. Rynn MA, Siqueland L, Rickels K. Placebo-controlled trial of sertraline in the treatment of children with generalized anxiety disorder. Am J Psychiatry 2001;158:2008–14.

28. Birmaher B, Axelson DA, Monk K, et al. Fluoxetine for the treatment of childhood anxiety disorders. J Am Acad Child Adolesc Psychiatry 2003;42:415–23.

29. Wagner KD, Berard R, Stein MB, et al. A multicenter, randomized, double-blind, placebo-controlled trial of paroxetine in children and adolescents with social anxiety disorder. Arch Gen Psychiatry 2004;61:1153–62.

30. Beidel DC, Turner SM, Sallee FR, et al. SET-C versus fluoxetine in the treatment of childhood social phobia. J Am Acad Child Adolesc Psychiatry 2007;46:1622–32.

31. Compton SN, Walkup JT, Albano AM, et al. Child/Adolescent Anxiety Multimodal Study (CAMS): rationale, design, and methods. Child Adolesc Psychiatry Ment Health 2010;4:1.

32. Ginsburg GS, Kendall PC, Sakolsky D, et al. Remission after acute treatment in children and adolescents with anxiety disorders: findings from the CAMS. J Consult Clin Psychol 2011;79:806–13.

33. March JS, Entusah AR, Rynn M. A randomized controlled trial of venlafaxine ER versus placebo in pediatric social anxiety disorder. Biol Psychiatry 2007;62: 1149–54.

34. Rynn MA, Riddle MA, Yeung PP, et al. Efficacy and safety of extended-release venlafaxine in the treatment of generalized anxiety disorder in children and adolescents: two placebo-controlled trials. Am J Psychiatry 2007;164:290–300.

35. Gittelman-Klein R, Klein DF. Controlled imipramine treatment of school phobia. Arch Gen Psychiatry 1971;25:204–7.

36. Berney T, Kolvin I, Bhate SR, et al. School phobia: a therapeutic trial with clomipramine and short-term outcome. Br J Psychiatry 1981;138:110–8.

37. Klein RG, Koplewicz HS, Kanner A. Imipramine treatment of children with separation anxiety disorder. J Am Acad Child Adolesc Psychiatry 1992;31:21–8.

38. Bernstein GA, Borchardt CM, Perwein AR, et al. Imipramine plus cognitive-behavioral therapy in the treatment of school refusal. J Am Acad Child Adolesc Psychiatry 2000;39:276–83.

39. Bernstein GA, Hektner JM, Borchardt CM, et al. Treatment of school refusal: one-year follow-up. J Am Acad Child Adolesc Psychiatry 2001;40:206–13.

40. Layne AE, Bernstein GA, Egan EA, et al. Predictors of treatment response in anxious-depressed adolescents with school refusal. J Am Acad Child Adolesc Psychiatry 2003;42:319–26.

41. Bernstein GA, Garfinkel BD, Borshardt CM. Comparative studies of pharmacotherapy for school refusal. J Am Acad Child Adolesc Psychiatry 1990;29: 773–81.

42. Simeon JG, Ferguson HB, Knott V, et al. Clinical, cognitive, and neurophysiological effects of alprazolam in children and adolescents with overanxious and avoidant disorders. J Am Acad Child Adolesc Psychiatry 1992;31:29–33.

43. Graae F, Milner J, Rizzotto L, et al. Clonazepam in childhood anxiety disorders. J Am Acad Child Adolesc Psychiatry 1994;33:372–6.

44. Renaud J, Birhamer B, Wassick SC, et al. Use of selective serotonin reuptake inhibitors for the treatment of childhood panic disorder: a pilot study. J Child Adolesc Psychopharmacol 1999;9:73–83.

45. Simeon JG. Use of anxiolytics in children. Encephale 1993;19:71–4.

46. Salazar DE, Frackiewicz EJ, Dockens R, et al. Pharmacokinetics and tolerability of buspirone during oral administration to children and adolescents with anxiety disorder and normal healthy adults. J Clin Pharmacol 2001;41:1351–8.

47. Masi G, Toni C, Mucci M, et al. Paroxetine in child and adolescent outpatients with panic disorder. J Child Adolesc Psychopharmacol 2001;11:151–7.

48. Fisman SN. Pharmacological treatment of major depressive disorder in children and adolescents: the paroxetine controversy. Can J Clin Pharmacol 2004;11: e214–7.

49. Nestadt G, Samuels J, Bienvenu JO, et al. A family study of obsessive compulsive disorder. Arch Gen Psychiatry 2000;57:358–63.

50. American Academy of Child and Adolescent Psychiatry. Practice parameter for the assessment and treatment of children and adolescents with obsessive-compulsive disorder. J Am Acad Child Adolesc Psychiatry 2012;51:98–113.

51. Swedo SE, Leonard HL, Garvey M, et al. Pediatric autoimmune neuropsychiatric disorders associated with streptococcal infections: clinical description of the first 50 cases. Am J Psychiatry 1998;155:264–71.

52. Swedo SE, Leonard HL, Rapoport JL. The Pediatric Autoimmune Neuropsychiatric Disorders Associated with Streptococcal Infection (PANDAS) subgroup: separating fact from fiction. Pediatrics 2004;113:907–11.

53. Leslie DL, Kozma L, Martin A, et al. Neuropsychiatric disorders associated with streptococcal infection: a case-control study among privately insured children. J Am Acad Child Adolesc Psychiatry 2008;47:1166–72.
54. Kurlan R, Johnson D, Laplan EL, Tourette Syndrome Study Group. Streptococcal infection and exacerbations of childhood tics and obsessive-compulsive symptoms: a prospective blinded cohort study. Pediatrics 2008;121:1188–97.
55. Leckman JF, King RA, Gilbert DL, et al. Streptococcal upper respiratory tract infections and exacerbations of tic and obsessive-compulsive symptoms: a prospective longitudinal study. J Am Acad Child Adolesc Psychiatry 2011;50:108–18.
56. Storch EA, Merlo LJ, Larson MJ, et al. Impact of comorbidity on cognitive-behavioral therapy response in pediatric obsessive-compulsive disorder. J Am Acad Child Adolesc Psychiatry 2008;47:583–92.
57. Franklin ME, Sapyta J, Freeman JB, et al. Cognitive behavior therapy augmentation of pharmacotherapy in pediatric obsessive-compulsive disorder: the Pediatric OCD Treatment Study II (POTS II) randomized controlled trial. JAMA 2011;306(11):1224–32.
58. Leonard HL, Swedo SE, Rapoport JL, et al. Treatment of obsessive-compulsive disorder with clomipramine and desipramine in children and adolescents. A double-blind crossover comparison. Arch Gen Psychiatry 1989;46:1088–92.
59. DeVeaugh-Geiss J, Moroz G, Biederman J, et al. Clomipramine hydrochloride in childhood and adolescent obsessive-compulsive disorder—a multicenter trial. J Am Acad Child Adolesc Psychiatry 1992;31:45–9.
60. Leonard HL, Swedo SE, Lenane MC, et al. A double-blind desipramine substitution during long-term clomipramine treatment in children and adolescents with obsessive-compulsive disorder. Arch Gen Psychiatry 1991;48:922–7.
61. March JS, Biederman J, Wolkow R, et al. Sertraline in children and adolescents with obsessive-compulsive disorder: a multicenter randomized controlled trial. JAMA 1998;280:1752–6.
62. Riddle MA, Scahill L, King RA, et al. Double-blind, crossover trial of fluoxetine and placebo in children and adolescents with obsessive-compulsive disorder. J Am Acad Child Adolesc Psychiatry 1992;31:1062–9.
63. Geller DA, Hoog SL, Heiligenstein JH, et al. Fluoxetine treatment for obsessive-compulsive disorder in children and adolescents: a placebo-controlled clinical trial. J Am Acad Child Adolesc Psychiatry 2001;40:773–9.
64. Liebowitz MR, Turner SM, Piacentini J, et al. Fluoxetine in children and adolescents with OCD: a placebo-controlled trial. J Am Acad Child Adolesc Psychiatry 2002;41:1431–8.
65. Riddle MA, Reeve EA, Yaryura-Tobias JA, et al. Fluvoxamine for children and adolescents with obsessive-compulsive disorder: a randomized, controlled, multicenter trial. J Am Acad Child Adolesc Psychiatry 2001;40:222–9.
66. Geller DA, Wagner KD, Emslie G, et al. Paroxetine treatment in children and adolescents with obsessive-compulsive disorder: a randomized, multicenter, double-blind, placebo-controlled trial. J Am Acad Child Adolesc Psychiatry 2004;43:1387–96.
67. Geller DA, Biederman J, Stewart SE, et al. Which SSRI? A meta-analysis of pharmacotherapy trials in pediatric obsessive-compulsive disorder [see comment]. Am J Psychiatry 2003;160:1919–28.
68. Franklin M, Foa E, March JS. The pediatric obsessive-compulsive disorder treatment study: rationale, design, and methods. J Child Adolesc Psychopharmacol 2003;13(Suppl 1):S39–51.

69. Pediatric OCD Treatment Study (POTS) Team. Cognitive-behavior therapy, sertraline, and their combination for children and adolescents with obsessive-compulsive disorder: the Pediatric OCD Treatment Study (POTS) randomized controlled trial. JAMA 2004;292:1969–76.

70. Leonard HL, Topol D, Bukstein O, et al. Clonazepam as an augmenting agent in the treatment of childhood-onset obsessive-compulsive disorder. J Am Acad Child Adolesc Psychiatry 1994;33:792–4.

71. Costello EJ, Erkanli A, Fairbank JA, et al. The prevalence of potentially traumatic events in childhood and adolescence. J Trauma Stress 2002;15:99–112.

72. American Academy of Child and Adolescent Psychiatry. Practice parameter for the assessment and treatment of children and adolescents with posttraumatic stress disorder. J Am Acad Child Adolesc Psychiatry 2010;49:414–30.

73. Breslau N, Davis GC, Andreski P, et al. Traumatic events and posttraumatic stress disorder in an urban population of young adults. Arch Gen Psychiatry 1991;48: 216–22.

74. Carrion VG, Weems CF, Ray R, et al. Toward an empirical definition of pediatric PTSD: the phenomenology of PTSD in youth. J Am Acad Child Adolesc Psychiatry 2002;41:166–73.

75. Seedat S, Lockhat R, Kaminer D, et al. An open trial of citalopram in adolescents with post-traumatic stress disorder. Int Clin Psychopharmacol 2001;16:21–5.

76. Seedat S, Stein DJ, Ziervogel C, et al. Comparison of response to a selective serotonin reuptake inhibitor in children, adolescents, and adults with posttraumatic stress disorder. J Child Adolesc Psychopharmacol 2002;12:37–46.

77. Yorbik O, Dikkatli S, Cansever A, et al. The efficacy of fluoxetine treatment in children and adolescents with posttraumatic stress disorder symptoms [in Turkish]. Klin Psikofarmakol Bulteni 2001;11:251–6.

78. Robb AS, Cueva JE, Sporn J, et al. Sertraline treatment of children and adolescents with posttraumatic stress disorder: a double-blind, placebo-controlled trial. J Child Adolesc Psychopharmacol 2010;20:463–71.

79. Cohen JA, Mannarino AP, Perel JM, et al. A pilot randomized trial of combined trauma-focused CBT and sertraline for childhood PTSD symptoms. J Am Acad Child Adolesc Psychiatry 2007;46:811–9.

80. Perry BD. Neurobiological sequelae of childhood trauma: PTSD in children. In: Murburg MM, editor. Catecholamine function in posttraumatic stress disorder: emerging concepts. Washington, DC: American Psychiatric Press; 1994. p. 223–55.

81. Harmon RJ, Riggs PD. Clinical perspectives: clonidine for posttraumatic stress disorder in preschool children. J Am Acad Child Adolesc Psychiatry 1996;35: 1247–9.

82. De Bellis MD, Keshevan MS, Harenski KA. Case study: anterior cingulate N-acetylaspartate/creatine ratios during clonidine treatment in a maltreated child with posttraumatic stress disorder. J Child Adolesc Psychopharmacol 2001;11: 311–6.

83. Famularo R, Kinscherff R, Fenton T. Propranolol treatment for childhood posttraumatic stress disorder, acute type: a pilot study. Am J Dis Child 1988;142:1206–19.

84. Horrigan JP, Barnhill LJ. Risperidone and PTSD in boys. J Neuropsychiatry Clin Neurosci 1999;11:126–7.

85. Murphy TK, Segarra A, Storch EA, et al. SSRI adverse events: how to monitor and manage. Int Rev Psychiatry 2008;20:203–8.

86. Bridge JA, Iyengar S, Salary CB, et al. Clinical response and risk for reported suicidal ideation and suicide attempts in pediatric antidepressant treatment: a meta-analysis of randomized controlled trials. JAMA 2007;297:1683–96.

87. Labellarte M, Biederman J, Emslie G, et al. Multiple-dose pharmacokinetics of flu-voxamine in children and adolescents. J Am Acad Child Adolesc Psychiatry 2004;43:1497–505.

88. Gleason MM, Egger HL, Emslie GJ, et al. Psychopharmacological treatment for very young children: contexts and guidelines. J Am Acad Child Adolesc Psychiatry 2007;46:1532–72.

89. Massanari M, Novitsky J, Reinstein LJ. Paradoxical reactions in children associated with midazolam during endoscopy. Clin Pediatr 1997;36:681–4.

90. Ista E, van Dijk M, Gamel C, et al. Withdrawal symptoms in children after long-term administration of sedatives and/or analgesics: a literature review: assessment remains troublesome. Intensive Care Med 2007;33:1396–406.

91. Birchley G. Opioid and benzodiazepine withdrawal syndromes in the pediatric intensive care unit: a review of recent literature. Nurs Crit Care 2009;14:26–37.

92. Yeh HH, Chen CY, Fang SY, et al. Five-year trajectories of long-term benzodiazepine use by adolescents: patient, provider, and medication factors. Psychiatr Serv 2011;62:900–7.

93. Pine DS. Treating children and adolescents with selective serotonin reuptake inhibitors: how long is appropriate? J Child Adolesc Psychopharmacol 2002; 12:189–203.

Depression

Christine J. Choe, MD[a],*, Graham J. Emslie, MD[b,c],
Taryn L. Mayes, MS[a]

KEYWORDS

- Depression • Youth depression • Antidepression treatment • MDD
- Psychopharmacotherapy

KEY POINTS

- Substantial clinical acumen is required to synthesize information from multiple informants (patient, parents, school, other health care providers) to diagnose depression.
- Treatment of depression in youth consists of social, psychological, and pharmacologic interventions, and is carefully tailored to the circumstances of each patient and family.
- Many youth will respond to brief nonmedication supportive care given over a few weeks before initiating antidepressant treatment.
- Once the decision to initiate medication is made, monotherapy with a selective serotonin reuptake inhibitor (SSRI) is the primary psychopharmacologic strategy.
- In youth with treatment-refractory depression, a reevaluation to confirm diagnosis and assess for comorbid conditions, treatment adherence, and the adequacy of psychosocial interventions is necessary.
- For patients who do not respond to 2 different SSRIs, monotherapy with a non-SSRI antidepressant or augmentation strategies are recommended.
- Management of depression may require additional strategies for more complex cases, such as brief adjunctive medication, management of comorbid conditions, and augmentation.
- Relapse is common, and therefore continuing medication for 6 to 9 months after remission is essential.

Disclosures: Dr Graham Emslie discloses that he received research/grant support from the National Institute of Mental Health; BioMarin Pharmaceutical Inc; Eli Lilly and Company; Forest Laboratories, Inc; and GlaxoSmithKline, and is a consultant for Biobehavioral Diagnostics, Inc; Bristol-Myers Squibb; Eli Lilly and Company; INC Research LLC; Lundbeck; Pfizer Inc; Seaside Therapeutics, Inc; Shire; and Valeant. Dr Choe and Ms. Mayes have no financial relationships to disclose.
[a] Department of Psychiatry, University of Texas Southwestern Medical Center, 5323 Harry Hines Boulevard, Dallas, TX 75390-8589, USA; [b] Department of Psychiatry and Pediatrics, University of Texas Southwestern Medical Center, 5323 Harry Hines Boulevard, Dallas, TX 75390-8589, USA; [c] Department of Psychiatry, Children's Medical Center, University of Texas Southwestern Medical Center, 5323 Harry Hines Boulevard, Dallas, TX 75390-8589, USA
* Corresponding author.
E-mail address: christine.choe@utsouthwestern.edu

Child Adolesc Psychiatric Clin N Am 21 (2012) 807–829
http://dx.doi.org/10.1016/j.chc.2012.07.002
1056-4993/12/$ – see front matter © 2012 Elsevier Inc. All rights reserved.

childpsych.theclinics.com

INTRODUCTION

Depressive disorders in the *Diagnostic and Statistical Manual of Mental Disorders* (Fourth Edition, Text Revision) include diagnoses of major depressive disorder (MDD), dysthymic disorder, and depression not otherwise specified. Epidemiologic studies using clinical interview have shown depression rates from 2% to 8%. Most youth recover from the initial depressive episode; however, recurrence is common, with 40% to 70% of youth experiencing a relapse or recurrence within 3 to 5 years.[1] Although the diagnostic criteria are similar for children and adolescents, typical symptom presentations differ by age group. Kovacs[2] noted that adolescents report more hypersomnia, fewer appetite and weight changes, and fewer reported delusions than children. Recent research has also attempted to delineate how depression presents in preschoolers. Luby and colleagues[3] reported that depressed preschool children show typical symptoms of depression, such as mood disturbance and anhedonia, but have less "masked" symptoms (eg, sleep problems, appetite changes). Similar to adults, children and adolescents also have negative cognitive functioning, such as cognitive distortions, negative attributions, hopelessness, and low self-esteem. Depression in youth results in functional impairment, including increased difficulties with schoolwork, peer and family relationships, and alcohol or substance abuse and dependence. Recurrence of depression in later years (even into adulthood) is also common.[1]

Psychopharmacologic studies of depression treatments have shown that data gathered among adults cannot be automatically extrapolated and applied to youth. A particular example is the failure to show efficacy of tricyclic antidepressants (TCAs) among depressed youth.[4] Another example is the increased risk of selective serotonin reuptake inhibitor (SSRI)–associated suicidality, which the U.S. Food and Drug Administration (FDA) has determined particularly affects young people up to the age of 24 years.[5,6] Efforts have been made toward increasing the number and quality of trials conducted among children,[7] leading to the development of guidelines based on direct empiric evidence and expert clinical consensus.[1,8–10]

Despite increasing evidence of effective treatments in the pediatric age group, many children and adolescents with depression (MDD, dysthymia, depression not otherwise specified or "minor depression," and adjustment disorder with depressed mood) receive inadequate treatment. Although no data are available on specific treatments except for MDD, the strategies used and described here are appropriate for youth with depression in general. This article reviews the process of assessment and research on available treatments, emphasizing overall strategies for implementing evidence-based treatments into clinical care.

ASSESSMENT
Initial Assessment

Diagnosis of depression in children and adolescents requires clinical interviews of the child and parent separately, using both open-ended questions and specific symptom review. In addition to assessing for symptoms of depression, the evaluation will also include assessment of comorbid conditions (both general medical conditions and psychiatric illnesses), and assessment of contextual factors (eg, peer and family relationships, school/work, stressors). A rational approach to treatment is based on accurate diagnosis and a detailed family history.

Ongoing Assessment

The goal of treatment is remission of depression, and therefore ongoing systematic monitoring of symptoms and suicidal ideation is important. Thus, once a diagnosis of depression has been made, assessment of symptoms and contextual factors does not end at the initial diagnostic evaluation. It has been established that measured care, or ongoing systematic assessment of symptoms alone, can improve outcome.[11] Unfortunately, clinicians treating psychiatric illnesses such as depression commonly fail to assess each symptom systematically. A variety of clinician-rated scales and self-report scales are available for clinicians to use that will provide ongoing assessment of symptom improvement and worsening. **Box 1** provides a list of rating scales that are often used to assess depressive symptoms. Response is often defined as a 50% decrease on clinician-rated scales (eg, the Children's Depression Rating Scale - Revised [CDRS-R] and the Quick Inventory of Depressive Symptoms [QIDS]), or a 1 or 2 ("very much" or "much" improved) on the Clinical Global Impressions Improvement Scale (CGI-I), whereas remission is often defined by a cutoff score (eg, CDRS-R ≤28).

Assessing adverse events at each visit is also important. Youth who are experiencing significant adverse effects from medication may choose to stop treatment prematurely. In addition, some uncommon but serious adverse effects must be assessed regularly, and particularly when initiating treatment or changing doses. Additional details about adverse effects associated with antidepressants are described later.

Brief Psychosocial Intervention

Medication management of depression in children and adolescents can include psychological and social interventions even when no medication is prescribed. In acute 8- to 12-week clinical trials of depressed children and adolescents, 30% to 50% of participants responded to pill placebo, a treatment arm that also included careful clinical management and regular visits.[12] Similarly, the Adolescent Depression Antidepressant and Psychotherapy Trial showed that approximately 1 in 4 adolescents will respond to a brief 2-session intervention plus standard clinical management.[13] Thus, before starting specific interventions for depression, providing supportive clinical care for 1 to 4 weeks may be sufficient to reduce depression.[1,8,9] Generally, supportive clinical care includes psychoeducation and therapeutic skills of listening empathetically, reflecting, giving advice, and general problem-solving. General problem-solving may include providing suggestions about sleep hygiene, eating, and staying active, or may include working with the school to help develop an individual education plan. This initial intervention period can last for 1 to 4 weeks depending on the severity and initial response to supportive care.[8,9]

Box 1
Common depression severity rating scales

Self-Reports

- Beck Depression Inventory; Children's Depression Inventory
- Mood and Feelings Questionnaire
- Patient Health Questionnaire
- QIDS
- Reynolds Adolescent Depression Scale

Clinician-Rated Measures

- CDRS-R
- CGI-I
- QIDS

If the child continues to have significant depressive symptoms after brief clinical supportive care, additional treatment with specific psychotherapy and/or pharmacologic treatment is warranted. The nature and intensity of the treatment depends on many factors, including the particular clinical features of the case, the resources available, the history of response to treatment, and the preferences of the patient and family.

Patients with mild depression or those with moderate depression who have decided with their clinician to initiate treatment without medications may be started on psychotherapy alone. Psychotherapy modalities with the strongest evidence base for youth are cognitive behavioral therapy (CBT) and interpersonal therapy.[14-16]

Decisions to initiate medication treatment are based on patient preference, inadequate response to supportive or specific psychotherapy, or depression severity (eg, chronic or recurrent depression, psychosis, suicidality). The remainder of this article focuses specifically on the pharmacologic management of depression in children and adolescents.

PHARMACOLOGIC TREATMENT OF DEPRESSION

The pharmacologic treatment of depression consists of an acute, continuation, and maintenance phase of treatment. Acute treatment focuses on reducing symptoms and achieving full remission of symptoms. Studies of antidepressants have generally used response to treatment as the outcome; however, remission (being symptom-free) is the goal. Although response rates to antidepressants in clinical trials range from 55% to 65%, remission rates are considerably lower (around 35%–40%). The acute phase generally lasts 2 to 4 months, and is the best-studied among the phases of treatment. Once remission is achieved, the next phase of treatment is the continuation phase. Continuation treatment is used to consolidate and build on the improvements of the acute phase, and lasts approximately 6 to 9 months. After the completion of the continuation phase, some patients will need maintenance treatment, which is used to prevent future episodes of depression, and may last 1 to 5 years.

Acute Treatment

SSRIs

Patients who are naive to antidepressant medications or have had previous inadequate trials of antidepressants would initiate pharmacologic treatment with SSRI monotherapy. Available SSRIs include citalopram, escitalopram, fluoxetine, sertraline, paroxetine, and fluvoxamine (**Table 1**). Fluoxetine is approved by the FDA for treatment of MDD in children age 8 years and older. Escitalopram is FDA approved for MDD in adolescents aged 12 years and older. Paroxetine is generally not recommended as a first-line treatment because of equivocal findings regarding efficacy,[17-19] higher rates of adverse effects in prepubertal children,[19] and its short half-life, which is associated with more severe discontinuation symptoms. Fluvoxamine has been studied primarily in anxiety disorders and obsessive compulsive disorder (OCD), and although its antidepressant effect in youth is not clear, it is generally not used to treat depression.

Although several positive trials of SSRIs have been conducted in youth, studies have tended to differ on outcome measures used and the definitions of response and remission, which complicates the comparison of trials and different SSRIs. Some trials of SSRIs and other antidepressants have also shown evidence of greater efficacy among adolescents compared with children.

Fluoxetine studies Fluoxetine has been most extensively studied, with 3 positive randomized controlled trials.[20-22] The first was a single-site study of 96 patients aged 7 to 17 years who were randomized to 20 mg of fluoxetine or placebo over 8 weeks.

Table 1
Efficacy, interaction effects, and pharmacokinetics of SSRIs

Medication	Level of Evidence[a]	Half-Life	Time to Steady State	Cytochrome P450 Enzyme Inhibited[b]	Kinetics
Fluoxetine	A+	4–6 d	>4 wk	1A2 (weak) 2B6 (moderate) 2C9 (moderate) 3A4 (moderate) 2C19 (potent) 2D6 (potent)	Nonlinear
Escitalopram	A (adolescents only)	27–33 h	7 d	2D6 (weak)	Linear
Citalopram	A	20 h	6–10 d	2D6 (weak)	Linear
Sertraline	A	26 h	5–7 d	1A2 (weak) 3A4 (moderate) 2B6 (moderate) 2D6 (moderate at low doses, potent at high doses)	
Paroxetine	B	21 h	7–14 d	1A2 (weak) 2C9 (weak) 2C19 (weak) 3A4 (moderate) 2B6 (potent) 2D6 (potent)	Nonlinear

[a] Levels of evidence: A: Positive double-blind, randomized, placebo-controlled trial; B: Positive prospective open-label study, no positive randomized controlled trial; C: Positive retrospective case series or case reports.
[b] Potent inhibition is in bold type.

Among the subjects, 56% receiving fluoxetine and 33% receiving placebo showed a response, defined by a CGI-I score of 1 or 2 ("very much" or "much" improved; $P<.02$).[20] A multisite replication trial of 219 patients, using a maximum of 20 mg of fluoxetine over 9 weeks, showed similar results based on CGI response (52.3% vs 36.8%; $P = .028$). Remission rates (defined as CDRS-R ≤28) were also significantly higher with fluoxetine compared with placebo (41% vs 20%; $P<.01$).[23] The most recent randomized controlled trial[22] is a multisite study in which 439 depressed adolescents were randomized to 1 of 4 arms for 12 weeks: CBT with fluoxetine (10–40 mg/d), fluoxetine alone (10–40 mg/d), CBT alone, or placebo (equivalent to 10–40 mg/d). Response rates for the 4 treatment arms, as measured by a CGI-I score of 1 or 2, were 71.0%, 60.6%, 43.2%, and 34.8%, respectively. The response rates of the 2 arms containing fluoxetine were statistically greater than those of CBT alone (combination: $P = .001$; fluoxetine: $P = .01$) or placebo (combination: $P = .001$; fluoxetine: $P = .001$). Based on these trials, 2 of which included children, fluoxetine is the only FDA-approved medication for depression in both children and adolescents (aged 8–17 years) with MDD. Fluoxetine has the longest half-life of all the SSRIs, which minimizes discontinuation effects if stopped abruptly and avoids rapid drops in serum levels with occasional missed doses. The long half-life also requires a longer "wash-out" period (approximately 5 weeks) before starting any subsequent medications that can cause a problematic interaction (eg, a monoamine oxidase inhibitor [MAO-I]). The initial dosage is usually 10 mg/d, with an increase after 1 week to a target dosage of 20 mg/d in children and 20 to 40 mg/d in adolescents. The maximum dosage is 60 mg/d.

Escitalopram studies Escitalopram is the only other antidepressant with an FDA indication for adolescents (≥12 years of age) with MDD. Two randomized controlled trials of escitalopram have been conducted. The first randomized 264 patients aged 6 to 17 years to either escitalopram at 10 to 20 mg or placebo. The overall response rates of 62.8% (escitalopram) and 52.3% (placebo) were not statistically different (P = .14; defined by a CGI-I of 1 or 2), but a post hoc analysis by age group showed a significant effect of medication among adolescents on all outcome measures.[24] The second study included adolescents only, and showed modest efficacy of escitalopram, with response rates of 64.3% for escitalopram and 52.9% for placebo (P = .03; defined by CGI-I of 1 or 2). Remission rates were not significantly different between groups.[25] Escitalopram is the active S-enantiomer of racemic citalopram and has twice the potency of citalopram to inhibit the serotonin transporter. Escitalopram is less likely to cause drug-drug interactions because of its low protein binding (56%) and minimal effects on cytochrome P450 (CYP) isoenzymes.[26] Starting dosages in children and adolescents are 5 to 10 mg/d, which would be increased after 1 week to a target dosage of 10 to 20 mg/d, and can be increased further to a maximum dosage of 30 mg/d.

Citalopram studies Citalopram has one published positive trial in children and adolescents.[27] In this trial, 174 patients aged 7 to 17 years were randomized to citalopram (20–40 mg/d) or placebo. Remission rates at week 8, defined by CDRS-R score of 28 or less, were higher in the escitalopram group (36% vs 24%; P<.05). Another trial of adolescents compared citalopram and placebo, and participants were allowed to receive concurrent psychotherapy. The overall study showed no difference in response rates, although in participants who did not receive any psychotherapy, citalopram was significantly more effective than placebo (response rates: 52% vs 45%; P = .019, defined as 50% reduction in Montgomery-Asberg Depression Scale [MADRS] score; remission rates: 22% vs 19%; P = .034, defined as MADRS score ≤12).[28] Like escitalopram, citalopram also has negligible CYP inhibition. Due to potential for QT prolongation with doses higher than 40 mg, the recommended dosing strategy for citalopram is to start with 10 mg/d, with an initial target dosage of 20 mg/d and a maximum dosage of 40 mg/d.

Sertraline studies Two identically designed studies in sertraline in a total of 376 youth ages 6 to 17 years did not individually show significant differences between placebo and active medication. When the 2 studies were pooled, a modest but significant difference was seen in the primary outcome measure of improvement in CDRS-R total score (-30.24 vs -25.83, respectively; P = .001). Response rates (CGI-I ≤2) were greater in the sertraline group (63% vs 53% placebo; P = .05).[29] The study was not powered to differentiate children from adolescents, but a trend was seen toward greater improvement in CDRS-R scores among adolescents compared with children. Sertraline has moderate CYP interactions. It is started at 12.5 to 25 mg/d in children and adolescents, and is increased after 1 week to an initial target dosage of 50 mg/d. The dosage can be increased further to 100 to 150 mg/d for inadequate responses, with a maximum dosage of 200 mg/d.

Paroxetine studies Three randomized controlled trials have been conducted with paroxetine, only one of which was positive.[17–19] In a study of 275 adolescents randomized to paroxetine 20 to 40 mg/d or placebo over 8 weeks (a separate imipramine arm was also included), more patients on paroxetine achieved a treatment response than those on placebo (65.6% vs 48.3%; P = .02). Several secondary outcome measures were also positive.[17] Paroxetine is generally not recommended as a first-line treatment for adolescents with depression, and is generally not recommended at all for children younger than 12 years because of the higher dropout rate with paroxetine in this age group. Paroxetine has nonlinear kinetics and shows considerable variation in half-life among individual pediatric patients.[30] It has potent inhibition of CYP2D6 and CYP2B6. Paroxetine is associated with more severe discontinuation effects among SSRIs because of its short half-life.[31] The starting dosage is 10 mg/d, with a target dosage of 20 to 40 mg/d and a maximum dosage of 50 mg/d.

Fluvoxamine studies Fluvoxamine is a 2-aminoethyloxime ether of aralkyl-ketone, with a mechanism of action similar to that of other SSRIs. However, it is not generally used to treat depression, and no studies of fluvoxamine in youth with depression are available. Fluvoxamine does have an FDA indication for treatment of youth with OCD, and is considered safe for treatment of children and teenagers younger than 18 years.

SSRI study conclusions Thus, evidence seems to exist of improvement in depression with several SSRIs, although fluoxetine and escitalopram are currently the only 2 antidepressants with FDA approval for treatment of depression in youth. Working with families to determine which medication to try is important, and selecting which antidepressant to use will be based on the individual patient. Some factors to consider when selecting which antidepressant to use include pharmacokinetic features, the side-effect profile, prior exposure (and response) to a particular antidepressant, and cost.

Clinical use of antidepressants during the acute phase
When starting an antidepressant, the initial target dose is generally at the lower end of the therapeutic range and continued for a minimum of 4 weeks before a treatment change is considered (ie, increasing the dose or changing the medication). **Table 2** provides formulations and dosing suggestions for SSRIs. If at any time full or partial remission is achieved (eg, 50% decrease on depression severity rating scale), the continuation phase would be started. Minimal responses can be treated through increasing the dose if tolerated. Patients with partial responses can continue to be observed for further improvement, but if the patient continues to show only a partial response by 12 weeks, a change in treatment is warranted. For patients who are having difficulty tolerating the side effects of a medication during the acute phase, the medication would generally be discontinued and a different medication initiated.

Table 2 Formulations and dosage of SSRIs				
Medication	**Formulations**	**Initial Dose**	**Target Dose**	**Maximum Dose**
Fluoxetine	Cap: 10 mg, 20 mg, 40 mg Tab: 10 mg Sol: 20 mg/5 mL	10 mg	20–40 mg	60 mg
Escitalopram	Tab: 5 mg, 10 mg, 20 mg Sol: 5 mg/5 mL	5–10 mg	10–20 mg	30 mg
Citalopram	Tab: 10 mg, 20 mg, 40 mg Sol: 10 mg/5 mL	10 mg	20–40 mg	40 mg
Sertraline	Tab: 25 mg, 50 mg, 100 mg Sol: 20 mg/mL	12.5–25 mg	50–150 mg	200 mg
Paroxetine	Tab: 10 mg, 20 mg, 30 mg, 40 mg Tab CR: 12.5 mg, 25 mg, 37.5 mg Susp: 10 mg/5 mL	10 mg	20–40 mg	50 mg

Abbreviations: Cap, capsule; CR, controlled-release; Tab, tablet; Sol, solution; Susp, suspension.

The frequency of monitoring visits depends on the factors of the individual case. Patients should be seen frequently early in treatment (eg, every 1–2 weeks) to assess for response to treatment, worsening of symptoms, suicidal thoughts and behaviors, and the presence of side effects. However, such frequent monitoring may be neither necessary nor realistic for all patients.[32] Morrato and colleagues[32] found that the FDA recommendations (weekly visits for the first month, biweekly for the second month, and another visit at 3 months) were followed in fewer than 5% of cases in youth. Furthermore, no significant increase in frequency of follow-up visits was seen after the FDA issued the warning for antidepressant-associated suicidality in 2004.[32] Visit frequency may also be increased during dose and medication changes. Systematic symptom assessment at each visit is necessary to determine whether the current treatment must be modified.

Treatment for Refractory Depression

Approximately 35% to 40% of youth will not respond to the initial antidepressant. For youth who have responded inadequately or experienced medication intolerance to the first antidepressant within 8 to 12 weeks, a treatment change is warranted. It is also important to reevaluate the patient's clinical status and psychosocial circumstances when an adequate trial of an antidepressant has been used. Specifically, one should

1. Confirm the original diagnosis,
2. Assess for continuing or unrecognized comorbidity, and
3. Determine if psychotherapeutic interventions are adequate.

Psychotherapeutic interventions can be initiated or intensified, or the mode of psychotherapy may be adjusted (eg, from supportive therapy to CBT). Recent stressors, family functioning, school interventions, and medication adherence are all areas that can be explored.

SSRIs

Currently, guidelines recommend switching to an alternate SSRI as second-line treatment.[8,9] Only one trial to date has examined treatment-resistant depression in adolescents. In the Treatment of SSRI-Resistant Depression in Adolescents (TORDIA) trial, 334 patients who had not responded to 8 weeks of SSRI treatment were randomly switched to an alternate SSRI, an alternate SSRI with CBT, venlafaxine, or venlafaxine with CBT. CBT with either medication was associated with a higher response rate than medication alone (54.8% vs 40.5%; $P = .009$). No difference was seen in response rate between SSRIs and venlafaxine, although venlafaxine resulted in greater increases in diastolic blood pressure and pulse and a higher incidence of skin reactions.[33] A later analysis of suicidal events found that, among patients with higher baseline suicidal ideation, venlafaxine was associated with a higher rate of self-harm events.[34] In summary, adding CBT to a medication switch was superior to switching medications alone. Switching to an alternate SSRI was equally efficacious to switching to venlafaxine and was associated with fewer side effects.

Non-SSRIs

To date, non-SSRI antidepressants have not been shown to be effective for acute treatment of youth with depression. However, treatment guidelines for early-onset depression recommend using non-SSRIs (eg, venlafaxine, duloxetine, bupropion, mirtazapine) as a third-line treatment, because they may be effective in youth with treatment-refractory depression. **Table 3** provides efficacy, interaction effects, and

Table 3
Efficacy, interaction effects, and pharmacokinetics of non-SSRIs

Medication	Level of Evidence[a]	Half-Life	Time to Steady State	Cytochrome P450 Enzyme Inhibited[b]	Kinetics
Bupropion	B	Biphasic: 1.5 h 14 h	8 d	2D6 (potent)	Linear
Bupropion SR	B	21 h	8 d	2D6 (potent)	Linear
Venlafaxine XR	B	10.3 h	3 d	2D6 (weak) 3A4 (weak)	Linear
Mirtazapine	B	20–40 h	4 d	No known inhibition. Substrate for: 1A2, 2D6, 3A4	Linear
Duloxetine	C	12.5 h	3 d	1A2 (potent) 2D6 (potent)	Linear

Abbreviations: SR, sustained release; XR, extended release.
[a] Levels of evidence: A: Positive double-blind, randomized, placebo controlled trial; B: Positive prospective open-label study, no positive RCT; C: Positive retrospective case series or case reports.
[b] Potent inhibition is in bold type.

pharmacokinetics of non-SSRI antidepressants, and **Table 4** details formulations and dosing recommendations for these medications.

Venlafaxine
Venlafaxine, a selective norepinephrine serotonin reuptake inhibitor (SNRI), has received the most research among non-SSRIs in early-onset depression. Venlafaxine

Table 4
Formulations and dosage of non-SSRIs

Medication	Formulations	Initial Dose	Target Dose	Max. Dose
Bupropion Bupropion SR	Tab IR: 75 mg, 100 mg Tab ER: 100 mg, 150 mg, 200 mg	IR: 100 mg SR: 150 mg	300 mg (3 divided doses for IR)	IR: max single dose = 150 mg; max total dose = 450 mg SR: max single dose = 200 mg; max total dose = 400 mg
Bupropion XL	Tab ER: 150 mg, 300 mg	150 mg	300 mg	450 mg
Venlafaxine XR	Cap: 37.5 mg, 75 mg, 150 mg	37.5 mg	150–225 mg	300 mg
Mirtazapine	Tab: 15 mg, 30 mg, 45 mg	7.5–15 mg	15–45 mg	45 mg
Duloxetine	Cap: 20 mg, 30 mg, 60 mg	20 mg bid	40–60 mg	60 mg

Abbreviations: Cap, capsule; ER, extended-release; IR, immediate-release; max, maximum; Tab, tablet; SR, sustained release.

has been shown to be modestly more efficacious for MDD than SSRIs in adults,[35] but not necessarily in youth.[33,36] As noted, the TORDIA study suggests that treatment refractory youth are equally responsive to venlafaxine as to another SSRI.[33] Two similarly designed, multicenter RCTs of venlafaxine extended release were conducted in a total of 334 children and adolescents for a total of 8 weeks. Neither study showed statistical significance on the primary outcome measure, which was a reduction in CDRS-R score from baseline. A post hoc analysis of age subgroups showed no significant effects of medication among children, but a significant difference in CDRS-R score by week 8 was seen among adolescents (change scores: -24.4 vs -20 for venlafaxine and placebo, respectively; $P = .022$). Several secondary outcome measures were also significant in adolescents, including a difference in response rates as measured by a decrease in CDRS-R score of 35% or greater (71% active vs 55% placebo; $P = .018$).[36] Venlafaxine shows few drug-drug interactions. The half-lives of venlafaxine and its extended-release version are short, which can increase the likelihood and severity of discontinuation symptoms. The initial dosage for immediate-release venlafaxine is 75 mg/d in divided doses, and for extended-release the dosage is 37.5 to 75.0 mg/d. Dosages can be increased by 75 mg/d every 4 to 7 days, to a target dosage of 150 to 225 mg/d, with maximum dosages of 225 to 400 mg/d.

Duloxetine

Duloxetine is another SNRI but with little research among youth. An open-label study of the safety and pharmacokinetics of duloxetine in children and adolescents (ages 7–17 years) indicated that the medication was generally well tolerated, and that dosing is similar to that used for adults.[37] Two large RCTs were recently completed comparing duloxetine, fluoxetine, and placebo, although results were not yet published at the time of writing (ClinicalTrials.gov Identifier: NCT00849693 and NCT00849901). Unlike venlafaxine, duloxetine has significant cytochrome actions (potent inhibition of CYP1A2 and CYP2D6). Typically, it is started at 20 mg in 2 divided doses, with target dosages of 40 to 60 mg/d, and a maximum dosage of 60 mg/d.

Bupropion

Bupropion's antidepressant actions are not well understood but are thought to be mediated through noradrenergic and dopaminergic mechanisms. One open study of bupropion sustained release in 24 adolescents with a depressive disorder and comorbid attention deficit hyperactivity disorder (ADHD) reported a global response rate of 88% in depressive symptoms, 63% for ADHD, and 58% in both disorders.[38] The average final dosage was 2.2 mg/kg each morning and 1.7 mg/kg each night, with a maximum dosage of 3 mg/kg twice daily. In adults, the immediate-release and sustained-release forms are started at 100 to 150 mg/d, and are increased 3 days later to a target dosage of 300 mg/d, with a total maximum dosage of 400 to 450 mg/d (see **Table 4**). The extended release form (XL) is started at 150 mg/d for 3 days, and is increased to a target dosage of 300 mg/d. The maximum daily dosage is 450 mg. No double-blind RCT has been conducted for bupropion in children and adolescents with MDD.

Mirtazapine

Mirtazapine is an atypical antidepressant that can cause sedation and weight gain, but has fewer of the sexual and gastrointestinal side effects of SSRI and SNRIs. Two multicenter RCTs of mirtazapine in depressed youth showed no significant differences between active treatment and placebo in any of the outcome variables.[23] Mirtazapine is started at 7.5 to 15 mg nightly and can be increased by 15 mg every 1 to 2 weeks, to target dosages of 15 to 45 mg/d. The maximum dosage is 45 mg/d.

Tricyclic Antidepressants

Tricyclic antidepressants are not commonly used in youth because of questionable efficacy in this population and an adverse side effect profile, including cardiotoxicity, anticholinergic effects, and high lethality with overdose. A recent systemic review of 13 randomized controlled trials of tricyclics in children and adolescents found no overall improvement.[38] A subgroup analysis showed moderate benefit among adolescents (effect size, -0.47, 95% CI, -0.92 to -0.02) and no benefit in children (effect size, 0.15; 95% CI, -0.34–0.64).[4]

MAO-Is

Use of MAO-Is is limited by the difficulty for youth to adhere to the tyramine-free diet; however, the selegiline transdermal system may be an option for youth who have not responded to other antidepressants. The selegiline patch does not usually require a special diet and has shown efficacy in adults.[39] A recent RCT examining selegiline transdermal patch in adolescents with MDD showed that the medication is generally safe and well tolerated. Youth treated with selegiline and placebo showed significant improvement in depressive symptoms, with a mean CDRS-R total score improvement of -21.4 ±16.6 for selegiline, and -21.5 ± 16.5 for placebo. Thus, the study did not show a positive benefit of selegiline compared with placebo.[40]

ADVERSE EFFECTS AND SAFETY OF ANTIDEPRESSANTS

SSRIs are generally well-tolerated and adverse effects usually occur early in treatment. Common side effects of SSRIs include headache, dizziness, nausea, diarrhea, somnolence or insomnia, tremors, sweating, rash, jitteriness, increased anxiety, vivid dreams, and sexual dysfunction. Some side effects, especially headache and jitteriness, often subside after approximately a week of treatment. Behavioral activation and vomiting are more common in children than in adolescents, whereas somnolence is more common in adolescents.[41] More rare side effects include a prolonged QT interval, hyponatremia, increased bleeding, seizures, worsening depression, psychosis, suicidality, manic symptoms, and serotonin syndrome.

Side effects of SNRIs are similar to those of SSRIs because of common serotonergic actions. Additional side effects of SNRIs that may be attributed to their noradrenergic effects include hypertension, increased heart rate, sweating, dizziness, loss of appetite, dry mouth, and jitteriness. Blood pressure should always be monitored with venlafaxine and duloxetine, especially at higher doses, and electrocardiograms can be considered in patients with cardiac risk factors. Venlafaxine may be more likely than SSRIs to cause an increase in suicidal ideation and self-harming events in youth.[5] Mirtazapine has fewer sexual and gastrointestinal side effects than SSRIs, but antihistaminergic actions can cause somnolence and increased appetite. Somnolence is more commonly associated with lower doses of mirtazapine.

Possible drug interactions should always be considered in patients taking multiple medications. Most SSRIs are moderate to potent inhibitors of various CYP enzymes (see **Tables 2** and **4**). Escitalopram and citalopram have the least effect on the CYP system. SSRIs are also highly protein-bound, which may increase the serum level of other protein-bound agents. Contraindications for SSRI use include concomitant use of MAO-Is (cardiotoxicity, serotonin syndrome), pimozide (bradycardia, somnolence, and cardiotoxicity), or thioridazine (cardiotoxicity). Use of SSRIs and tramadol can increase the risk of seizures and serotonin syndrome, and may increase the serum concentration of tramadol. Bupropion is a potent inhibition of CYP2D6. Bupropion is contraindicated in patients with eating or seizure disorders or at high risk for seizures, and with concomitant MAO-I use. Mirtazapine has no known effects on CYP. Venlafaxine is a weak inhibitor of the CYP2D6 and CYP3A4 systems, whereas duloxetine is a potent inhibitor of the CYP1A2 and CYP2D6 systems. Duloxetine is also contraindicated in uncontrolled narrow-angle glaucoma. Mirtazapine, venlafaxine, and duloxetine are contraindicated for combined use with MAO-Is.

Suicidality

Concerns about increased suicidal thinking and behavior with the use of antidepressants during the acute treatment phase among children and adolescents led the FDA to publish a black box warning in October 2004 for all antidepressants. A metaanalysis of 24 trials of antidepressant treatment in 4582 youth with primarily depressive and anxiety disorders found an overall relative risk for suicidal behaviors and ideation was 1.95 (95% CI, 1.28–2.98), with an overall risk difference of 0.02 (95% CI, 0.01–0.03). As noted by the authors, this indicates that among 100 patients treated with antidepressants, 1 to 3 may show an increase in suicidality (beyond the risk of suicidality from the illness alone). The relative risk of suicidality for SSRIs in depression trials was lower, at 1.66 (95% CI, 1.02–2.68).[5] Another meta-analysis included 3 more unpublished and published trials in addition to the 24 trials in the above study and found a smaller but significant overall risk difference of 0.7% (95% CI, 0.1–1.3).[12]

The risk of increased suicidal and self-harming events with antidepressant medication treatment must be balanced with the real risks of suicide as a result of inadequately treated depression. Suicide is the third leading cause of death among youth,[42] and is most frequently associated with unipolar or bipolar depression.[43] Despite the concerns about increased risk of suicidal behaviors with antidepressants, epidemiologic studies have shown an inverse correlation between the rate of newer antidepressant prescriptions and suicide rates.[43–45]

The FDA has recommended monitoring for symptoms of "anxiety, agitation, panic attacks, insomnia, irritability, hostility, impulsivity, akathisia, hypomania, or mania" as possible precursors to suicide, with possible discontinuation of the medication when the presentation of these adverse events are new for the patient, sudden in onset, or severe.[46]

Manic Switching/Activation Syndrome

The potential for antidepressants to induce hypomania or mania is well-known, although rates of manic induction in RCTs of youth with depression have generally been low. In adults, TCAs have been shown to be the most likely to induce mania among antidepressant classes, but some research has indicated that this may not be the case in youth.[47] Youth at risk of developing a bipolar disorder (eg, those with family histories of bipolar disorder, and those with psychosis, mood dysregulation with ADHD symptoms, very early-onset depression, or a history of antidepressant-induced mania) should be carefully monitored throughout antidepressant therapy.

Antidepressants can also cause a syndrome of behavioral activation, which usually presents in the first few weeks of treatment, and is characterized by an increased level of activity, irritability, insomnia, and disinhibition.[41,48] Activation rates in placebo-controlled trials have occurred in an average of 11% of children but only 2% to 4% of adolescents and adults.[49] Little research has been done on the activation phenomenon, but some concern has been expressed that activation may be one of the mechanisms leading to the suicidality associated with antidepressants.[48] Starting medications at low doses and titrating upwards gradually is thought to decrease the likelihood of activation.

Serotonin Syndrome

Serotonin syndrome results from an overstimulation of central and peripheral serotonin receptors, and can be characterized by tremor and diarrhea in mild cases to confusion, agitation, fever, sweating, shivering, increased blood pressure and pulse, muscular hypertonicity and hyperreflexia, and death in more severe cases. It usually occurs from a high dose or overdose of a single serotonergic agent, when multiple serotonergic agents are used simultaneously (eg, SSRI and an MAO-I), or through drug-drug interactions that increase the serum level of the serotonergic medication.[50] Patients who are switching from fluoxetine to an MAO-I must discontinue the fluoxetine for at least 5 weeks before starting the MAO-I. Otherwise, SSRIs usually must be discontinued for 2 weeks before starting a MAO-I or any other medications that cannot be used in combination.

Discontinuation Syndrome

Discontinuation syndromes have been associated with abrupt discontinuation of all classes of antidepressants. Symptoms associated with abrupt discontinuation of SSRIs include dizziness, headache, muscle aches, sweating, gastrointestinal symptoms, insomnia, irritability, electric shock–like sensations, and vivid dreaming. Symptoms begin 1 to 4 days after discontinuation and can persist for up to 3 weeks.[51] Discontinuation syndrome can occur with any SSRI, but those with shorter half-lives such as paroxetine, fluvoxamine, and venlafaxine (an SNRI) have the most prominent effects.[52] Most SSRIs should be discontinued slowly over 2 to 3 weeks, whereas fluoxetine may not need to be tapered at all because of its long half-life. If discontinuation symptoms do occur, the medication can be restarted and tapered off more slowly. Tapering off antidepressants more rapidly than over 2 weeks not only may cause discontinuation symptoms but also has been associated with a shorter time to recurrence of a mood episode in adults.[53]

ADDITIONAL STRATEGIES FOR TREATING COMPLEX CASES OF DEPRESSION

The medication management strategies described earlier focus specifically on treatment of depression. However, many youth present with more complex issues, such as symptoms associated with depression (eg, agitation, cognitive distortions, significant insomnia) or comorbid conditions (medical or psychiatric). Likewise, some youth will show improvement with the initial medication strategies, but will continue to exhibit residual symptoms that do not resolve. Medication strategies that may be used in these more complex cases include brief adjunctive medication to address associated features of depression, comorbid conditions, or augmentation.

Brief Adjunctive Medication

In evaluating what treatment change is needed, it is important to assess the level of improvement in symptom change with the initial treatment and to identify factors that may be impeding improvement. If associated symptoms are the predominant concern, an additional consideration is whether these symptoms must be specifically targeted with adjunctive treatment. Adjunctive treatments, which are generally used for only as long as the associated symptom is present, may be initiated at the start of depression treatment or within a few weeks of the antidepressant. One example would be the specific targeting of insomnia. Commonly used agents for insomnia in children and adolescents include α-agonists, melatonin, trazodone, antihistamines, hypnotics (eg, zolpidem, eszopiclone), and atypical antipsychotics.[54] Depressed adolescents with insomnia may be less responsive to antidepressant treatment, which may indicate the importance of targeting insomnia in this population.[55] Although further study is needed, the use of trazodone for insomnia during treatment with SSRIs or venlafaxine has been associated with a lower rate of depressive response.[56]

Aggression and agitation are also common in youth with depression, particularly adolescents. Pharmacologic treatment of aggression or agitation would initially target depression, because oppositional and aggressive behaviors frequently complicate the presentation of depressed youth.[57] Of course, the focus of treatment would be modified in the presence of severe aggression or other dangerous behaviors. Monitoring is needed for emergent or worsening aggression or agitation with the use of antidepressants. Antipsychotic medications are frequently used as adjunctive treatment for aggression.[58] Other adjunctive medications that have been used for aggression and disruptive behavior disorders are mood stabilizers and stimulants.[59,60] **Table 5** provides some common potential adjunctive medication strategies.

Comorbid Conditions

Comorbid psychiatric conditions in depressed children and adolescents are exceedingly common. In fact, most youth with depression will also have another psychiatric diagnosis, with anxiety disorders and disruptive disorders being the most common.[1] Treatment of comorbidity is essential, because these conditions have been

Table 5
Brief adjunctive medication strategies

Adjuncts for Associated Symptoms	Options	Medication	Usual Dosage Range (mg/d)	Usual Dosage Schedule
Insomnia	Benzodiazepines	Lorazepam	0.5–2	qhs (not for chronic use; taper after 1–2 wk)
	Antidepressants	Trazodone	25–100	
	Hypnotics	Zolpidem	5–10	qhs
		Zaleplon	5–10	qhs
	Over-the-counter	Melatonin	3–6	qhs
		Diphenhydramine	0.5 mg/kg (maximum: 25 mg/d)	qhs
Anxiety or panic attacks	Benzodiazepines	Lorazepam	0.5–6	bid–tid, as needed
		Clonazepam	0.25–3	bid, as needed
Anxiety, if BZD contraindicated	Serotonin 1A partial agonist	Buspirone	15–60	bid–tid
Agitation/ aggression	Benzodiazepine	See above	See above	See above
	Low-dose antipsychotic	Risperidone	1–4	qhs–bid
		Haloperidol	1–5	qhs–bid
		Quetiapine	50–300	qhs
		Aripiprazole	5–15	qd
	Mood stabilizer	Valproic acid	500–1500	qhs
		Oxcarbazepine	300–1200	bid
Extrapyramidal side effects	Anticholinergic	Benztropine	2–6	qhs–tid

Abbreviations: BZD, benzodiazepines; qhs, every evening.

associated with treatment resistance,[61] overall worse outcome,[62,63] and an increased risk of suicide.[43] The approach to treatment usually consists of assessing the severity of the respective disorders and treating the most severe disorder first.[1,8] Alternatively, a particular disorder may be treated first if it is preventing effective treatment of the other disorders. Specific treatments for common comorbid conditions are discussed here.

MDD with psychotic features

Treatment of MDD with psychotic features generally consists of an SSRI with the addition of an antipsychotic medication.[8] The antidepressant would be managed within the same algorithm of treatment as MDD without psychotic features. American Academy of Child and Adolescent Psychiatry (AACAP) guidelines state that monotherapy with an antidepressant may be adequate for the treatment of "vague or mild" psychotic symptoms.[1] Atypical antipsychotics are recommended because of the decreased incidence of neurologic side effects compared with typical antipsychotics. The ACAAP Practice Parameters for the Use of Atypical Antipsychotic Medications in Children and Adolescents provides a review on their use (http://www.aacap.org/cs/root/member_information/practice_information/practice_parameters/practice_parameters). After remission of the psychotic symptoms, the antipsychotic is slowly tapered off, with continuation of the antidepressant. Caution should be exercised regarding possible interactions between the antidepressant and antipsychotic medications, and the potential acute and long-term side effects of antipsychotics. Another option may consist of initial treatment with an antipsychotic alone, followed by the addition of an antidepressant if improvement is not seen.

Anxiety disorder Several RCTs have been conducted in pediatric anxiety disorders showing efficacy of SSRIs in OCD and non-OCD anxiety disorders.[64] The pharmacologic recommendation would be to use an SSRI to treat both conditions; however, because CBT has also been found to be effective in anxiety disorders, including OCD, its addition to treatment should be strongly considered.[65,66]

ADHD The recommendation is again to treat the most severe disorder first, but with the awareness that the response to stimulant treatment of ADHD occurs more quickly than antidepressant treatment of depression. Atomoxetine can also be used safely with SSRIs but with careful monitoring for side effects, because inhibitors of CYP2D6, such as fluoxetine and paroxetine, can increase plasma levels of atomoxetine.[67] Another option is monotherapy with bupropion, as indicated by a previously mentioned open study that showed a response of one or both disorders in adolescents.[38]

Substance use disorders A reasonable approach here would be simultaneous treatment of both conditions. Studies in adult and adolescents have generally shown that antidepressants are well tolerated in this population, but improvement in depressive symptoms is modestly to poorly correlated with decreases in substance use.[68–70] In 3 placebo-controlled trials of SSRIs in adolescents with MDD and alcohol use disorders, overall reductions in depressive symptoms and alcohol use occurred, but no group differences between SSRIs and placebo were seen.[71–73] In 2 of these studies, both the active and placebo groups were receiving psychotherapeutic interventions, which may have diminished any medication effect.[71,73] Therefore, another reasonable approach may be to initiate treatment with psychotherapeutic interventions targeting depression and substance use, with the addition of antidepressant medication only if a response does not occur.

Augmentation

In youth with insufficient response to antidepressant treatment, determining whether to switch to a different antidepressant or whether additional treatments are needed is based on several factors. Generally, youth showing minimal or no response to treatment are recommended to switch antidepressants. The data from the Treatment of SSRI-Resistant Depression in Adolescents (TORDIA) study suggest that an additional 50% to 60% of youth will respond to changing antidepressants, with a greater chance of improvement in those who also add therapy. Augmentation, however, is generally used for children and adolescents who are exhibiting at least some response to the antidepressant, and the augmenting agent may be added rather than switching to another monotherapy antidepressant.

Augmentation has the advantage of avoiding an interruption of the initial antidepressant, but has the risks and inconveniences of polypharmacy. Augmentation may be preferable to switching in patients who tolerated the initial antidepressant and experienced a response but not remission.[74] Unlike adjunctive medication, which is continued only as long as the associated symptom is present, augmentation medications are considered an integral component of the treatment leading to remission, and are therefore continued throughout primary treatment.

Research on augmentation strategies in youth is scarce and limited to adolescents.[75–77] Data from adults show additional improvement in patients augmented with lithium, atypical antipsychotics, other antidepressants (eg, bupropion), and buspirone. A large adult study showed efficacy of bupropion as an augmenting agent after monotherapy with citalopram failed.[55] Addition of buspirone also resulted in remission rates similar to those of bupropion alone, but a smaller reduction in number and severity of symptoms and more frequent side effects occurred with buspirone.[78] The addition of atypical antipsychotics to antidepressant treatment has been fairly well established among depressed adults.[79] A post hoc analysis from the TORDIA study (of adolescents with treatment-resistant depression) showed that the addition of a mood stabilizer (atypical antipsychotic, lithium, divalproex, or topiramate) led to higher remission rates when added to an SSRI during the first 12 weeks of treatment (50% vs 17% with no mood stabilizer; $P = .03$).[80] Lithium showed positive effects when added to TCAs in 2 small open studies in adolescents.[75,76] Augmenting agents such as thyroid hormone, bupropion, and buspirone have not been systematically studied in youth.

CONTINUATION AND MAINTENANCE TREATMENT

The continuation phase is used to consolidate and continue to build on the improvements of the acute phase, and lasts approximately 6 to 9 months.[1,8,9] Unless precluded by side effects, the medications used in the acute phase are continued at the same doses. Follow-up of both the Treatment for Adolescents with Depression Study (TADS) and TORDIA study showed that continuation treatment with medication and/or CBT after completion of the acute phase resulted in further improvements in response rate for all conditions.[80,81] In one of the few randomized studies of continuation treatment in children and adolescents, 102 patients who had responded to 12 weeks of open treatment with fluoxetine were randomly assigned to 6 months of continuation therapy or placebo. Significantly fewer patients on fluoxetine experienced a relapse compared with those on placebo (42.0% vs 69.2%, respectively; $P = .009$). The median time to relapse in the placebo group was 8 weeks, whereas in the fluoxetine group, it was greater than 24 weeks.[82] Among responders to acute pharmacologic treatment, adding CBT to medication during the continuation phase may provide additional protection against relapse.[83]

Residual symptoms are common in youth with depression,[82,84,85] and increase risk of relapse and recurrence.[82,86] In the continuation study by Emslie and colleagues,[82] youth with residual symptoms were significantly more likely to experience relapse than those with no residual depressive symptoms (46.3% vs 22.9%; P = .014). Thus, addressing specific residual symptoms is important to reduce risk of relapse in youth.

After completion of the continuation phase, the decision must be made whether to initiate maintenance treatment. This decision would depend primarily on an assessment of the risk of depression recurrence in the individual and the potential severity of the recurrence. Factors to consider would be the number and severity of past recurrences, the presence of comorbidity, suicidality, or psychosis during the episode, the presence of social stressors, and the level of social support. Maintenance studies in depressed youth have been few, but naturalistic follow-up of adolescents who completed acute and continuation treatment with antidepressants has shown further improvement during

---

CLINICAL VIGNETTE

The patient is a 15-year-old girl who lives with her parents and 13-year-old brother. She attends the 10th grade in a suburban public school. She was referred to you by her pediatrician because of recent concerns about increased suicidal thoughts. Patient and parents were interviewed separately.

Patient had generally done well at home and at school apart from some persistent difficulties with organization around school work and social difficulties. Problems with school worsened when she began high school, and during the fall of her 9th grade year, she was seen by her pediatrician because of increasing irritability and arguing with family, changes in sleep, and low self-esteem. She was treated by her pediatrician with 20 mg of fluoxetine, which was later increased to 40 mg because of insufficient improvement. She showed substantial improvement in symptoms on the higher dose. She completed 9th grade, with plans to attend a new school starting in 10th grade. Although she was initially very positive about the new school, after 2 months she had a recurrence of symptoms, including problems with school performance, sleep problems, and again increased irritability and arguing with family around rules and limits. During your interview she states that she "hates the new school" because her peers "are mean and always making fun of me." She reports her parents argue with her about various issues, such as keeping her room clean and completing her homework. She makes self-deprecating statements such as "I'm an idiot." She denies any suicidal ideation, but does endorse death wishes. Parents report frequent conflict with her because of her forgetfulness and disorganization, which has worsened over the past several months. They describe her as having tendency to daydream and space out when spoken to.

After your evaluation, you determine that she is experiencing a relapse of major depressive disorder and has comorbid attention deficit/hyperactivity disorder inattentive type, which had not been addressed previously. After a discussion of the diagnosis and treatment options, the patient and her parents agree to the plan of continuing the fluoxetine at the current dose and adding a stimulant medication for her attention difficulties. You discuss the plan of continuing the medication for a few weeks to see if her symptoms improve with the addition of the stimulant, but suggest that if her mood difficulties continue or worsen, a change in antidepressant treatment may be needed. In addition, you provide a safety plan in the case of suicidality. At subsequent visits, the parents report significant improvement in her attention and note that her depression has also improved somewhat, but continue to be concerned about some irritability. The patient is pleased with her improved ability to focus on schoolwork, and feels that she is better able to follow the conversations of her peers; however, she continues to endorse thoughts consistent with a poor self-esteem, especially regarding feeling accepted by her peers, and reports continued relational difficulties with her parents. You recommend individual psychotherapy with cognitive behavioral therapy to target her residual symptoms. If her depression continues, pharmacologic augmentation strategies may be considered.

maintenance treatment.[87-89] In the TORDIA trial, in which adolescents were treated with an SSRI or venlafaxine, with or without the addition of CBT, the overall remission rate increased from 38.9% at the end of 24 weeks of active treatment to 61% at 72 weeks, as observed through naturalistic follow-up.[80,89] One small study in 22 adolescents randomized to 12-month maintenance with sertraline or placebo suggested that those on maintenance treatment had a lower rate of relapse compared with those on placebo (0% vs 38%), but the results were not significant.[90] Primarily based on research in adults, the general recommendation is to provide maintenance treatment for 1 year or more in youth with a history of at least 2 depressive episodes or 1 severe or chronic episode.[91] Treatment should aim for complete or near-complete resolution of symptoms, because youth with residual symptoms may be at greater risk of recurrence.

SUMMARY

Educational, psychological, social, and pharmacologic interventions are important elements to consider in formulating a treatment plan for depressed youth. Pharmacologic treatment should be conducted in a methodical and rational manner, ensuring that medication doses are maximized and maintained for an adequate length of time before moving on to the next trial. Clinicians who treat youth now have a body of empiric research to help guide treatment decisions; however, personalized treatment based on associated symptoms, comorbid conditions, contextual factors, and psychiatric history is essential.

A major advancement has been studies that have incorporated both psychotherapy and pharmacology in large, placebo-controlled, randomized trials. Clearly, further work must be done in many areas in the pediatric population, including expanding the study of non-SSRI antidepressants and augmentation strategies. A need also exists for research in populations that are commonly encountered in clinical practice, such as patients with comorbid psychiatric conditions or medical illness, or who are on concurrent medications. Another important development would be standardization of measures of efficacy and safety in randomized trials, which would enable easier comparison among trials and agents, and allow the pooling of data from several sources.[7] Long-term safety data are particularly needed, because the effects of antidepressant exposure on physical growth and the developing brain are largely unknown.

REFERENCES

1. Birmaher B, Brent D, Bernet W, et al. Practice parameter for the assessment and treatment of children and adolescents with depressive disorders. J Am Acad Child Adolesc Psychiatry 2007;46(11):1503–26.
2. Kovacs M. Presentation and course of major depressive disorder during childhood and later years of the life span. J Am Acad Child Adolesc Psychiatry 1996;35(6):705–15.
3. Luby J, Heffelfinger AK, Mrakotsky C, et al. The clinical picture of depression in preschool children. J Am Acad Child Adolesc Psychiatry 2003;42(3):340–8.
4. Hazell P, O'Connell D, Heathcote D, et-al. Tricyclic drugs for depression in children and adolescents. Cochrane Database of Systematic Reviews 2002, Issue 2. Art. No.: CD002317. DOI: 10.1002/14651858.CD002317.
5. Hammad TA, Laughren T, Racoosin J. Suicidality in pediatric patients treated with antidepressant drugs. Arch Gen Psychiatry 2006;63:332–9.
6. Stone M, Laughren T, Jones ML, et al. Risk of suicidality in clinical trials of antidepressants in adults: analysis of proprietary data submitted to US Food and Drug Administration. BMJ 2009;339:b2880.

7. DeVeaugh-Geiss J, March JS, Shapiro M, et al. Child and adolescent psychopharmacology in the new millennium: a workshop for academia, industry, and government. J Am Acad Child Adolesc Psychiatry 2006;45(3):261-70.
8. Hughes CW, Emslie GJ, Crismon ML, et al. Texas children's medication algorithm project: update from texas consensus conference panel on medication treatment of childhood major depressive disorder. J Am Acad Child Adolesc Psychiatry 2007;46(6):667-86.
9. Cheung A, Zuckerbrot RA, Jensen PS, et al. Guidelines for Adolescent Depression in Primary Care (GLAD-PC): II. Treatment and ongoing management. Pediatrics 2007;120(5):e1313-26.
10. Zuckerbrot RA, Cheung A, Jensen PS, et al. Guidelines for Adolescent Depression in Primary Care (GLAD-PC): I. Identification, assessment, and initial management. Pediatrics 2007;120(5):e1299-312.
11. Trivedi MH, Daly EJ. Measurement-based care for refractory depression: a clinical decision support model for clinical research and practice. Drug Alcohol Depend 2007;88(Suppl 2):S61-71.
12. Bridge J, Iyengar S, Salary CB, et al. Clinical response and risk for reported suicidal ideation and suicide attempts in pediatric antidepressant treatment treatment: a meta-analysis of randomized controlled trials. JAMA 2007;297(15): 1683-96.
13. Goodyer IM, Dubicka B, Wilkinson P, et al. Selective serotonin reuptake inhibitors (SSRIs) and routine specialists care with and without cognitive behaviour therapy in adolescents with major depression: randomised controlled trial. BMJ 2007; 335(7611):142.
14. Mufson L, Dorta KP, Wickramaratne P, et al. A randomized effectiveness trial of interpersonal psychotherapy for depressed adolescents. Arch Gen Psychiatry 2004;61:577-84.
15. Weisz JR, McCarty CA, Valeri SM. Effects of psychotherapy for depression in children and adolescents: a meta-analysis. Psychol Bull 2006;132(1):132-49.
16. David-Ferdon C, Kaslow NJ. Evidence-based psychosocial treatments for child and adolescent depression. J Clin Child Adolesc Psychol 2008;37(1):62-104.
17. Keller MB, Ryan ND, Strober M, et al. Efficacy of paroxetine in the treatment of adolescent major depression: a randomized, controlled trial. J Am Acad Child Adolesc Psychiatry 2001;40(7):762-72.
18. Berard R, Fong R, Carpenter DJ, et al. An international, multicenter, placebo-controlled trial of paroxetine in adolescents with major depressive disorder. J Child Adolesc Psychopharmacol 2006;16(1-2):59-75.
19. Emslie GJ, Wagner KD, Kutcher S, et al. Paroxetine treatment in children and adolescents with major depressive disorder: a randomized, multicenter, double-blind, placebo-controlled trial. J Am Acad Child Adolesc Psychiatry 2006;45(6):709-19.
20. Emslie GJ, Rush AJ, Weinberg WA, et al. A double-blind, randomized, placebo-controlled trial of fluoxetine in children and adolescents with depression. Arch Gen Psychiatry 1997;54(11):1031-7.
21. Emslie GJ, Heiligenstein JH, Wagner KD, et al. Fluoxetine for acute treatment of depression in children and adolescents: a placebo-controlled, randomized clinical trial. J Am Acad Child Adolesc Psychiatry 2002;41(10):1205-15.
22. TADS Team. Fluoxetine, cognitive-behavioral therapy, and their combination for adolescents with depression: Treatment for Adolescents with Depression Study (TADS) randomized controlled trial. JAMA 2004;292(7):807-20.
23. Cheung A, Emslie GJ, Mayes TL. Review of the efficacy and safety of antidepressants in youth depression. J Child Psychol Psychiatry 2005;46(7):735-54.

24. Wagner KD, Jonas J, Findling RL, et al. A double-blind, randomized, placebo-controlled trial of escitalopram in the treatment of pediatric depression. J Am Acad Child Adolesc Psychiatry 2006;45(3):280–8.

25. Emslie GJ, Ventura D, Korotzer A, et al. Escitalopram in the treatment of adolescent depression: a randomized placebo-controlled multisite trial. J Am Acad Child Adolesc Psychiatry 2009;48(7):721–9.

26. Rao N. The clinical pharmacokinetics of escitalopram. Clin Pharm 2007;46(4):281–90.

27. Wagner KD, Robb AS, Findling RL, et al. A randomized, placebo-controlled trial of citalopram for the treatment of major depression in children and adolescents. Am J Psychiatry 2004;161(6):1079–83.

28. Von Knorring AL, Olsson GI, Thomsen PH, et al. a randomized, double-blind, placebo-controlled study of citalopram in adolescents with major depressive disorder. J Clin Psychopharmacol 2006;26(3):311–5.

29. Wagner KD, Ambrosini PJ, Rynn M, et al. Efficacy of sertraline in the treatment of children and adolescents with major depressive disorder: two randomized controlled trials. JAMA 2003;290(8):1033–41.

30. Findling RL, Reed MD, Myers C, et al. Paroxetine pharmacokinetics in depressed children and adolescents. J Am Acad Child Adolesc Psychiatry 1999;38(8):952–9.

31. Tint A, Haddad PM, Anderson IM. The effect of rate of antidepressant tapering on the incidence of discontinuation symptoms: a randomised study. J Psychopharmacol 2008;22(3):330–2.

32. Morrato EH, Libby AM, Orton HD, et al. Frequency of provider contact after FDA advisory on risk of pediatric suicidality with SSRIs. Am J Psychiatry 2008;165(1):42–50.

33. Brent D, Emslie G, Clarke G, et al. Switching to another SSRI or to venlafaxine with or without cognitive behavioral therapy for adolescents with SSRI-resistant depression: the TORDIA randomized controlled trial. JAMA 2008;299(8):901–13.

34. Brent DA, Emslie GJ, Clarke GN, et al. Predictors of spontaneous and systematically assessed suicidal adverse events in the treatment of SSRI-resistant depression in adolescents (TORDIA) study. Am J Psychiatry 2009;166(4):418–26.

35. Papakostas GI, Thase ME, Fava M, et al. Are antidepressant drugs that combine serotonergic and noradrenergic mechanisms of action more effective than the selective serotonin reuptake inhibitors in treating major depressive disorder? A meta-analysis of studies of newer agents. Biol Psychiatry 2007;62(11):1217–27.

36. Emslie GJ, Findling RL, Yeung PP, et al. Venlafaxine ER for the treatment of pediatric subjects with depression: results of two placebo-controlled trials. J Am Acad Child Adolesc Psychiatry 2007;46(4):479–88.

37. Prakash A, Lobo E, Kratochvil CJ, et al. An open-label safety and pharmacokinetics study of duloxetine in pediatric patients with major depression. J Child Adolesc Psychopharmacol 2012;22(1):48–55.

38. Daviss WB, Bentivoglio P, Rascusin R, et al. Bupropion sustained release in adolescents with comorbid attention-deficit/hyperactivity disorder and depression. J Am Acad Child Adolesc Psychiatry 2001;40(3):307–14.

39. Nandagopal JJ, DelBello MP. Selegiline transdermal system: a novel treatment option for major depressive disorder. Expert Opin Pharmacother 2009;10(10):1665–73.

40. DelBello MP, Hochadel TJ, Portland KB, et al. A double-blind, placebo-controlled study of selegiline transdermal system (STS) in depressed adolescents. Paper presented at: 38th Annual Meeting of the American Academy of Child and Adolescent Psychiatry; October 18–23, 2011; Toronto, Ontario, Canada.

41. Safer DJ, Zito JM. Treatment-emergent adverse events from selective serotonin reuptake inhibitors by age group: children versus adolescents. J Child Adolesc Psychopharmacol 2006;16(1–2):159–69.
42. Kochanek KD, Kirmeyer SE, Martin JA, et al. Annual summary of vital statistics: 2009. Pediatrics 2012;129(2):338–48.
43. Bridge J, Goldstein TR, Brent DA. Adolescent suicide and suicidal behavior. J Child Psychol Psychiatry 2006;47(3–4):372–94.
44. Gibbons RD, Brown CH, Hur K, et al. Early evidence on the effects of regulators' suicidality warnings on SSRI prescriptions and suicide in children and adolescents. Am J Psychiatry 2007;164(9):1356–63.
45. Gibbons RD, Hur K, Bhaumik DK, et al. The relationship between antidepressant prescription rates and rate of early adolescent suicide. Am J Psychiatry 2006; 163(11):1898–904.
46. Worsening depression and suicidality in patients being treated with antidepressants. U.S. Food and Drug Administration Web site. Available at: http://www.fda.gov/Drugs/DrugSafety/PostmarketDrugSafetyInformationforPatientsandProviders/DrugSafetyInformationforHeathcareProfessionals/PublicHealthAdvisories/ucm161696.htm. Accessed April 24, 2012.
47. Goldsmith M, Singh M, Chang K. Antidepressants and psychostimulants in pediatric populations: is there an association with mania? Paediatr Drugs 2011;13(4): 225–43.
48. Goodman WK, Murphy T, Storch EA. Risk of adverse behavioral effects with pediatric use of antidepressants. Psychopharmacology 2007;191:87–96.
49. Safer DJ. Age-grouped differences in adverse drug events from psychotropic medication. J Child Adolesc Psychopharmacol 2011;21(4):299–309.
50. Boyer EW, Shannon M. The serotonin syndrome. N Engl J Med 2005;352(11): 1112–20.
51. Zajecka J, Tracy KA, Mitchell S. Discontinuation symptoms after treatment with serotonin reuptake inhibitors: a literature review. J Clin Psychiatry 1997;58(7):291–7.
52. Rosenbaum JF, Fava M, Hoog SL, et al. Selective serotonin reuptake inhibitor discontinuation syndrome: a randomized clinical trial. Biol Psychiatry 1998; 44(2):77–87.
53. Baldessarini RJ, Tondo L, Ghiani C, et al. Illness risk following rapid versus gradual discontinuation of antidepressants. Am J Psychiatry 2010;167(8):934–41.
54. Owens JA, Moturi S. Pharmacologic treatment of pediatric insomnia. Child Adolesc Psychiatr Clin N Am 2009;18(4):1001–16.
55. Emslie GJ, Kennard BD, Mayes TL, et al. Insomnia moderates outcome of serotonin-selective reuptake inhibitor treatment in depressed youth. J Child Adolesc Psychopharmacol 2012;22(1):21–8.
56. Shamseddeen W, Clarke G, Keller MB, et al. Adjunctive sleep medications and depression outcome in the treatment of serotonin-selective reuptake inhibitor resistant depression in adolescents study. J Child Adolesc Psychopharmacol 2012;22(1):29–36.
57. Knox M, King C, Hanna GL, et al. Aggressive behavior in clinically depressed adolescents. J Am Acad Child Adolesc Psychiatry 2000;39(5):611–8.
58. Schur SB, Sikich L, Findling RL, et al. Treatment recommendations for the use of antipsychotics for aggressive youth (TRAAY). Part I: a review. J Am Acad Child Adolesc Psychiatry 2003;42(2):132–44.
59. Malone RP, Delaney MA, Luebbert JF, et al. A double-blind placebo-controlled study of lithium in hospitalized aggressive children and adolescents with conduct disorder. Arch Gen Psychiatry 2000;57(7):649–54.

60. Klein RG, Abikoff H, Klass E, et al. Clinical efficacy of methylphenidate in conduct disorder with and without attention deficit hyperactivity disorder. Arch Gen Psychiatry 1997;54(12):1073–80.
61. Brent DA, Kolko DJ, Birmaher B, et al. Predictors of treatment efficacy in a clinical trial of three psychosocial treatments for adolescent depression. J Am Acad Child Adolesc Psychiatry 1998;37(9):906–14.
62. Fombonne E, Wostear G, Harrington R, et al. The Maudsley long-term follow-up of child and adolescent depression. 1. psychiatric outcomes in adulthood. Br J Psychiatry 2001;179(3):210–7.
63. McCauley E, Myers K, Mitchell J, et al. Depression in young people: initial presentation and clinical course. J Am Acad Child Adolesc Psychiatry 1993;32(4):714–22.
64. Kodish I, Rockhill C, Ryan S, et al. Pharmacotherapy for anxiety disorders in children and adolescents. Pediatr Clin North Am 2011;58(1):55–72, x.
65. POTS Team. Cognitive-behavior therapy, sertraline, and their combination for children and adolescents with obsessive-compulsive behavior. JAMA 2004;292(3):1969–76.
66. Hudson JL. Short term CBT and sertraline, alone or in combination, reduce anxiety in children and adolescents. Evid Based Ment Health 2009;12(3):88.
67. Kratochvil C, Newcorn J, Arnold LE, et al. Atomoxetine alone or combined with fluoxetine for treating ADHD with comorbid depressive or anxiety symptoms. J Am Acad Child Adolesc Psychiatry 2005;44(9):915–24.
68. Nunes EV, Levin FR. Treatment of depression in patients with alcohol or other drug dependence: a meta-analysis. JAMA 2004;291(15):1887–96.
69. Riggs PD, Mikulich-Gilbertson SK, Davies RD, et al. A randomized controlled trial of fluoxetine and cognitive behavioral therapy in adolescents with major depression, behavior problems, and substance use disorder. Arch Pediatr Adolesc Med 2007;161(11):9.
70. Goldstein BI, Shamseddeen W, Spirito A, et al. Substance use and the treatment of resistant depression in adolescents. J Am Acad Child Adolesc Psychiatry 2009;48(12):1182–92.
71. Deas D, Randall CL, Roberts JS, et al. A double-blind, placebo controlled trial of sertraline in depressed adolescent alcoholics: a pilot study. Hum Psychopharmacol 2000;15:461–9.
72. Findling RL, Pagano ME, McNamara NK, et al. The short-term safety and efficacy of fluoxetine in depressed adolescents with alcohol and cannabis use disorders: a pilot randomized placebo-controlled trial. Child Adolesc Psychiatry Ment Health 2009;3(1):11.
73. Cornelius JR, Bukstein OG, Wood DS, et al. Double-blind placebo-controlled trial of fluoxetine in adolescents with comorbid major depression and an alcohol use disorder. Addict Behav 2009;34(10):905–9.
74. Gaynes BN, Dusetzina SB, Ellis AR, et al. Treating depression after initial treatment failure: directly comparing switch and augmenting strategies in STAR*D. J Clin Psychopharmacol 2012;32(1):114–9.
75. Ryan ND, Meyer V, Dachille S, et al. Lithium antidepressant augmentation in TCA-refractory depression in adolescents. J Am Acad Child Adolesc Psychiatry 1988;27(3):6.
76. Strober M, Freeman R, Rigali J, et al. The pharmacotherapy of depressive illness in adolescence: II. Effects of lithium augmentation in nonresponders to imipramine. J Am Acad Child Adolesc Psychiatry 1992;31(1):16–20.
77. Pathak S, Johns ES, Kowatch RA. Adjunctive quetiapine for treatment-resistant adolescent major depressive disorder: a case series. J Child Adolesc Psychopharmacol 2005;15(4):696–702.

78. Trivedi MH, Fava G, Wisniewski SR, et al. Medication augmentation after the failure of SSRIs for depression. N Engl J Med 2006;354(12):1243–52.
79. Nelson JC, Papakostas GI. Atypical antipsychotic augmentation in major depressive disorder: a meta-analysis of placebo-controlled randomized trials. Am J Psychiatry 2009;166(9):980–91.
80. Emslie GJ, Mayes T, Porta G, et al. Treatment of resistant depression in adolescents (TORDIA): week 24 outcomes. Am J Psychiatry 2010;167(7):782–91.
81. TADS Team. The Treatment for Adolescents with Depression Study (TADS): long-term effectiveness and safety outcomes. Arch Gen Psychiatry 2007;64(10):1132–44.
82. Emslie GJ, Kennard BD, Mayes TL, et al. Fluoxetine versus placebo in preventing relapse of major depression in children and adolescents. Am J Psychiatry 2008;165(4):459–67.
83. Kennard BD, Emslie GJ, Mayes TL, et al. Cognitive-behavioral therapy to prevent relapse in pediatric responders to pharmacotherapy for major depressive disorder. J Am Acad Child Adolesc Psychiatry 2008;47(12):1395–404.
84. Kennard B, Silva S, Vitiello B, et al. Remission and residual symptoms after short-term treatment in the Treatment of Adolescents with Depression Study (TADS). J Am Acad Child Adolesc Psychiatry 2006;45(12):1404–11.
85. Tao R, Emslie GJ, Mayes TL, et al. Symptom improvement and residual symptoms during acute antidepressant treatment in pediatric major depressive disorder. J Child Adolesc Psychopharmacol 2010;20(5):423–30.
86. Brent DA, Birmaher B, Kolko D, et al. Subsyndromal depression in adolescents after a brief psychotherapy trial: course and outcome. J Affect Disord 2001;63(1–3):51–8.
87. Kennard BD, Silva SG, Tonev S, et al. Remission and recovery in the Treatment for Adolescents with Depression Study (TADS): acute and long-term outcomes. J Am Acad Child Adolesc Psychiatry 2009;48(2):186–95.
88. Curry J, Silva S, Rohde P, et al. Recovery and recurrence following treatment for adolescent major depression. Arch Gen Psychiatry 2011;68(3):263–9.
89. Vitiello B, Emslie G, Clarke G, et al. Long-term outcome of adolescent depression initially resistant to selective serotonin reuptake inhibitor treatment: a follow-up study of the TORDIA sample. J Clin Psychiatry 2011;72(3):388–96.
90. Cheung A, Kusumakar V, Kutcher S, et al. Maintenance study for adolescent depression. J Child Adolesc Psychopharmacol 2008;18(4):389–94.
91. Kennard BD, Emslie GJ, Mayes TL, et al. Relapse and recurrence in pediatric depression. Child Adolesc Psychiatr Clin N Am 2006;15:1057–79.

Psychopharmacologic Treatment of Obesity and Eating Disorders in Children and Adolescents

Pauline S. Powers, MD[a],*, Nancy L. Cloak, MD[b,c]

KEYWORDS

- Obesity • Eating disorders • Psychopharmacologic treatment • Adolescents

KEY POINTS

- Most evidence-based treatments for eating disorders are psychosocial.
- No medications are approved by the Food and Drug Administration (FDA) for the treatment of eating disorders in children and adolescents and only one is approved for the treatment of adults.
- Selective serotonin reuptake inhibitors are not effective for anorexia but may be helpful for comorbid conditions.
- Fluoxetine (Prozac) is FDA-approved for treatment of bulimia in adults, and there is a single positive open-label trial in adolescents.
- Orlistat (Xenical, Alli) is FDA approved for the treatment of obesity in children aged 12 years and older.
- Issues associated with psychiatric comorbidity in eating disorders and obesity relate to (1) accurate diagnosis and effective treatment, (2) medical complications, (3) potential for medications to exacerbate eating disorders and obesity, (4) risks of medication nonadherence or misuse, and (5) the impact of eating disorders and gastric bypass surgery on pharmacokinetics.

OVERVIEW

Obesity and eating disorders are common conditions that usually begin in childhood or adolescence and are difficult to treat. More than 110 million children are overweight or obese worldwide[1] and they have at least a 70% chance of becoming obese adults.[2] The lifetime prevalence of eating disorders is about 11% in the United States.[3] One

Funding sources: None.

Conflict of interest: None.

[a] Department of Pediatrics, Center for Eating and Weight Disorders, College of Medicine, University of South Florida, 3515 East Fletcher Avenue, Tampa, FL 33613, USA; [b] Oregon Center for Clinical Investigations, 2232 NW Pettygrove Street, Portland, OR 97210, USA; [c] Private Practice, 2455 Northwest Marshall Street, Suite 7, Portland, OR 97210, USA

* Corresponding author.

E-mail address: ppowers@health.usf.edu

recent surveillance study in Britain[4] found that the overall incidence of eating disorders in children younger than 13 years was 3.01 per 100 000 and that 50% of these children required hospital admission.

The rates of premature mortality are significant for adolescents and children with obesity and eating disorders. The long-term consequences of obesity (diabetes, hypertension, and cardiac disease) may shorten lifespans by an average of up to 7 years,[5] although younger people may be more at risk for premature mortality.[6] Even those who lose weight are still at risk for a host of physiologic and psychological complications.[7] Standardized mortality ratios (SMRs) for obesity vary by age and sex. (The SMR is the ratio between the observed number of deaths in a study population and the number of deaths expected based on the age- and sex-specific rates in a standard population. If the ratio is more than 1, there is said to be excess deaths in the study population.) Overall, the SMR for obesity for men is 1.67 and 1.45 for women, indicating a significant excess risk of death; the SMR for young men aged 18 to 29 years is the highest at 2.46.[8] A recent meta-analysis also found elevated SMRs for anorexia nervosa (AN), bulimia nervosa (BN), and eating disorders not otherwise specified (ED NOS).[9] Thus, in addition to their high prevalence, eating disorders and obesity carry significant risks for mortality (for example, the SMR for AN is 5.86), which are comparable to mortality risks for other serious diseases of youth, such as asthma[10] and type 1 diabetes (**Fig. 1**).[11]

Most of the evidence-based treatments for eating disorders are psychotherapies (**Table 1**); only one medication is approved by the US Food and Drug Administration (FDA) for the treatment of an eating disorder (fluoxetine [Prozac] at 60 mg/d for adults with bulimia); and only one medication is approved for the treatment of obesity in youth (orlistat [Xenical, Alli]). However, other medications are frequently used off-label. In this review, the authors summarize the evidence base for medications that are currently used for obesity and eating disorders. The existing evidence in children and adolescents are reviewed, but most of the data derives from studies in adults. The authors also discuss the FDA approval status for the most commonly used medications and review their contraindications and major adverse effects (**Table 2**). Investigational agents currently being considered, issues related to psychiatric and medical comorbidity, and limitations of pharmacologic strategies are addressed, and recommendations for treatment are provided.

PHARMACOTHERAPY FOR AN

AN is associated with an intense fear of gaining weight or becoming fat that leads to energy restriction and significantly low body weight (**Table 3**). Affecting 0.3% of US adolescents,[12] AN is associated with multiple medical complications and has the

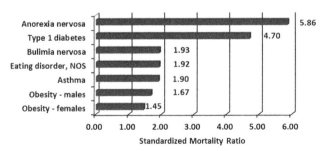

Fig. 1. Standardized mortality ratios for selected diseases in children and adolescents (references in text).

Table 1
Major evidence-based treatments for eating disorders

| Disorder | Intervention | Outcome Measure | Control | Percentage Achieving | | NNT[a] |
				Treatment (%)	Control (%)	
AN	Family based treatment[130] (adolescents only)	Full weight restoration, normal EDE scores	Individual therapy	41.8	22.6	5
BN	CBT[131]	Abstinence from bingeing and purging	Nonspecific therapy	56.0	24.0	3
	Interpersonal psychotherapy[132]	Abstinence from bingeing and purging	Behavior therapy	44.0	20.0	4
	Self-help (CBT based)[133]	≥50% decrease in bingeing and purging	Wait list	56.3	31.0	4
	Fluoxetine[44]	≥50% decrease in bingeing and purging	Pill placebo	63.0	43.0	5
Binge-eating disorder	CBT[134]	Abstinence from binge eating	Behavioral weight loss	51.0	36.0	7
	Topiramate[84]	Abstinence from binge eating	Pill placebo	58.0	29.0	3
	Self-help (CBT based)[135]	Abstinence from binge eating	Wait list	43.0	8.0	3

Abbreviations: CBT, cognitive-behavioral psychotherapy; EDE, Eating Disorder Examination; NNT, number needed to treat.
[a] Number needed to treat is the average number of patients who need to be treated for one additional patient to benefit compared with a control or no treatment. It is calculated as the reciprocal of the absolute percentage difference between the treatment group and the control group.

Table 2
Selected medications used to treat eating disorders and obesity[a]

Medication	Drug Class	Diagnosis	FDA Approved for ED, Obesity	Dose[b]	FDA Approved for Other Dx in Children or Adolescents	Side Effects	Black-Box Warnings
Aripiprazole	Atypical antipsychotic	AN	No	2–10 mg	Schizophrenia (13 y and older); bipolar I (10 y and older); irritable autism (6 y and older)	Sedation, possible metabolic syndrome, akathisia	Suicidality in patients younger than 24 y, increased mortality in elderly with dementia
Atomoxetine	SNRI	BED	No	80–110 mg	ADHD (6 y and older)	Dry mouth, nausea, hepatotoxicity (rare)	Suicidality
Bupropion SR	Antidepressant (aminoketone class)	Obesity	No	50–400 mg	No	Seizure risk (1%), increased in patients with ED	Suicidality
Citalopram	SSRI	BED	No	60 mg[c]	No	Gastrointestinal, sexual dysfunction, risk for serotonin syndrome	Suicidality
Cyproheptadine	Antihistamine	AN	No	2–16 mg	Rhinitis (2 y and older)	Sedation	None
Diethylpropion	Appetite suppressant	Obesity	Yes	25 mg bid	Obesity (16 y and older)	Arrhythmias, gastrointestinal, addictive	Pulmonary hypertension, valvulopathy

Drug	Class	Use		Dose	Pediatric indication	Side effects	Serious adverse effects
Duloxetine	SSNRI	BED	No	60–90 mg	No	Gastrointestinal, sexual dysfunction, risk for hepatotoxicity (rare), risk for serotonin syndrome	Suicidality
Escitalopram	SSRI	BED	No	30 mg	Depression (12 y and older)	Gastrointestinal, sexual dysfunction, risk for serotonin syndrome	Suicidality
Exenatide	Glucagonlike peptide agonist	Obesity	No	5–10 mcg SQ bid	No	Nausea	Pancreatitis
Fluoxetine	SSRI	BN, BED	Yes, BN in adults	60 mg	Depression (8 y and older); OCD (6 y and older)	Gastrointestinal, sexual dysfunction, risk for serotonin syndrome	Suicidality
Fluvoxamine	SSRI	BN, BED	No, No	100 mg bid	OCD (8 y and older)	Gastrointestinal, sexual dysfunction, risk for serotonin syndrome	Suicidality
Liraglutide	Glucagon-like peptide agonist	Obesity	No	0.6–1.8 mcg SQ	No	Nausea	C-cell tumors in animals
Lorcaserin	5-HT-2C receptor agonist	Obesity	Yes	10 mg bid	No	Headache, dizziness, fatigue, nausea	None
Metformin	Biguanide insulin sensitizer	Obesity	No	500–1000 mg bid	Type 2 diabetes mellitus (10 y and older)	Gastrointestinal symptoms	Lactic acidosis (rare but can be lethal)

(continued on next page)

Table 2
(continued)

Medication	Drug Class	Diagnosis	FDA Approved for ED, Obesity	Dose[b]	FDA Approved for Other Dx in Children or Adolescents	Side Effects	Black-Box Warnings
Naltrexone	Opioid antagonist	BN	No	200 mg	No	Avoid with opioids	Hepatotoxicity
Olanzapine	Atypical antipsychotic	AN	No	1.25–10.0 mg	Schizophrenia (13 y and older)	Sedation, possible metabolic syndrome	Increased mortality in dementia
Ondansetron	Selective 5-HT-3 antagonist	BN	No	8 mg tid	Nausea, vomiting associated with chemotherapy (4 y and older)	Visual, possible QT prolongation	None
Orlistat	Reversible lipase inhibitor	Obesity	Yes, 12 y and older	120 mg tid		Gastrointestinal, vitamin D supplement needed	Contraindicated in cholelithiasis
Phendimetrazine	Appetite suppressant	Obesity	Yes	35 mg tid	No	Tachycardia, glaucoma, addictive	Pulmonary hypertension, valvulopathy
Phentermine	Appetite suppressant	Obesity	Yes	37.5 mg	No	Cardiovascular, tachycardia, hypertension, addictive	Pulmonary hypertension, valvulopathy
Phentermine-topiramate ER	Appetite suppressant/ anticonvulsant	Obesity	Yes	7.5/46 mg– 15/92 mg	No	Paraesthesias, dizziness, dysgeusia	None

Pramlintide	Amylin analogue	Obesity	No	60–240 mcg SQ tid before meal	No	Hypoglycemia, gastrointestinal	Hypoglycemia (with insulin)
Quetiapine	Atypical antipsychotic	AN	No	25–300 mg	No	Sedation, possible metabolic syndrome	Suicidality, increased mortality in dementia
Sertraline	SSRI	BN BED	No	100 mg (BN), 200 mg (BED)	No	Gastrointestinal, sexual dysfunction, risk for serotonin syndrome	Suicidality
Topiramate	Anticonvulsant	BN BED	No No	100–250 mg 200–300 mg	Seizure disorder (2 y and older)	Nausea, odd taste, cognitive problems; rare: metabolic acidosis, kidney stones	None
Venlafaxine XR	SSNRI	Atypical AN	No	75 mg	No	Gastrointestinal, sexual dysfunction, risk for serotonin syndrome	Suicidality

Abbreviations: ADHD, attention-deficit/hyperactivity disorder; BED, binge-eating disorder; BN, bulimia nervosa; Dx, diagnosis; ED, eating disorder; OCD, obsessive-compulsive disorder; SNRI, selective norepinephrine reuptake inhibitor; SSNRI, selective serotonin/norepinephrine reuptake inhibitor; SSRI, selective serotonin reuptake inhibitor; SQ, subcutaneously.

[a] Fluoxetine is FDA approved for BN in adults in a dosage of 60 mg/d. No other medication is approved for any eating disorder. Orlistat is the only medication that is FDA approved for obesity in children and adolescents (aged 12 years and older).

[b] Dosages are once per day unless otherwise indicated. Dosages shown are those found to be effective in clinical trials, most of which were done with adults. Clinicians should review prescribing information and use judgment when prescribing for pediatric patients.

[c] Use of citalopram at doses greater than 40 mg/day is not recommended, due to the potential for QT prolongation. Source: http://www.fda.gov/Safety/MedWatch/SafetyInformation/SafetyAlertsforHumanMedicalProducts/ucm297624.htm. Accessed August 4, 2012.

Data from www.drugs.com; www.FDA.gov; www.dailymed.nlm.nih.gov/. Accessed March 27, 2012.

Table 3
DSM-IV TR diagnostic criteria for eating disorders and proposed DSM-V revisions[a]

	Current Criteria (DSM-IV-TR)	Proposed Changes in Criteria (DSM-V)
General	Two sections: (1) eating disorders and (2) feeding and eating disorders of infancy and early childhood	Combined into one section entitled "Eating Disorders Diagnoses"
AN	Refusal to maintain a minimally normal weight (at least 85% of ideal body weight)	Restricted intake leading to significantly low body weight for age, sex, developmental trajectory, and physical health
	Intense fear of gaining weight	Intense fear of gaining weight or persistent behavior to avoid weight gain, despite underweight
	Disturbance in way body is experienced, undue influence of body shape/weight on self-evaluation, or denial of the seriousness of current low body weight.	Disturbance in way body is experienced, undue influence of body shape/weight on self-evaluation, or persistent lack of recognition of the seriousness of low body weight
	In females, primary amenorrhea or 3 mo or more of secondary amenorrhea	Removal of amenorrhea criterion
BN	Recurrent binge eating (large amounts of food in discrete time period coupled with feeling of loss of control)	Recurrent binge eating (large amounts of food in discrete time period coupled with feeling of loss of control)
	Recurrent compensatory behavior	Recurrent compensatory behavior
	Self-evaluation unduly influenced by shape or weight	Self-evaluation unduly influenced by shape or weight
	Does not occur during episodes of AN	Does not occur during episodes of AN
	Occurs 3 times per week for last 3 mo	Occurs 1 time per week for last 3 mo
	Two types (purging and nonpurging)	Removal of 2 types
Binge-Eating Disorder	Falls under ED-NOS with research criteria for further study	Established as independent diagnosis in DSM-V
	Recurrent episodes of binge eating	Recurrent episodes of binge eating
	Binge eating is associated with 3 or more of following:	Binge-eating is associated with 3 or more of following:
	1. Eating more rapidly than normal	1. Eating more rapidly than normal
	2. Eating until uncomfortably full	2. Eating until uncomfortably full
	3. Eating large amounts when not physically hungry	3. Eating large amounts when not physically hungry
	4. Eating alone because of embarrassment	4. Eating alone because of embarrassment
	5. Feeling guilty or disgusted with self after eating	5. Feeling guilty or disgusted with self after eating
	Marked distress about binge eating	Marked distress about binge eating
	Occurs at least 2 d a wk for 6 mo	Occurs at least weekly for 3 mo

[a] Proposed revisions are indicated by italics.

highest mortality rate of any psychiatric disorder.[13] At present, no medication is approved by the FDA for the treatment of AN, although a wide variety of medications have been studied,[14] primarily antidepressants and atypical antipsychotics. However, despite initial promise in open-label studies, double-blind placebo-controlled trials have been disappointing for both classes of drugs.

Antidepressants

Initial reports indicating that the selective serotonin reuptake inhibitors (SSRIs) were effective for the core symptoms of AN were promising,[15] particularly those suggesting that fluoxetine might prevent relapse.[16] However, subsequent well-controlled studies have shown no benefit of fluoxetine for the treatment of AN, or for prevention of relapse.[17,18] SSRIs are also ineffective for the treatment of depression in acutely ill patients with AN,[19] probably because the antidepressant effect depends on adequate intake of tryptophan.[20] They may have a role in treating patients who have made progress with nutritional rehabilitation.

Antipsychotics

With the advent of atypical antipsychotics, most in the first group to be approved have been studied for the treatment of AN, at least with case reports or open-label studies. Two that have not been assessed are clozapine (Clozaril) and ziprasidone (Geodon) because of their associations with leukopenia and QT prolongation, respectively. Similar to the experience with antidepressants, early case reports and open-label studies suggested improvement with olanzapine[21] (Zyprexa) and quetiapine (Seroquel),[22] but double-blind placebo-controlled trials were less positive. One study found that among adult patients with AN already in structured treatment, there was a slightly more rapid weight gain and a lessening of obsessive compulsive symptoms with olanzapine compared with placebo.[23] Later studies with adolescents did not find a benefit for olanzapine.[24,25] Similarly, a follow-up double-blind placebo-controlled trial of quetiapine in adults found that there was no difference between quetiapine and placebo.[26] A double-blind placebo-controlled study of risperidone (Risperdal) in adolescents and young adults was also negative.[27] Case reports of aripiprazole (Abilify) are promising,[28] but a randomized trial has not yet been completed. Thus far, the antipsychotics most recently approved (asenapine [Saphris], lurasidone [Latuda], iloperidone [Fanapt], and paliperidone [Invega]) have not been studied.

There are reasons to think that antipsychotics might be helpful. For example, the common body image disturbance (the fixed false belief that one is fat when actually semistarved) meets the criteria for a psychotic symptom. For some patients, scores on the Positive and Negative Syndrome Scale are elevated and similar to those of patients with schizophrenia.[29] Also, there are studies suggesting that there are dopamine D2/D3 receptor binding abnormalities among patients with AN.[30,31] Despite these interesting observations, thus far, no antipsychotic medication has been demonstrated to be systematically effective for adult patients with AN in randomized double-blind placebo-controlled trials.[32] Results with adolescents have usually been clearly negative.

However, individual patients may benefit from atypical antipsychotics and, thus far, the evidence is slightly better for olanzapine than for the other atypical antipsychotics. A suitable patient might be an adolescent with severe AN who is hospitalized and has slightly odd thinking or a blunted or inappropriate affect or who describes what might be command hallucinations telling her (or him) not to eat. Even in this situation, very careful monitoring and discontinuation of the medication as soon as possible is wise.

Other Agents

Although there are no clearly efficacious medications for AN, anecdotally, it has been found that patients may benefit from low doses of minor tranquilizers before meals during the initial refeeding phase. Treatments for some of the physiologic complications of AN have been studied. Bone loss begins soon after the onset of the illness and is distinct from and more severe than postmenopausal osteoporosis.[33] Estrogen has not been as effective as expected,[34] although a recent study of the transdermal preparation suggested that it may be marginally helpful.[35] One problem with administering estrogen is that menses may return and obscure the positive prognostic value of a spontaneous return of menses. Hormonally induced menses may reinforce the denial that is so commonly part of AN. Neither calcium nor vitamin D has been demonstrated to be effective in treating osteoporosis associated with AN, but daily intakes of 1000 to 1300 mg of calcium and 600 IU of vitamin D are recommended for children and adolescents.[36] Bisphosphonates may be useful in some patients, particularly if they have already had a fracture, but recent reports of jaw necrosis[37] and atypical hip fractures[38] make this a questionable treatment if patients have not had a fracture. The long-term consequences of bisphosphonates in young women are unknown. New methods of diagnosing osteoporosis and new guidelines (FRAX, the WHO's fracture risk assessment tool)[39] for deciding if treatment should begin may be helpful in the future. Although it is well established that many patients have delayed gastric emptying[40] and treatment with metoclopramide may alleviate this problem, the risk for extrapyramidal symptoms or tardive dyskinesia is high, particularly in semistarved patients and, therefore, other strategies (eg, use of fluids for nutrition rather than solids at the beginning of the refeeding phase) may be more prudent.

Investigational Agents

Table 4 lists studies that are registered on the Clinical Trials Web site (http:// clinicaltrials.gov/) for which results are not yet available or that are still underway. Most are studies of atypical antipsychotics or various treatments of bone loss. One exception on the list is hydroxyzine, long FDA approved for anxiety, which might help some of the common anxiety disorders that occur in AN.

PHARMACOTHERAPY FOR BN

BN is characterized by recurrent episodes of binge eating followed by compensatory behavior to avoid weight gain in an individual who is not underweight (seeTable 3). Unlike AN, BN is very rare in prepubertal children. However, it affects 0.9% of adolescents in the United States and is associated with significant psychiatric comorbidity; social impairment; suicidal ideation[12]; and serious medical complications, including fluid and electrolyte disturbances and esophageal rupture.[41] Unlike AN, BN responds to pharmacotherapy, which can be an effective component of a treatment program for patients with BN, particularly for patients with comorbid symptoms of anxiety or depression, or as an initial treatment of patients who lack access to cognitive-behavioral psychotherapy (CBT) or who have failed to respond to it.[42]

Antidepressants

Because they are generally safe and well tolerated, the SSRI antidepressants are currently recommended as the pharmacotherapy of choice for BN; among these, fluoxetine is the only agent that has FDA approval for the treatment of BN (in adults), at a dosage of 60 mg/d. The exact mechanism of action is unknown but probably relates to disturbances of monoamines, particularly serotonin, that are seen in both

Table 4
Selected agents in clinical trials for treatment of eating disorders and obesity

AN	BN	Binge-Eating Disorder	Obesity
Olanzapine[a]	Topiramate[a]	Topiramate[a]	Topiramate[a]
Risperidone[a]	CCK-1 Agonist	Bupropion	Orlistat[a]
Aripiprazole[a]	Baclofen	Lisdexamfetamine	Metformin[a]
Hydroxyzine[a]	Memantine	Orlistat	Exenatide[a]
Alprazolam[a]	N-acetylcysteine	Duloxetine	Liraglutide
Dronabinol	Erythromycin	Pramipexole	Tesofensine (monoamine reuptake inhibitor)
		Baclofen	Bupropion-naltrexone[b]
		Armodafinil	Bupropion-zonisamide[b]
			Beloranib (angiogenesis inhibitor)
			GSK 1521498 (opioid inverse agonist)
			MK 0557 (neuropeptide Y antagonist)
			SCH 497079 (histamine antagonist)
			SR 14778 (cannabinoid antagonist)
			V 24343 (cannabinoid antagonist)
			CP 866 087 (opioid antagonist)

Italicized agents are currently FDA approved for other indications.
  [a] Under study for children and/or adolescents.
  [b] Individual components are currently FDA approved for obesity (phentermine) or other indications.
  Data from www.clinicaltrials.gov. Accessed March 28, 2012.

ill and recovered individuals.[43] In the study leading to the FDA approval of fluoxetine for the treatment of BN, the proportion of patients responding, as defined by a 50% or greater decrease in binge-eating or self-induced vomiting episodes, in the 60-mg/d fluoxetine and placebo treatment groups was 63% and 43%, respectively, for binge-eating episodes per week and 57% and 26%, respectively, for vomiting episodes per week. This finding represents a number needed to treat (NNT) of 5 to achieve at least a 50% reduction in both binge-eating and vomiting behaviors.[44] A 20-mg/d dosage of fluoxetine was not effective. In this and other trials of fluoxetine for BN, there were concomitant improvements in measures of depression, eating disorder psychopathology, and global severity of symptoms. Compared with its use in the treatment of depression, the treatment of BN with fluoxetine requires higher doses, but the time to response is generally quicker; most eventual responders attain a response by 3 weeks.[45] A response seems to be independent of the presence or absence of comorbid depression.[46] Continuation of the medication after treatment response reduces but does not eliminate the probability of relapse; at the end of a 12-month placebo-controlled extension trial, previous responders to fluoxetine who continued the medication had a 33% relapse rate compared with 51% of those who were switched to placebo.[47] In this study, relapse was defined as a return to the baseline binge/purge frequency. For this reason, it is recommended that treatment be continued for at least 6 months after a response.[48]

Because fluoxetine is FDA approved for BN in adults and is FDA approved for the treatment of depression and obsessive-compulsive disorder in children and adolescents, it should be the first choice if pharmacologic treatment is considered. Support for its use in children and adolescents with BN consists of a single 8-week open trial with 10 adolescents aged 12 to 18 years in which fluoxetine (60 mg daily) was combined with supportive psychotherapy. The average weekly binges decreased from 4.1 to 0, the average weekly purges decreased from 6.4 to 0.4, and a significant improvement was noted on standard measures of eating disorder psychopathology. There were no discontinuations caused by adverse effects.[49] Although SSRIs other than fluoxetine should theoretically be of benefit, there are no trials in adolescents, and supporting evidence in adults is limited to one small placebo-controlled trial each of fluvoxamine (Luvox; 200 mg/d)[50] and sertraline (Zoloft; 100 mg/d),[51] both showing statistically and clinically significant reductions in bingeing and vomiting in comparison with placebo. However, a larger controlled trial of flexibly dosed fluvoxamine was negative,[52] as was a trial of citalopram (Celexa) up to 40 mg/d.[53] Paroxetine (Paxil) has not been studied.

The most common adverse effects of fluoxetine and other SSRIs are gastrointestinal disturbances (nausea, loose stools, or constipation), insomnia, jitteriness or agitation, and sexual dysfunction. To enhance compliance, patients should be informed that these medications are generally weight neutral. Although a recent reanalysis of the data has questioned the connection between antidepressants and suicidality,[54] at this time, informed consent should include a discussion of the black-box warning regarding the increased risk of suicidal ideation and behaviors (although not actual suicides) associated with the use of newer antidepressants in children, adolescents, and young adults,[55,56] and clinicians should follow FDA guidelines for monitoring.[57]

Other Agents

Topiramate (Topamax) is FDA approved for the treatment of partial-onset or secondarily generalized seizure disorders in children (aged 2 years and older), adolescents, and adults. Its association with appetite suppression and weight loss, probably mediated by the blockade of AMPA (α-amino-3-hydroxy-5-methyl-4-isoxazolepropionic acid)/kainate glutamate receptors in the hypothalamus,[58] has led to several trials in adult patients with BN. Two 10-week trials have shown a benefit of topiramate at dosages of 100 to 250 mg/d for reducing binge/purge episodes, weight, and overall clinical severity. Compared with placebo, 27.4%[59] and 33.4%[60] more patients experienced a response, which was defined as a 50% or greater reduction in binge/purge episodes; there were also improvements in measures of eating disorder psychopathology and quality of life. Because of its potential to induce weight loss, topiramate should be avoided in low-weight individuals with BN and patients with binge/purge-type AN. There have been reports of misuse by patients with eating disorders who are seeking weight loss.[61]

Based on observations in animals that opioid antagonists decrease stress-induced eating and a positive study of intravenous naloxone (Narcan) in patients with BN, several small trials have been conducted with naltrexone (Revia), which is approved for the treatment of opioid and alcohol dependence in adults. Dosages of 200 mg/d or more were beneficial in reducing bingeing and purging,[62,63] but it was not effective at the usual prescribed dosage of 50 mg/d,[64] and there have been concerns about hepatotoxicity at the higher doses. Ondansetron (Zofran) is a serotonin 3 receptor (5-HT-3) antagonist approved for the prevention of nausea and vomiting associated with chemotherapy or anesthesia in children and widely used for nausea and vomiting associated with other medical conditions. A single small (N = 26) randomized trial showed efficacy in patients with BN who had not responded to antidepressants or psychotherapy[65]; the medication was well tolerated, but the expense and frequency of administration have limited its use.

Investigational Agents and Light Therapy

Based on emerging evidence for the involvement of the gamma-aminobutyric acid (GABA) and glutamate systems in the reward process and the regulation of food intake,[66] the GABA-B receptor agonist baclofen (Lioresal), the NMDA receptor antagonist memantine (Namenda),[67] and the glutamate release inhibitor N-acetylcysteine[68] are being investigated (see **Table 4**). Bright-light therapy has been studied in 3 small controlled trials (total N = 69), all of which found efficacy for 30-minute exposure to 2500 to 10 000 lux per day.[69-71] Effects were seen as early as 1 week and seemed greatest in individuals who reported a seasonal pattern for their symptoms.

PHARMACOTHERAPY FOR BINGE-EATING DISORDER

Like BN, binge-eating disorder is characterized by recurrent episodes of binge eating accompanied by distress and lack of control over eating, but unlike bulimia, individuals do not compensate for their behavior (see **Table 3**). Currently, binge-eating disorder is classified in the appendix of the *Diagnostic and Statistical Manual of Mental Disorders* (Fourth Edition, Text Revision) (DSM-IV-TR) as a research diagnosis but it will be formally included as a disorder in DSM-V, with some modifications in criteria.[72] It is the most prevalent eating disorder in US adolescents, affecting 1.6% of the population between the ages of 13 and 18; like BN, it is associated with high levels of psychiatric comorbidity, social impairment, and suicidal ideation.[12] Because untreated binge-eating disorder is associated with the development of obesity over time,[73] identifying and treating children and adolescents with binge-eating disorder are important components of obesity-prevention efforts in this population. In general, treatment recommendations for binge-eating disorder are similar to those for bulimia, encompassing primarily CBT and antidepressant medications,[42] although no medications are currently FDA approved for the treatment of binge-eating disorder.

SSRIs

SSRI antidepressant medications have been studied for binge-eating disorder based on their efficacy in BN and likely work via similar actions on monoamine systems. There have been 7 randomized placebo-controlled trials of SSRIs in the treatment of adults with binge-eating disorder: 2 each of fluoxetine[74,75] and fluvoxamine[76,77] and one each of escitalopram (Lexapro),[78] citalopram,[79] and sertraline.[80] Target doses were at the higher end of the usual range (eg, 60–80 mg/d of fluoxetine, 30 mg/d of escitalopram, 300 mg/d of fluvoxamine, 200 mg/d of sertraline, and 60 mg/d of citalopram). All medications were effective in reducing binge-eating behavior and also improved other outcome measures, such as eating disorder psychopathology and depression. Although placebo-corrected binge-eating abstinence rates ranged from 12% to 39%, weight loss was modest, averaging 1.7 kg greater than placebo across the trials.

Other Monoaminergic Agents

Sibutramine (Meridia), a serotonin-norepinephrine reuptake inhibitor that was formerly approved for the treatment of obesity, was effective in reducing binge eating and weight but was removed from the market in 2010 because of concerns about cardiovascular toxicity. Another serotonin-norepinephrine inhibitor, duloxetine, was recently found to be effective in a 12-week randomized placebo-controlled trial. With an average dosage of 79 mg/d, 56% of patients on medication achieved remission of binge eating versus 30% of those taking placebo; average weight loss was 3.2 kg versus 0.3 kg.[81] A 10-week randomized placebo-controlled trial of the selective norepinephrine reuptake inhibitor atomoxetine (average dose 106 mg/d) yielded remission rates of 70% for medication versus 32% for placebo, an average weight loss of 2.7 kg versus 0 kg, and significantly greater improvements on measures of eating disorder psychopathology.[82]

Anticonvulsants

There have been 3 short-term (14–21 week) randomized placebo-controlled trials of topiramate in adults with binge-eating disorder, with each showing efficacy.[83–85] Rates of placebo-corrected binge abstinence ranged between 22.7% and 34.0%, with placebo-corrected weight losses ranging between 4.3 and 5.9 kg. A benefit for decreasing binge eating was seen by the second week of treatment. Dropout rates ranged from 30% to 42%, and there were frequent adverse effects, mainly paresthesias, taste alterations, and problems with cognitive functioning. Placebo-controlled studies of other anticonvulsants that affect the glutamatergic system, zonisamide (Zonegran)[86] and lamotrigine (Lamictal),[87] have not shown benefit.

Investigational Agents and Bariatric Surgery

As for BN, several initial investigations have focused on existing modulators of the glutamate and GABA systems, including the glutamate receptor antagonists memantine[67] and acamprosate (Campral).[88] Other existing agents that are currently being investigated include the stimulant lisdexamfetamine (Vyvanse); the stimulantlike agent armodafinil (Nuvigil); the dopamine agonist pramipexole (Mirapex); and the GABA-B agonist baclofen, which is also being evaluated for the treatment of bulimia (see **Table 3**).

Binge-eating disorder is not a contraindication to bariatric surgery,[89] although clinicians are advised to assess its severity and the need for treatment both preoperatively and postoperatively. In appropriately selected patients, bariatric surgery seems to result in the improvement of binge eating[90–92]; in a 1-year prospective follow-up study of patients undergoing bariatric surgery who were diagnosed by clinical interview based on DSM-V criteria, the presence of binge-eating disorder did not adversely impact weight loss.[93] Gastric bypass was the procedure used in each of these studies, and results may not apply with other bariatric procedures.

PHARMACOTHERAPY FOR OBESITY

Because of its increasing prevalence and growing recognition of its health consequences, obesity in children and adolescents has become a major focus in both clinical and public-policy settings.[94] Treatment guidelines focus on lifestyle changes, including diet, physical activity, and reduced screen time.[95] These interventions are of limited efficacy; one meta-analysis found effect sizes for a significant reduction in body mass index (BMI) of .02 for physical activity alone and 0.22 for diet alone. Behavioral interventions that involve the family were more effective (effect size 0.64).[96] Therefore, treatment guidelines encourage consideration of pharmacotherapy for obese children and adolescents who do not respond to lifestyle interventions.[95]

However, finding safe and effective pharmacologic interventions for obesity has been challenging. This work is probably challenging because the neurobiological systems that control food intake and energy balance are highly redundant and highly interrelated with the systems involved in the regulation of mood and the response to reward. Despite an explosion in basic research, the anatomy, chemistry, and functions of these elaborate neural systems and their interactions with the gastrointestinal system and adipose tissue remain poorly characterized.[97] The development of medications for obesity has also been hampered by the frequent occurrence of adverse effects. For example, one analysis of the proposed naltrexone-bupropion combination antiobesity agent found that to achieve a weight loss of at least 10% from baseline, 6 additional patients would need to be treated for one to benefit (NNT of 6); but 1 patient among 5 to 8 patients would withdraw because of adverse events (number needed to harm of 5–8).[98] Several agents have been removed from the market because of serious adverse effects, including phentermine-fenfluramine (cardiac valvulopathy), sibutramine (cardiovascular events), and rimonabant (withdrawn from the market in Europe and never approved in the United States because of mood changes and suicidality). For these reasons, the number of medications presently approved for the treatment of obesity is small, although there are several drugs in development.

Medications Approved for Treatment of Obesity in Children and Adolescents

Currently, orlistat is the only medication that is FDA approved for the treatment of obesity in adolescents aged 12 and older, in combination with lifestyle interventions. It is a reversible lipase inhibitor that blocks the absorption of approximately 30% of dietary fat at the prescription dosage of 120 mg 3 times a day and about 25% of fat absorption at the over-the-counter dosage of 60 mg 3 times a day. In the multicenter randomized placebo-controlled trial leading to its approval for use in adolescents, 67% of patients aged 12 to 16 years who took orlistat for 1 year in combination with diet and exercise lost 5% or more of their initial body weight compared with 21% of patients treated with diet and exercise alone (NNT of 2), although the actual difference in weight was small (2.6 kg) and the orlistat-treated patients began to regain weight at the same rate as the placebo-treated patients, beginning at about week 24 of the study. Other than decreases in waist circumference and diastolic blood pressure, and a trend toward lower fasting blood sugar, there were no significant differences in cardio-metabolic parameters. The most common adverse effects are bloating, abdominal discomfort, flatulence, and oily stools. Limiting dietary fat to 15 g per meal can minimize these adverse effects. Orlistat has been associated with reduced absorption of fat-soluble vitamins and significant decreases in serum vitamin D levels, so vitamin supplementation and monitoring of serum vitamin D is advised.[99] Clinicians should screen patients for the presence of eating disorder psychopathology because there have been several case reports of orlistat misuse as a purging agent by individuals with eating disorders.[100–102]

Medications Approved in Children and Adolescents for Other Indications and Studied for Treatment of Obesity

Among the medications approved in pediatric populations for other uses, metformin (Glucophage) has been studied for the treatment of obesity in children and adolescents, and topiramate has been evaluated in obese adults. Neither is currently FDA approved for the treatment of obesity. Metformin is a biguanide that increases sensitivity of various tissues (muscle, liver, adipose) to the uptake and action of insulin. It is FDA approved for the treatment of type 2 diabetes in adults and children aged 10 years and older. In 2008, a meta-analysis was conducted of 5 placebo-controlled trials with a total of 365 obese patients aged 6 to 19 years. All trials lasted 6 months and 3 used lifestyle interventions in both arms. Metformin at dosages of 1000 to 2000 mg/d reduced BMI by an average of 1.42 kg/m^2. Overall, because its benefits for both weight loss and diabetes prevention are modest in comparison with lifestyle interventions,[103] it should probably be reserved for obese adolescents who also have diabetes or insulin resistance.

Although it has not been studied in obese children and adolescents, several investigators have studied topiramate for obesity in adults. A meta-analysis of 10 trials involving 3320 adults showed significant efficacy, with an average placebo-corrected weight loss of 5.3 kg.[104] Topiramate dosages ranged from 64 mg/d to 400 mg/d, and both weight loss and adverse effects were dose dependent. Topiramate may be an effective alternative to orlistat for obese children and adolescents who have comorbid seizure disorders or who fail to respond to orlistat or do not tolerate it.

Medications Approved for Treatment of Obesity in Adults

In addition to orlistat, the appetite suppressants phentermine (Adipex-P, Ionamin), diethylpropion (Durad, Tenuate), and phendimetrazine (Bontril) are FDA approved for short-term (12 weeks) use in adults. All are controlled substances with addiction potential, and all carry FDA warnings regarding the potential for development of pulmonary hypertension and valvular heart disease if used for more than 12 weeks. A meta-analysis found average placebo-adjusted weight losses of 3.6 kg for phentermine and 3.0 kg for diethylpropion; phendimetrazine was not included because of limited data.[105] With one exception,[106] these agents have not been studied in children and adolescents and because of their potentials for addiction and serious cardiovascular side effects, they should probably not be used. Two newly FDA-approved medications (lorcaserin [Belviq] and phentermine-topiramate ER [Qsymia]; see **Table 5**) have not been studied in children or adolescents.

Medications Approved in Adults for Other Indications and Studied for Treatment of Obesity

Among these medications are one antidepressant and several agents used to treat diabetes. Bupropion is approved for depression and smoking cessation in adults and has some structural similarity to older agents used for weight loss. However, a meta-analysis showed a modest average placebo-corrected weight loss of 2.77 kg.[107] Pramlintide (Symlin), a synthetic analogue of amylin, a peptide that is cosecreted by islet cells with insulin, reduces postprandial glucose and increases satiety. A meta-analysis of 8 adult studies that reported effects on weight showed modest placebo-adjusted weight losses of 2.57 kg in obese patients with type 2 diabetes and 2.27 kg in obese patients without diabetes.[108] Two glucagonlike peptide 1 agonists, exenatide (Byetta) and liraglutide (Victoza), have been approved for the treatment of type 2 diabetes in adults and are being evaluated for the treatment of obesity (**Table 5**).

Medications in Development

In addition to the existing antidiabetic agents liraglutide and exenatide, antiobesity medications in advanced stages of development include one novel monoaminergic agent, tesofensine, and two combinations of existing medications: Contrave, a combination of sustained-release bupropion and naltrexone; and Empatic, a combination of sustained-release bupropion and zonisamide. Details are provided in **Table 5**.

As reviewed elsewhere,[109,110] many of the medications in earlier stages of development target known components of the complex systems that regulate appetite and weight (see **Table 4**). Bariatric surgery is increasingly used in adolescents and results in much greater weight losses than behavioral interventions or medications but can be associated with significant medical complications and, in some patients, adverse psychological outcomes.[111] A detailed discussion of this topic is beyond the scope of this article, but reviews of guidelines,[112] outcomes,[113] and adverse effects[114] are available.

COMORBIDITY

Issues associated with psychiatric comorbidity in eating disorders and obesity relate to (1) the negative impacts of the eating disorder on accurate diagnosis and effective treatment, (2) implications of medical complications of eating disorders for choices of pharmacotherapeutic agents, (3) the potential for some psychotropic medications to exacerbate eating disorders and obesity, (4) the risk of medication nonadherence or misuse in patients with eating disorders, and (5) the impact of eating disorders and gastric bypass surgery on pharmacokinetics.

Diagnosis and Treatment

Many psychiatric conditions are commonly comorbid with eating disorders; for example, among adolescents with BN, 50%, 66%, and 19% met criteria for a mood disorder, anxiety disorder, and/or substance use disorder, respectively.[12] However, accurate diagnosis is a key issue: starvation alone can produce anxiety, depression, cognitive impairment, and obsessive-compulsive symptoms.[115] Despite being at normal weight, patients with bulimia also show metabolic signs of starvation,[116] which can produce depression and mood lability in combination with chaotic eating patterns. All patients can have adjustment reactions related to the significant impact of their symptoms on school, work, and relationships. Therefore, most patients should have a period of 4 to 6 weeks of normal eating before treatment is initiated.[117]

There is very limited evidence regarding the effectiveness of pharmacotherapy for comorbid conditions in individuals with eating disorders because improvement in comorbid conditions has been assessed only as a secondary outcome. As discussed, SSRIs are not effective for depression or anxiety in acute AN, but most studies of SSRIs in BN and binge-eating disorder have shown improvement in depression scores. Venlafaxine has been shown to be superior to fluoxetine in reducing anxiety in a small trial of patients with atypical AN,[118] but there has not been a double-blind placebo-controlled trial in patients with typical AN. Obsessive compulsive disorder that is not just related to food and eating and that does not resolve when patients are weight restored[119] may respond to SSRIs and clomipramine, although the latter should be avoided until patients are weight restored because of the potential for worsening of hypotension, constipation, and cardiac conduction abnormalities in underweight patients.

Medical Complications of Eating Disorders and Choice of Pharmacotherapy

Although eating disorders are associated with many medical complications, cardiovascular problems are the most immediately life threatening. These problems include bradycardia, hypotension, and arrhythmias, especially those related to the prolongation of the QT interval.[120] Clinicians should use caution when administering medications that also affect the cardiovascular system. For example, agents that have alpha-receptor blocking actions, such as trazodone (Desyrel), risperidone, clozapine, low potency typical antipsychotics, and tricyclics, can exacerbate hypotension; and lithium, carbamazepine (Tegretol), tricyclics, and many antipsychotics can worsen cardiac conduction abnormalities. Baseline electrocardiograms (EKGs) should be considered for all patients with eating disorders and obesity, and practice guidelines specifically recommend EKG monitoring for more severely ill patients who are significantly underweight and/or purging frequently.[42] Because electrolyte abnormalities are also associated with arrhythmias, electrolytes should be monitored in patients with known or suspected purging. Dehydration and constipation are other conditions frequently seen in patients with eating disorders. Therefore, lithium should be avoided in patients who purge because of the potential for toxicity with fluid shifts, and patients who are likely to have malnutrition-related gastrointestinal slowing should probably not receive medications with anticholinergic properties.

Medication-related Weight Changes and Eating Disorders

Clinicians have long observed that weight changes caused by external factors (eg, oral surgery,[121] pancreatitis[122]) can be associated with new onset or worsening of eating disorders. As reviewed elsewhere,[123] this has also been reported in the context of

Table 5
Medications for obesity that are newly approved or in advanced stages of development

Agent	Mechanism	Study: Placebo-Adjusted Weight Loss (Duration)	Adverse Effects	Status
Exenatide (Byetta)	Glucagonlike peptide 1 agonist	Rosenstock et al,[136] 2010: 3.3 kg (24 wk) Dushay et al,[137] 2012: 2.9 kg (35 wk) Kely et al,[138] 2012: 3.9 kg (26 wk)[a]	Nausea, warning regarding pancreatitis	Phase III trial completed
Liraglutide (Victoza)	Glucagon-like peptide 1 agonist	Astrup et al,[139] 2009: 4.4 kg (20 wk)	Nausea, warnings about pancreatitis, increased C-cell tumors in animals	Phase III trial in process
Lorcaserin (Belviq)	Serotonin 2C receptor agonist	Smith et al,[140] 2010: 3.6 kg (52 wk) Fidler et al,[141] 2011: 3.1 kg (52 wk) O'Neil et al,[142] 2012: 4.5–5.0 kg (52 wk)	Fatigue, dizziness, headache, nausea	FDA approved for adults on June 27, 2012; release for marketing is pending DEA review
Tesofensine	Dopamine, serotonin, and norepinephrine reuptake inhibitor	NeuroSearch: 4.5, 9.1, and 10.6 kg with doses of 0.25, 0.5, and 1.0 mg, respectively[143] (24 wk)	Dry mouth, nausea, dizziness, dose-dependent increases in heart rate and blood pressure	Phase III studies planned

Drug	Mechanism	Study/doses	Side effects	Status
Phentermine-topiramate ER (Qsymia)	Monoamine releaser, NMDA receptor antagonist	Vivus, Inc: 7.5 kg[144] (28 wk) Allison et al,[145] 2012: 10.9 kg (52 wk) Gadde et al,[146] 2011: 8.9 kg (52 wk)	Paresthesias, dry mouth, disturbed taste, constipation, poor concentration	FDA approved for adults on July 17, 2012
Bupropion-naltrexone (Contrave)	α-melanocyte-stimulating hormone releaser; opioid antagonist	Greenway et al,[147] 2009: 5.4–5.9 kg (24 wk) Greenway et al,[148] 2010: 6.1 kg (56 wk) Wadden et al,[149] 2011: 4.2 kg (approximate[b], 56 wk)	Nausea, headache, constipation, dizziness, dry mouth, transient increase in blood pressure	NDA not approved because of concerns about long-term cardiovascular safety in February 2012 Manufacturer will be conducting a large randomized cardiovascular outcomes trial with anticipated resubmission in about 2 y
Bupropion-zonisamide (Empatic)	α-melanocyte-stimulating hormone releaser; NMDA receptor antagonist	Orexigen[150]: 360 mg bupropion/120 mg zonisamide: 5.3 kg (24 wk) 360 mg bupropion/360 mg zonisamide: 7.8 kg (24 wk)	Insomnia, headache, nausea	Phase IIb trial completed

Abbreviation: NDA, New Drug Application.
a Trial conducted in pediatric patients (aged 9–16 years).
b Weight losses in this study were reported only as percentages of baseline weight.

weight changes associated with various medications, including many psychotropics. The association is often indirect; weight gain associated with medication will lead to intensified restricting and/or purging, but 2 atypical antipsychotics have also been directly associated with new onset of binge eating.[124] Although not studied specifically in individuals with eating disorders, medication-related weight gain is an important contributor to nonadherence in psychiatric patients in general.[125] Patients with strong drives for thinness are also at risk for misusing medications to produce weight loss. Insulin omission is the most well-known and dangerous example,[126] but there are also reports of topiramate[61] and fluoxetine[127] overuse for the purpose of weight loss. Clinicians should be mindful of the potential impact of psychotropic medications on eating behavior and weight when choosing pharmacologic interventions, discuss this openly with patients, and closely monitor weight, adherence, and the appropriate use of weight-altering medications after they are initiated.

Eating Disorders, Obesity Surgery, and Pharmacokinetics

There have been no studies of pharmacokinetics in patients with eating disorders. However, patients with AN frequently have delayed gastric emptying,[128] which could

---

Summary of psychopharmacologic treatment of obesity and eating disorders in children and adolescents

Most evidence-based treatments for eating disorders are psychosocial. No medications are FDA approved for the treatment of eating disorders in children and adolescents and only one is approved for the treatment of adults (fluoxetine 60 mg/d for BN).

For AN, although clinical trials in adolescents have been negative, olanzapine anecdotally may be helpful for severely ill patients whose symptoms have delusional and hallucinatory qualities and interfere with the benefits from usual treatment. SSRIs are not effective for anorexia either acutely or for relapse prevention and are not beneficial for depression in acutely ill patients, but they may be helpful for comorbid conditions after nutritional rehabilitation is well underway. Oral estrogen is of no benefit for bone loss and may reinforce patients' denial by restoring menses.

For bulimia, fluoxetine at 60 mg/d is the pharmacotherapy of choice because it is approved in adults and there is a small positive trial in adolescents. Topiramate may be an alternative because it has been shown to be effective in adults and is approved for seizure disorders in children.

For binge-eating disorder, the SSRIs are effective in reducing binge eating but not weight in adults. Topiramate is effective in reducing both binge eating and weight, but tolerability has been an issue. There have been promising small trials of duloxetine and atomoxetine, which is approved for the treatment of attention-deficit/hyperactivity disorder in children aged 6 years and older. There are no clinical trials to date in children or adolescents.

Orlistat is FDA approved for the treatment of obesity in children aged 12 years and older. Most adolescents lose more than 5% of body weight, but compliance can be an issue because of gastrointestinal side effects and 3-times-daily dosing. Topiramate has been effective in adults and is approved for another indication in children (see earlier discussion). Metformin is approved for children and adolescents with diabetes and has been studied for obesity, but weight loss is modest. There are several agents in the late stages of development, many of which are new applications of currently marketed medications.

Issues associated with psychiatric comorbidity in eating disorders and obesity relate to (1) the negative impact of the eating disorder on accurate diagnosis and effective treatment, (2) implications of medical complications of eating disorders for choices of pharmacotherapeutic agents, (3) the potential for some psychotropic medications to exacerbate eating disorders and obesity, (4) the risks of medication nonadherence or misuse in patients with eating disorders, and (5) the impact of eating disorders and gastric bypass surgery on pharmacokinetics.

theoretically prolong absorption and time to peak drug concentrations. Patients who purge by self-induced vomiting are at risk for malabsorption if they purge within several hours of taking their medications, and this should be assessed when patients seem not to respond to a medication. Immediately following gastric bypass surgery, patients are at risk for decreased absorption of medications; one study of SSRIs found that the area under the concentration/time curve decreased to an average of 54% of preoperative values, and about half of the patients had depressive relapses.[129] Their drug levels returned to baseline by 6 months.

REFERENCES

1. Cali AM, Caprio S. Obesity in children and adolescents. J Clin Endocrinol Metab 2008;93:s31–6.
2. U.S. Department of Health and Human Services. Overweight and obesity: health consequences. Available at: http://www.surgeongeneral.gov/topics/obesity/calltoaction/fact_consequences.htm. Accessed February 28, 2012.
3. Hudson JI, Hiripi E, Pope HG, et al. The prevalence and correlates of eating disorders in the National Comorbidity Survey Replication. Biol Psychiatry 2007;61:348–58.
4. Nicolls DE, Lynn R, Viner RM. Childhood eating disorders: British national surveillance study. Br J Psychiatry 2011;198:295–301.
5. Peeters A, Barendregt J, Willekens F, et al. Obesity in adulthood and its consequences for life expectancy: a life-table analysis. Ann Intern Med 2003;138:24–32.
6. Reuser M, Bonneux L, Willekens F. The burden of mortality of obesity at middle and old age is small. A life table analysis of the US Health and Retirement Survey. Eur J Epidemiol 2008;23:601–7.
7. Must A, Jacques PF, Dallal GE, et al. Long-term morbidity and mortality of overweight adolescents. A follow-up of the Harvard Growth Study of 1922 to 1935. N Engl J Med 1992;327:1350–5.
8. Bender R, Jockel KH, Trautner C, et al. Effect of age on excess mortality in obesity. JAMA 1999;281:1498–504.
9. Arcelus J, Mitchell AJ, Wales J, et al. Mortality rates in patients with anorexia nervosa and other eating disorders: a meta-analysis of 36 studies. Arch Gen Psychiatry 2011;68:724–31.
10. Kuo C, Chen VC, Lee W, et al. Asthma and suicide mortality in young people: a 12-year follow-up study. Am J Psychiatry 2010;167:1092–9.
11. Feltbower RG, Bodansky HJ, Patterson CC, et al. Acute complications and drug misuse are important causes of death for children and young adults with type 1 diabetes: results from the Yorkshire Register of diabetes in children and young adults. Diabetes Care 2008;31:922–6.
12. Swanson SA, Crow SJ, Le Grange D, et al. Prevalence and correlates of eating disorders in adolescents: results from the national comorbidity survey replication adolescent supplement. Arch Gen Psychiatry 2011;68:714–23.
13. Harris EC, Barraclough B. Excess mortality of mental disorder. Br J Psychiatry 1998;173:11–53.
14. Crow SJ, Mitchell JE, Roerig JD, et al. What potential role is there for medication treatment in anorexia nervosa? Int J Eat Disord 2009;42:1–8.
15. Kaye WH, Weltzin TE, Husu LK, et al. An open trial of fluoxetine in patients with anorexia nervosa. J Clin Psychiatry 1991;52:464–71.
16. Kaye WH, Nagata T, Weltzin TE, et al. Double-blind placebo-controlled administration of fluoxetine in restricting- and restricting-purging-type anorexia nervosa. Biol Psychiatry 2001;49:644–52.

17. Attia E, Haiman C, Walsh BT, et al. Does fluoxetine augment the inpatient treatment of anorexia nervosa? Am J Psychiatry 1998;155:548–51.
18. Strober M, Pataki C, Freeman R, et al. No effect of adjunctive fluoxetine on eating behavior or weight phobia during the inpatient treatment of anorexia nervosa: an historical case-control study. J Child Adolesc Psychopharmacol 1999;9: 195–201.
19. Mischoulon D, Eddy KT, Keshaviah A, et al. Depression and eating disorders: treatment and course. J Affect Disord 2011;130:470–7.
20. Delgado PL, Miller HL, Salomon RM, et al. Tryptophan-depletion challenge in depressed patients treated with desipramine or fluoxetine: implications for the role of serotonin in the mechanism of antidepressant action. Biol Psychiatry 1999;46:212–20.
21. Powers PS, Santana CA, Bannon YS. Olanzapine in the treatment of anorexia nervosa: an open label trial. Int J Eat Disord 2002;32:146–54.
22. Powers PS, Bannon Y, Eubanks R, et al. Quetiapine in anorexia nervosa patients: an open label outpatient pilot study. Int J Eat Disord 2007;40:21–6.
23. Bissada H, Tasca G, Barber A, et al. Olanzapine in the treatment of low body weight and obsessive thinking in women with anorexia nervosa: a randomized, double-blind, placebo-controlled trial. Am J Psychiatry 2008;165:1281–8.
24. Kafantaris V, Leigh F, Hertz S, et al. A placebo-controlled pilot study of adjunctive olanzapine for adolescents with anorexia nervosa. J Child Adolesc Psychopharmacol 2011;21:207–12.
25. Norris M, Spettigue W, Buchholz A, et al. Olanzapine use for the adjunctive treatment of adolescents with anorexia nervosa. J Child Adolesc Psychopharmacol 2011;21:213–20.
26. Powers PS, Klabunde M, Kaye W. Double blind placebo-controlled trial of quetiapine in anorexia nervosa: a negative study. Eur Eat Disord Rev 2012;20: 331–4.
27. Hagman J, Gralla J, Sigel E, et al. A double-blind, placebo-controlled study of risperidone for the treatment of adolescents and young adults with anorexia nervosa: a pilot study. J Am Acad Child Adolesc Psychiatry 2011;50:854–6.
28. Trunko ME, Schwartz TA, Duvvuri V, et al. Aripiprazole in anorexia nervosa and low-weight bulimia nervosa: case reports. Int J Eat Disord 2011;44:269–75.
29. Powers PS, Simpson H, McCormick KT. Anorexia nervosa and psychosis. Prim Psychiatr 2005;45:39–45.
30. Frank GK, Bailer UF, Henry SE, et al. Increased dopamine D2/D3 receptor binding after recovery from anorexia nervosa measured by positron emission tomography and [11c]raclopride. Biol Psychiatry 2005;58:908–12.
31. Kaye WH, Frank GK, McConaha C. Altered dopamine activity after recovery from restricting-type anorexia nervosa. Neuropsychopharmacology 1999;21:503–6.
32. Kishi T, Kafantaris V, Sunday S, et al. Are antipsychotics effective for the treatment of anorexia nervosa? Results from a systematic review and meta-analysis. J Clin Psychiatry 2012;73(6):e757–66.
33. Mehler P, Clary BS, Gaudiani JL. Osteoporosis in anorexia nervosa. Eat Disord 2011;19:194–202.
34. Mehler PS, MacKenzie TD. Treatment of osteopenia and osteoporosis in anorexia nervosa: a systematic review of the literature. Int J Eat Disord 2009; 42:195–201.
35. Misra M, Katzman D, Miller KK, et al. Physiological estrogen replacement increases bone density in adolescent girls with anorexia nervosa. J Bone Miner Res 2011;26:2430–8.

36. Institute of Medicine Report Brief. Dietary reference intakes for calcium and vitamin D. 2010. Available at: http://www.iom.edu/~/media/Files/Report%20 Files/2010/Dietary-Reference-Intakes-for-Calcium-and-Vitamin-D/Vitamin%20D %20and%20Calcium%202010%20Report%20Brief.pdf. Accessed March 21, 2012.
37. Abrahamsen B. Bisphosphonate adverse effects, lessons from large databases. Curr Opin Rheumatol 2010;22:404–9.
38. Czerwinski E. Atypical subtrochanteric fractures after long-term bisphosphonate therapy. Endokrynol Pol 2011;62:84–7.
39. Silverman SL. Identifying patients at risk for osteoporotic fracture: FRAX and the new NOF guidelines. Menopause Management 2009;18:14–7.
40. Zipfel S, Sammet I, Rapps R, et al. Gastrointestinal disturbances in eating disorders: clinical and neurobiological aspects. Auton Neurosci 2006;129:99–106.
41. Mehler PS. Bulimia nervosa. N Engl J Med 2003;349:875–81.
42. Work group on eating disorders. Practice guideline for the treatment of eating disorders. 3rd edition. American Psychiatric Association; 2006. Available at: http://psychiatryonline.org/data/Books/prac/EatingDisorders3ePG_04-28-06.pdf. Accessed February 25, 2012.
43. Kaye WH. Neurobiology of anorexia and bulimia nervosa. Physiol Behav 2008; 94:121–35.
44. Fluoxetine Bulimia Nervosa Study Group. Fluoxetine in the treatment of bulimia nervosa: a multi-centered, placebo-controlled, double-blind trial. Arch Gen Psychiatry 1992;49:139–47.
45. Sysko R, Sha N, Wang Y, et al. Early response to antidepressant treatment in bulimia nervosa. Psychol Med 2010;40:999–1005.
46. Goldstein DH, Wilson MG, Ashcroft RC, et al. Effectiveness of fluoxetine therapy in bulimia nervosa regardless of comorbid depression. Int J Eat Disord 1999;25: 19–27.
47. Romano SH, Halmi KA, Sarkar NP, et al. A placebo-controlled study of fluoxetine in continued treatment of bulimia nervosa after successful acute fluoxetine treatment. Am J Psychiatry 2002;159:96–102.
48. Agras WS. Pharmacotherapy of bulimia nervosa and binge eating disorder: longer-term outcomes. Psychopharmacol Bull 1997;33:433–6.
49. Kotler LA, Devlin MJ, Davies M, et al. An open trial of fluoxetine for adolescents with bulimia nervosa. J Child Adolesc Psychopharmacol 2003;13:329–35.
50. Milano W, Siano C, Petrella C, et al. Treatment of bulimia nervosa with fluvoxamine: a randomized controlled trial. Adv Ther 2005;22:278–83.
51. Milano W, Petrella C, Sabatino C, et al. Treatment of bulimia nervosa with sertraline: a randomized controlled trial. Adv Ther 2004;21:232–7.
52. Schmidt U, Cooper PJ, Essers H, et al. Fluvoxamine and graded psychotherapy in the treatment of bulimia nervosa: a randomized, double-blind, placebo-controlled, multicenter study of short-term and long-term pharmacotherapy combined with a stepped care approach to psychotherapy. J Clin Psychopharmacol 2005;24:549–52.
53. Sundblad C, Landen M, Eriksson T, et al. Effects of the androgen antagonist flutamide and the serotonin reuptake inhibitor citalopram in bulimia nervosa: a placebo-controlled pilot study. J Clin Psychopharmacol 2005;25:85–8.
54. Gibbons RD, Brown H, Hur K, et al. Suicidal thoughts and behavior with antidepressant treatment: re-analysis of the randomized placebo-controlled trials with fluoxetine and venlafaxine. Arch Gen Psychiatry 2012;69:580–7. http://dx.doi.org/10.1001/archgenpsychiatry.2011.2048.

55. U.S. Food and Drug Administration (FDA). FDA launches a multi-pronged strategy to strengthen safeguards for children treated with antidepressant medications. 2004. Available at: http://www.fda.gov/NewsEvents/Newsroom/PressAnnouncements/2004/ucm108363.htm. Accessed February 25, 2012.

56. U.S.Food and Drug Administration. FDA proposes new warnings about suicidal thinking, behavior in young adults who take antidepressant medications. 2007. Available at: http://www.fda.gov/NewsEvents/Newsroom/PressAnnouncements/2007/ucm108905.htm. Accessed February 25, 2012.

57. U.S. Food and Drug Administration. Medication guide: about using antidepressant medications in children and teenagers. 2005. Available at: http://www.fda.gov/downloads/drugs/drugsafety/informationbydrugclass/UCM161646.pdf. Accessed February 26, 2012.

58. Stanley BG, Willett VL, Donias HW, et al. Lateral hypothalamic NMDA receptors and glutamate as physiological mediators of eating and weight control. Am J Physiol 1996;270(2 Pt 2):R443–9.

59. Hoopes SP, Reimherr FW, Hedges DW, et al. Treatment of bulimia nervosa with topiramate in a randomized, double-blind, placebo-controlled trial, part 1: improvement in binge and purge measures. J Clin Psychiatry 2003;64:1335–41.

60. Nickel C, Tritt K, Muehlbacher M, et al. Topiramate treatment in bulimia nervosa patients: a randomized, double-blind, placebo-controlled trial. Int J Eat Disord 2005;38:295–300.

61. Colom F, Vieta E, Benabarre A, et al. Topiramate abuse in a bipolar patient with an eating disorder. J Clin Psychiatry 2001;62:475–6.

62. Jonas JM, Gold MS. The use of opiate antagonists in treating bulimia: a study of low-dose versus high-dose naltrexone. Psychiatry Res 1988;24:195–9.

63. Marrazzi MA, Bacon JP, Kinzie J, et al. Naltrexone use in the treatment of anorexia nervosa and bulimia nervosa. Int Clin Psychopharmacol 1995;10:163–72.

64. Mitchell JE, Christenson G, Jennings J, et al. A placebo-controlled, double-blind crossover study of naltrexone hydrochloride in outpatients with normal weight bulimia. J Clin Psychopharmacol 1989;9:94–7.

65. Faris FL, Kim SW, Meller WH, et al. Effect of decreasing afferent vagal activity with ondansetron on symptoms of bulimia nervosa: a randomised, double-blind trial. Lancet 2000;355:792–7.

66. Guardia D, Rolland B, Karila L, et al. GABAergic and glutamatergic modulation in binge eating: therapeutic approach. Curr Pharm Des 2011;17:1396–409.

67. Brennan BP, Roberts JL, Fogarty KV, et al. Memantine in the treatment of binge eating disorder: an open-label, prospective trial. Int J Eat Disord 2008;41:520–6.

68. Grant JE, Odlaug BL, Kim SW. N-acetylcysteine, a glutamate modulator, in the treatment of trichotillomania: a double-blind, placebo-controlled study. Arch Gen Psychiatry 2009;66:756–63.

69. Braun DL, Sunday SR, Fornari VM, et al. Bright light therapy decreases winter binge frequency in women with bulimia nervosa: a double-blind, placebo-controlled study. Compr Psychiatry 1999;40:442–8.

70. Blouin AG, Blouin JH, Iversen H, et al. Light therapy in bulimia nervosa: a double-blind, placebo-controlled study. Psychiatry Res 1996;60:1–9.

71. Lam RW, Goldner EM, Solyom L, et al. A controlled study of light therapy for bulimia nervosa. Am J Psychiatry 1994;151:744–50.

72. DSM-V Work Group on Eating Disorders. Binge eating disorder proposed revision. Available at: http://www.dsm5.org/ProposedRevisions/Pages/proposedrevision.aspx?rid=372#. Accessed March 3, 2012.

73. Fairburn CG, Cooper Z, Doll HA, et al. The natural course of bulimia nervosa and binge eating disorder in young women. Arch Gen Psychiatry 2000;57: 659–65.

74. Arnold LM, McElroy SL, Hudson JI, et al. A placebo-controlled, randomized trial of fluoxetine in the treatment of binge-eating disorder. J Clin Psychiatry 2002;63: 1028–33.

75. Grilo CM, Masheb RM, Wilson GT. Efficacy of cognitive behavioral therapy and fluoxetine for the treatment of binge eating disorder: a randomized double-blind placebo-controlled comparison. Biol Psychiatry 2005;57:301–9.

76. Hudson JI, McElroy SL, Raymond NC, et al. Fluvoxamine in the treatment of binge-eating disorder: a multicenter placebo-controlled, double-blind trial. Am J Psychiatry 1998;155:1756–62.

77. Pearlstein T, Spurell E, Hohlstein LA, et al. A double-blind, placebo-controlled trial of fluvoxamine in binge eating disorder: a high placebo response. Arch Womens Ment Health 2003;6:147–51.

78. Guerdjikova AI, McElroy SL, Kotwal R, et al. High-dose escitalopram in the treatment of binge-eating disorder with obesity: a placebo-controlled monotherapy trial. Hum Psychopharmacol 2008;23:1–11.

79. McElroy SL, Hudson JI, Malhotra S, et al. Citalopram in the treatment of binge-eating disorder: a placebo-controlled trial. J Clin Psychiatry 2003;64:807–13.

80. McElroy SL, Casuto LS, Nelson EB, et al. Placebo-controlled trial of sertraline in the treatment of binge eating disorder. Am J Psychiatry 2000;157:1004–6.

81. Guerdjikova AI, McElroy SL, Winstanley ER, et al. Duloxetine in the treatment of binge eating disorder with depressive disorders: a placebo-controlled trial. Int J Eat Disord 2012;45:281–9.

82. McElroy SL, Guerdjikova A, Kotwal R, et al. Atomoxetine in the treatment of binge-eating disorder: a randomized placebo-controlled trial. J Clin Psychiatry 2007;68:390–8.

83. Claudino AM, de Oliveira IR, Appolinario JC, et al. Double-blind, randomized, placebo-controlled trial of topiramate plus cognitive-behavior therapy in binge-eating disorder. J Clin Psychiatry 2007;68:1324–32.

84. McElroy SL, Hudson JI, Capece JA, et al. Topiramate for the treatment of binge eating disorder associated with obesity: a placebo-controlled study. Biol Psychiatry 2007;61:1039–48.

85. McElroy SL, Arnold LM, Shapira NA, et al. Topiramate in the treatment of binge eating disorder associated with obesity: a randomized, placebo controlled trial. Am J Psychiatry 2003;160:255–61.

86. McElroy SL, Kotwal R, Guerdjikova AI, et al. Zonisamide in the treatment of binge eating disorder with obesity: a randomized controlled trial. J Clin Psychiatry 2006;67:1897–906.

87. Guerdjikova AI, McElroy SL, Welge JA, et al. Lamotrigine in the treatment of binge-eating disorder with obesity: a randomized, placebo-controlled monotherapy trial. Int Clin Psychopharmacol 2009;24:150–8.

88. McElroy SL, Guerdjikova AI, Winstanley EL, et al. Acamprosate in the treatment of binge eating disorder: a placebo-controlled trial. Int J Eat Disord 2011;44: 81–90.

89. Mechanick JI, Kushner RF, Sugerman HJ, et al. American Association of Clinical Endocrinologists, The Obesity Society, and American Society for Metabolic & Bariatric Surgery medical guidelines for clinical practice for the perioperative nutritional, metabolic, and nonsurgical support of the bariatric surgery patient. Obesity (Silver Spring) 2009;17(Suppl 1):S1–70.

90. Alger-Mayer S, Rosati C, Polimeni JM, et al. Preoperative binge eating status and gastric bypass surgery: a long-term outcome study. Obes Surg 2009;19: 139–45.
91. Boan J, Kolotkin RL, Westman EC, et al. Binge eating, quality of life and physical activity improve after Roux-en-Y gastric bypass for morbid obesity. Obes Surg 2004;14:341–8.
92. Kalarchian MA, Wilson GT, Brolin RE, et al. Effects of bariatric surgery on binge eating and related psychopathology. Eat Weight Disord 1999;4:1–5.
93. Wadden TA, Faulconbridge LF, Jones-Corneille LR, et al. Binge eating disorder and the outcome of bariatric surgery at one year: a prospective, observational study. Obesity (Silver Spring) 2011;19:1220–8.
94. Kersh R, Stroup DF, Taylor WC. Childhood obesity: a framework for policy approaches and ethical considerations. Prev Chronic Dis 2011;8(5):A93. Available at: http://www.cdc.gov/pcd/issues/2011/sep/10_0273.htm. Accessed March 9, 2012.
95. Barlow SE. Expert committee recommendations regarding the prevention, assessment, and treatment of child and adolescent overweight and obesity: summary report. Pediatrics 2007;120:S164.
96. McGovern L, Johnson JN, Paulo R, et al. Treatment of pediatric obesity: a systematic review and meta-analysis of randomized trials. J Clin Endocrinol Metab 2008;93:4600–5.
97. Lenard NR, Berthoud H. Central and peripheral regulation of food intake and physical activity: pathways and genes. Obesity (Silver Spring) 2008;16(Suppl 3): S11–22.
98. Cotrome L. Miracle pills for weight loss: what is the number needed to treat, number needed to harm and likelihood to be helped or harmed for naltrexone-bupropion combination? Int J Clin Pract 2010;64:1461–71.
99. McDuffie JR, Calis KA, Booth SL, et al. Effects of orlistat on fat-soluble vitamins in obese adolescents. Pharmacotherapy 2002;22:814–22.
100. Hagler RA. Orlistat misuse as purging in a patient with binge-eating disorder. Psychosomatics 2009;50:177–8.
101. Malhotra S, McElroy SL. Orlistat misuse in bulimia nervosa. Am J Psychiatry 2002;159:492–3.
102. Fernández-Aranda F, Amor A, Jiménez-Murcia S, et al. Bulimia nervosa and misuse of orlistat: two case reports. Int J Eat Disord 2001;30:458–61.
103. Diabetes Prevention Program Research Group. Reduction in the incidence of type 2 diabetes with lifestyle intervention and metformin. N Engl J Med 2002; 346:393–403.
104. Kramer CK, Leitão CB, Pinto LC, et al. Efficacy and safety of topiramate on weight loss: a meta-analysis of randomized controlled trials. Obes Rev 2011; 12:e338–47.
105. Haddock CK, Poston WS, Dill PL, et al. Pharmacotherapy for obesity: a quantitative analysis of four decades of published randomized clinical trials. Int J Obes Relat Metab Disord 2002;26:262–73.
106. Andelman MB, Jones C, Nathan S. Treatment of obesity in underprivileged adolescents. Comparison of diethylpropion hydrochloride with placebo in a double-blind study. Clin Pediatr (Phila) 1967;6:327–30.
107. Li Z, Maglione M, Tu W, et al. Meta-analysis: pharmacologic treatment of obesity. Ann Intern Med 2005;142:532–46.
108. Singh-Franco D, Perez A, Harrington C. The effect of pramlintide acetate on glycemic control and weight in patients with type 2 diabetes mellitus and in obese

patients without diabetes: a systematic review and meta-analysis. Diabetes Obes Metab 2011;13:169–80.

109. Witkamp RF. Current and future drug targets in weight management. Pharm Res 2011;28:1792–818.

110. Powell AG, Apovian CM, Aronne LJ. New drug targets for the treatment of obesity. Clin Pharmacol Ther 2011;90:40–51.

111. Järvholm K, Olbers T, Marcus C, et al. Short-term psychological outcomes in severely obese adolescents after bariatric surgery. Obesity (Silver Spring) 2012;20:318–23.

112. Aikenhead A, Lobstein T, Knai C. Review of current guidelines on adolescent bariatric surgery. Clinical Obesity 2011;1:3–11.

113. Bondada S, Jen HC, DeUgarte DA. Outcomes of bariatric surgery in adolescents. Curr Opin Pediatr 2011;23:552–6.

114. Treadwell JR, Sun F, Schoelles K. Systematic review and meta-analysis of bariatric surgery for pediatric obesity. Ann Surg 2008;248:763–6.

115. Keys A, Brozek J, Henschel A, et al. The biology of human starvation, vols. 1–2. Minneapolis (MN): University of Minnesota Press; 1950.

116. Pirke KM, Pahl J, Schweiger U, et al. Metabolic and endocrine indices of starvation in bulimia: a comparison with anorexia nervosa. Psychiatry Res 1985;15: 33–9.

117. Woodside BD, Staab R. Management of psychiatric comorbidity in anorexia nervosa and bulimia nervosa. CNS Drugs 2006;20:655–63.

118. Ricca V, Mannucci E, Paionni A, et al. Venlafaxine versus fluoxetine in the treatment of atypical anorectic outpatients: a preliminary study. Eat Weight Disord 1999;4:10–4.

119. Altman SE, Shankman SA. What is the association between obsessive-compulsive disorder and eating disorders. Clin Psychol Rev 2009;29:638–46.

120. Caserio D, Frishman WH. Cardiovascular complications of eating disorders. Cardiol Rev 2006;14:227–31.

121. Maine M, Goldberg MH. The role of third molar surgery in the exacerbation of eating disorders. J Oral Maxillofac Surg 2001;59:1297–300.

122. Zerbe KJ. Recurrent pancreatitis presenting as fever of unknown origin in a recovering bulimic. Int J Eat Disord 1992;12:337–40.

123. Powers PS, Cloak N. Medication-related weight changes: impact on treatment of eating disorder patients. In: Yager J, Powers P, editors. Clinical manual of eating disorders. Washington, DC: American Psychiatric Publishing, Inc; 2007. p. 143–61.

124. Kluge M, Schuld A, Himmerich H, et al. Clozapine and olanzapine are associated with food craving and binge eating: results from a randomized double-blind study. J Clin Psychopharmacol 2007;27:662–6.

125. Weiden PJ, Mackell JA, McDonnell DD. Obesity as a risk factor for antipsychotic noncompliance. Schizophr Res 2004;66:51–7.

126. Takii M, Uchigata Y, Tokunaga S, et al. The duration of severe insulin omission is the factor most closely associated with the microvascular complications of type 1 diabetic females with clinical eating disorders. Int J Eat Disord 2008;41: 259–64.

127. Wilcox JA. Abuse of fluoxetine by a patient with anorexia nervosa [letter]. Am J Psychiatry 1987;144:1100.

128. Benini L, Todesco T, Dalle Grave R, et al. Gastric emptying in patients with restricting and binge/purging subtypes of anorexia nervosa. Am J Gastroenterol 2004;99:1448–54.

129. Hamad GG, Helsel JC, Perel JM, et al. The effect of gastric bypass on the pharmacokinetics of selective serotonin reuptake inhibitors. Am J Psychiatry 2012; 169:256–63.

130. Lock J, Le Grange D, Agras WS, et al. Randomized clinical trial comparing family based treatment with adolescent-focused individual therapy for adolescents with anorexia nervosa. Arch Gen Psychiatry 2010;67:1025–32.

131. Agras WS, Schneider JA, Arnow B, et al. Cognitive-behavioral and response-prevention treatments for bulimia nervosa. J Consult Clin Psychol 1989;57: 215–21.

132. Fairburn CG, Jones R, Peveler RC, et al. Psychotherapy and bulimia nervosa: longer-term effects of interpersonal therapy, behavior therapy, and cognitive behavior therapy. Arch Gen Psychiatry 1993;50:419–28.

133. Carter JC, Olmsted MO, Kaplan AS, et al. Self-help for bulimia nervosa: a randomized controlled trial. Am J Psychiatry 2003;160:973–6.

134. Grilo CM, Masheb RM, Wilson GT, et al. Cognitive-behavioral therapy, behavioral weight loss, and sequential treatment for obese patients with binge-eating disorder: a randomized controlled trial. J Consult Clin Psychol 2011;79: 675–85.

135. Carter JC, Fairburn CG. Cognitive-behavioral self-help for binge eating disorder: a controlled effectiveness study. J Consult Clin Psychol 1998;66:616–23.

136. Rosenstock J, Klaff LJ, Schwartz S, et al. Effects of exenatide and lifestyle modification on body weight and glucose tolerance in obese subjects with and without pre-diabetes. Diabetes Care 2010;33:1173–5.

137. Dushay J, Gao C, Gopalakrishnan GS, et al. Short-term exenatide treatment leads to significant weight loss in a subset of obese women without diabetes. Diabetes Care 2012;35:4–11.

138. Kely AS, Metzig AM, Ridser KD, et al. Exenatide as a weight loss therapy in extreme pediatric obesity: a randomized, controlled pilot study. Obesity (Silver Spring) 2012;20:364–70.

139. Astrup A, Rössner S, Van Gaal L, et al. Effects of liraglutide in the treatment of obesity: a randomised, double-blind, placebo-controlled study. Lancet 2009; 374(9701):1606–16.

140. Smith SR, Weissman NJ, Andersen CM, et al. Multicenter, placebo-controlled trial of lorcaserin for weight management. N Engl J Med 2010;363:245–56.

141. Fidler MC, Sanchez M, Raether B, et al. A one-year randomized trial of lorcaserin for weight loss in obese and overweight adults: the BLOSSOM trial. J Clin Endocrinol Metab 2011;96:3067–77.

142. O'Neil P, Smith SR, Weissman NJ, et al. Randomized placebo-controlled clinical trial of lorcaserin for weight loss in type 2 diabetes mellitus: the BLOOM-DM study. Obesity (Silver Spring) 2012;20(7):1426–36. http://dx.doi.org/10.1038/oby2012.66.

143. NeuroSearch A/S. NeuroSearch reports on scientific advice received from the FDA and EMA concerning the clinical development programme for tesofensine. 2011. Available at: http://www.cisionwire.com/neurosearch-a-s-g/r/neurosearch-reports-on-scientific-advice-received-from-the-fda-and-ema-concerning-the-clinical-development-programme-for-tesofensine,e236452. Accessed March 17, 2012.

144. Vivus, Inc. Qnexa meets primary endpoint by demonstrating superior weight loss over components and placebo in the 28-week Equate study (OB-301). 2008. Available at: http://ir.vivus.com/releasedetail.cfm?ReleaseID=353965. Accessed March 7, 2012.

145. Allison DB, Gadde KM, Garvey WT, et al. Controlled-release phentermine/topiramate in severely obese adults: a randomized controlled trial (EQUIP). Obesity (Silver Spring) 2012;20:330–42.

146. Gadde KM, Allison DB, Ryan DH, et al. Effects of low-dose, controlled-release, phentermine plus topiramate combination on weight and associated comorbidities in overweight and obese adults (CONQUER): a randomised, placebo-controlled, phase 3 trial. Lancet 2011;377:1341–52.

147. Greenway FL, Dunayevich E, Tollefson G, et al. Comparison of combined bupropion and naltrexone therapy for obesity with monotherapy and placebo. J Clin Endocrinol Metab 2009;94:4898–906.

148. Greenway FL, Fujioka K, Plotkowski RA, et al. Effects of naltrexone plus bupropion on weight loss in overweight and obese adults (COR-I): a multicentre, randomised, double-blind, placebo-controlled, phase 3 trial. Lancet 2010;376: 595–605.

149. Wadden TA, Foreyt JP, Foster GD, et al. Weight loss with naltrexone SR/bupropion SR combination therapy as an adjunct to behavior modification: the COR-BMOD trial. Obesity (Silver Spring) 2011;19:110–20.

150. Orexigen Therapeutics Inc. Orexigen Therapeutics Phase 2b trial for Empatic meets primary efficacy endpoint demonstrating significantly greater weight loss versus comparators in obese patients. 2009. Available at: http://ir.orexigen.com/phoenix.zhtml?c=207034&p=irol-newsArticle&ID=1336796&highlight=. Accessed March 19, 2012.

Pediatric Sleep Pharmacology

Rafael Pelayo, MD*, Kin Yuen, MD, MS

KEYWORDS

- Sleep disorders • Sleep apnea • Narcolepsy • Insomnia • Sedation
- Off-label medications

KEY POINTS

- The most common pharmacologic options in the treatment of sleep disorders in youth are reviewed.
- Knowledge of sleep physiology and pathophysiology is necessary for the pharmacologic management of sleep disorders.
- Most children with sleep disorders improve with proper treatment.
- A key principal in sleep pharmacology is that sedation is not the equivalent of normal refreshing sleep.
- Behavioral treatment should be considered before initiating pharmacotherapy. A combined approach may be necessary.
- Clonidine is commonly prescribed despite the absence of randomized control trials supporting its use in youth and despite lacking an indication for insomnia in adults.
- Paradoxic drug reactions can occur from incorrect doses or incorrect timing of administration of medications.

OVERVIEW OF PEDIATRIC SLEEP DISORDERS

This article reviews common sleep disorders in children and pharmacologic options for them. Discussions of pediatric sleep pharmacology typically focus on treatment of insomnia.[1–3] Although insomnia is a major concern in this population, there are other conditions that warrant review. Narcolepsy, parasomnias, restless legs syndrome (RLS), and sleep apnea are also discussed here.

GENERAL PRINCIPLES OF PEDIATRIC SLEEP PHARMACOLOGY
Sleep Development in Youth

Although the need for sleep is biologic, the way people sleep is learned. Children learn how to sleep or form associations with sleep based on their families. As the child is

Stanford Sleep Medicine Center, Department of Psychiatry, Stanford University School of Medicine, 450 Broadway Street, Redwood City, CA 94063, USA
* Corresponding author.
E-mail address: pelayo@stanford.edu

Child Adolesc Psychiatric Clin N Am 21 (2012) 861–883
http://dx.doi.org/10.1016/j.chc.2012.08.001
1056-4993/12/$ – see front matter © 2012 Elsevier Inc. All rights reserved.

readied for bed, the child may associate sleep onset with particular events. If the child associates parental attention or activity with sleep, any awakenings during the night may then necessitate parental attention. If returning the child to sleep requires frequent parental assistance, the parents' sleep is disturbed and contributes to the family dreading the nighttime hours.

Parental Expectations and Sleep Disorders

All discussions of pediatric sleep pharmacology need to take into account the cultural background of the family. The parents need to agree about their expectations of the child's sleep, especially if the parents have different cultural backgrounds. The parents' own prior sleep experiences both in childhood and as adults should be explored. In addition, the influence of other family members, such as grandparents, in shaping the family's views should be considered. If the child lives in 2 separate households, as can typically occur with divorce, is the sleep problem present in both homes or are there differences? Will any prescribed medication be given in both homes?

The importance of a review of parental expectations and understanding of normal sleep cannot be overstated before starting a discussion of medication. A parent may be complaining about a child's sleep because it is exacerbating the parents' untreated sleep disorder. Parental referral for sleep issues may be most appropriate in diagnosing and treating the parent's sleep disorder.

Off-label Medications for Sleep

Various medications are used off-label to treat sleep disorders in youth, such as clonidine.[3–6] Clonidine does not carry an indication for insomnia nor is it typically prescribed for adult sleep disorders. However, clonidine is prescribed commonly for children with insomnia. This practice is almost routine despite the absence of any randomized control trials supporting its use. Stojanovski and colleagues[6] examined US outpatient trends in physician prescribing of medications for children with sleep difficulties using data from 18.6 million patient visits in the National Ambulatory Medical Care Survey (NAMCS). During the study period, 81% of children and only 48% of adults received a prescription medication. Most commonly prescribed to children were antihistamines and clonidine. More concerning is the practice of using antipsychotics, such as quetiapine, for sleep. Treatments for children should ideally be evidence based.

Special Considerations in Pediatric Sleep Medications

The paucity of evidence-based pharmacologic guidelines for sleep disorders in children may be caused by the inherent difficulty of the clinical situation. A key principal in sleep pharmacology is not to equate sedation with normal refreshing sleep. Alcohol is a good example, because consuming large amounts of alcohol can be sedating, but the user does not wake up feeling refreshed. There may be an overreliance on the effects of the medication without adequate understanding of the cause of the poor sleep or the appropriate application of behavioral techniques to help improve the child's sleep.

Pediatric Sleep Medication Reactions

A common scenario in clinical practice is a parent's complaint of a child's paradoxic reaction to a hypnotic medication. The parent may state, "He did not sleep at all" or "he became hyper." Insufficient dose or incorrect timing of administration are more likely causes for the absence of efficacy and/or adverse reactions. Humans have a circadian surge in alertness in the evening, the so-called second wind. If a sleep medication is given too early, then it has to counter this circadian alerting. The child may become disinhibited, behave inappropriately, or have frightening hypnagogic hallucinations but still remain awake.[2] Hypnotics should be given on an empty stomach, because food delays the absorption. If the medication is given too early in the evening, the child may not be sleepy enough for the medication to work or it may fail to be adequately absorbed.

Pediatric Sleep Medication Dosage

When prescribing a medication for a child, there is a natural inclination to give the lowest dose possible. However, children may have faster hepatic metabolism resulting in faster elimination of the medication.[7] If the dose of the agent is too low, the medication may alter the child's behavior, but not help the child fall asleep. If a medication only makes the child drowsy without inducing sleep, then frightening hypnagogic hallucinations may occur. This experience might be particularly disturbing in children with an underlying psychiatric or neurologic condition. Given the resulting confusion or disorientation caused by incorrect use of a sedating medication, parents may report paradoxic reactions.

Please refer to **Table 1** for a review of all medications discussed in this article. Unless otherwise indicated in the text, these medications are not US Food and Drug Administration (FDA) indicated for specific sleep disorders in children.

INSOMNIA

Insomnia is characterized in adults by difficulty falling asleep and/or staying asleep, with associated subjective daytime impairment. In children, it is the parent who leads the family to seek medical attention. The young child may awaken for any number of reasons and eventually falls asleep again; however, the parent's sleep schedule is disrupted. The medical history is incomplete without a discussion of what the parents' sleep was like before they were parents. If the parents had any prior sleep impairment, such as mild sleep apnea, they will have greater difficulty handling the typical sleep disruptions of parenthood. In general, behavior techniques should be the mainstay of treatment.[8] Medications may have a role as an adjunct in the insomnia management.

Pharmacologic Treatment of Insomnia in Children

Antihistamines

Among antihistamines, diphenhydramine is commonly used to treat insomnia. Other H_1 antihistamines are similarly used for their sedative effects because they are lipid soluble and pass through the blood-brain-barrier.[9] Ethanolamines and phenothiazines have marked sedative effects, whereas ethylenediamines cause moderate sedation, and alkylamines mild sedation.[10] However, centrally acting H_1 antagonists have also been shown to have convulsant effects, especially in young children, and overdosage has been associated with seizure and death.[11] These agents may worsen obstructive sleep apnea (OSA), and also may suppress rapid eye movement (REM) sleep.[12]

Diphenhydramine

Diphenhydramine is a competitive H_1-histamine receptor blocker and is rapidly absorbed. Peak blood and tissue levels are achieved within 2 hours of ingestion. When given shortly before bedtime, a significant decrease in sleep latency time and number of awakenings can be achieved. The duration of activity following an average

Table 1
Selected medications for sleep disorders in children

Medication	Dose	Side Effects	Potential Application	Contraindications	Clinical Trials
Diphenhydramine	Adults: 25–50 mg Children: 0.5 mg/kg, 25 mg maximum	Sedation, anticholinergic effects	Transient insomnia	Effects enhanced by other CNS depressants, should not be used in newborn infants, or glaucoma	Yes
Choral hydrate	25–50 mg/kg/dose, 1 g maximum	Sedation, respiratory suppression	Transient insomnia	Hepatic disease, drug interactions with fluoxetine and stimulants	No
Eszopiclone	1–3 mg	Sedation, bad taste, headaches	Insomnia	History of benzodiazepine abuse	Yes in adults only
Zolpidem	Immediate release, 5–10 mg; extended release, 6.25–12 mg	Sedation, headaches	Insomnia	History of benzodiazepine abuse	Yes in adults only
Zaleplon	5–10 mg	Sedation, dizziness	Insomnia	History of benzodiazepine abuse	Yes in adults only
Melatonin	0.3–5 mg	Headaches	Delayed sleep phase syndrome, sleep-onset insomnia	Autoimmune diseases	Yes

Pramipexole	0.125–1.0 mg	Nausea, sedation, hypotension	RLS	Known hypersensitivity	Yes in adults only
Ropinirole	0.25–1.0 mg	Nausea, sedation	RLS	Known hypersensitivity	Yes in adults only
Montelukast	15 y and older: one 10-mg tablet 6–14 y: one 5-mg chewable tablet 2–5 y: one 4-mg chewable tablet or 1 packet of 4-mg oral granules	Upper respiratory infection, fever, headache, pharyngitis, cough, abdominal pain	Adjunct for OSA	Develop neuropsychiatric symptoms	Yes
Sodium oxybate	4–9 g divided in 2 doses during the night	Sedation, enuresis, nausea	Narcolepsy	Associated with substance abuse; contraindicated in succinic semialdehyde dehydrogenase deficiency; sodium load is a relative contraindication for hypertension, heart, and kidney disease	Yes in adults only
Modafinil	50–200 mg	Headaches, drug rashes	Narcolepsy	Drug interactions with oral contraceptives	Yes

Abbreviation: CNS, central nervous system.

dose of diphenhydramine is 4 to 6 hours.[13] A plasma diphenhydramine level exceeding 30 ng/mL produces drowsiness.[13,14] The half-life in children is 5.4 ± 1.8 hours; shorter than reported in adults.[15] The recommended dosage for adults is 25 to 50 mg, whereas in children the effective dose is between 0.5 mg/kg and 25 mg.

A randomized controlled trial of infants' responses to diphenhydramine, the Trial of Infant Response to Diphenhydramine (TIRED) study,[16] was terminated early because of lack of effectiveness of diphenhydramine compared with placebo. Only 1 of 22 infants receiving diphenhydramine showed improvement, compared with 3 of 22 receiving placebo. The study concluded that, during 1 week of therapy and at follow-up 2 and 4 weeks later, diphenhydramine was no more effective than placebo in reducing nighttime awakening or improving overall parental satisfaction with sleep for infants.[16]

Adverse effects of diphenhydramine

The most common adverse reaction to diphenhydramine at therapeutic doses is impaired consciousness. The predominant features in an overdose are anticholinergic effects, including fever, mydriasis, blurred vision, dry mouth, constipation, urinary retention, tachycardia, dystonia, and confusion. Other common symptoms of diphenhydramine poisoning include catatonic stupor, anxiety, and visual hallucinations.[17] Rare presentations include respiratory insufficiency, rhabdomyolysis, cardiac rhythm disturbances, and seizures.[17–19]

Diphenhydramine toxicity

Fatal intoxications with diphenhydramine in 5 infants were reported in a case series by Baker and colleagues.[11] The infants were 6, 8, and 9 weeks old and 2 were 12 weeks old. Postmortem blood diphenhydramine levels were 1.6, 1.5, 1.6, and 1.1 mg/L, respectively. In 1 case, the child's father admitted giving the infant diphenhydramine in an attempt to induce the infant to sleep; in another case, a daycare provider admitted putting diphenhydramine in the baby's bottle.[11]

HYPNOTICS
Chloral Hydrate

Chloral hydrate (CH) is a commonly used sedative hypnotic, and it is often prescribed to both children and adults. It causes drowsiness and sedation, then sleep within 1 hour. The plasma half-life is 8 to 12 hours in older children and adults, but for neonates and infants is 3 to 4 times longer.[20] Usual doses ranges between 25 and 50 mg/kg/dose up to a maximum of 1 g per dose by mouth or as needed. Higher doses, 80 to 100 mg/kg, have been given to children younger than 5 years with good effect and minimal toxicity. Neonatal dosing may need adjustment, particularly when used in a multidose fashion.[20]

Adverse effects of CH

Therapeutic doses reduce blood pressure minimally and suppress respirations slightly, but protective airway reflexes are not affected. Children with OSA, wheezing, Leigh disease, or other encephalic white matter or brain stem disorders may be at increased risk for respiratory compromise.[20] CH may similarly be contraindicated in children who are also on stimulants, because of rare reports of malignant arrhythmias. Although coadministration with other classes of sedatives always acts synergistically on the central nervous system, taking CH with fluoxetine has also been reported to cause prolonged sedation, but for unclear reasons.[20] Tolerance to its sedating effects may occur. Chronic use of CH for insomnia should be discouraged given the potential for side effects and tolerance.

CH toxicity
Respiratory suppression may occur with overdose, resulting in deep stupor and coma. Cardiovascular instability, in the form of decreased myocardial contractility, shortened refractory period, and changes in myocardial sensitivity to endogenous catecholamines, accounts for most of the mortality at toxic levels.

Melatonin

Melatonin is a popular over-the-counter treatment of insomnia in children, with some clinical trials supporting its efficacy when properly used.[21–23] It is thought that the physiologic 10-fold to 15-fold increase in nocturnal blood melatonin concentration occurs 1 to 2 hours before bedtime and may be the final trigger for inducing sleep.[24] The circadian rhythm of melatonin usually develops between the second and third month of life. Neonates and infants depend on their mothers' melatonin circadian rhythm through their milk.[25]

A meta-analysis in the British Medical Journal concluded that "...no evidence that melatonin is effective in treating secondary sleep disorders or sleep disorders accompanying sleep restriction, such as jet lag and shift work disorder."[26] This meta-analysis was criticized for inclusions of poorly designed studies.[21,22] The main difference between the conflicting meta-analysis studies is whether the timing of exogenous melatonin administration was included in the assessment of effectiveness. The most effective time of administration is 5 to 6 hours before the dim light melatonin onset (DLMO),[21] which is roughly 9 to 10 hours after the patient has awakened.

The meta-analysis by van Geijlswijk and colleagues[23] confirmed that administration of melatonin before the DLMO (1.5–6.5 hours) was more effective in advancing circadian timing. Using randomized trials with stricter methodology, melatonin shortened sleep latency by about 16 minutes and increased total sleep time by 28 minutes using objective sleep measurements including polysomnography and actigraphy. The usual dose of melatonin used in these trials was 5 mg. If an adolescent is falling asleep 2 or 3 hours later than expected, shortening the sleep latency by 16 minutes on average may at first seem not clinically significant. However, combining melatonin with behavioral changes may allow incremental improvements in motivated patients over time.

Given its ability to enhance immune function, the National Sleep Foundation has warned against using melatonin in patients[25] with immune disorders, with lymphoproliferative disorders, and those taking corticosteroids or other immunosuppressants. Melatonin is still considered a diet supplement and the FDA does not regulate its safety, purity, or efficacy.[24]

The use of melatonin for children may be most effective in insomnia because of circadian factors. This use includes children with delayed sleep phase syndrome and also blind children. Children with midline brain defects, such as agenesis of corpus callosum, sometimes seem to respond to melatonin treatment of insomnia, presumably because of associated defects in the pineal region.[27,28] Smits and colleagues[28] conducted a double-blind placebo-controlled trial of 5 mg of melatonin in children age 6 to 12 years with sleep-onset insomnia. The melatonin-treated group reported falling asleep 63 minutes earlier and had an increased total sleep time of 41 minutes.

Melatonin for children with attention-deficit/hyperactivity disorder
Weiss and colleagues[29] reported on the use of sleep hygiene and melatonin treatment of initial insomnia in children with attention-deficit/hyperactivity disorder (ADHD), which is analogous to the use of a combination of hypnotics and cognitive behavior therapy for adults with insomnia. The results showed a significant improvement in

insomnia with a sleep-onset reduction time of 16 minutes with melatonin relative to placebo. The improved sleep had no demonstrable effect on ADHD symptoms.[29] A similar report by Van der Heijden and colleagues[30] investigated the effect of melatonin treatment on sleep, behavior, cognition, and quality of life in children with ADHD and chronic sleep-onset insomnia. Melatonin advanced circadian rhythms of sleep-wake and endogenous melatonin and enhanced total time asleep in children with ADHD and chronic sleep-onset insomnia. Similar to the Weiss and colleagues[29] study, improved sleep with melatonin had no effect on problem behavior, cognitive performance, or quality of life.

Melatonin for children with neurodevelopmental and spectrum disorders
A randomized, double-blind, placebo-controlled crossover trial of controlled-release melatonin (5 mg) in the treatment of delayed sleep phase syndrome and impaired sleep maintenance of children with neurodevelopmental disabilities, including autistic spectrum disorders, was published.[31] The sleep maintenance measures did not improve. There was additional improvement in sleep diary measures of sleep efficiency and the longest sleep episode in the open-label phase. Perhaps most importantly, the therapy was effective in reducing family stress.[31] In families with children with neurodevelopmental disabilities, even small improvements may have a large impact in the family.

A smaller randomized, double-blind, placebo-controlled trial of melatonin in children specifically with autism spectrum disorder and fragile X syndrome was published.[32] The investigators concluded that melatonin was effective and tolerated by children with autism spectrum disorder and fragile X syndrome.[32] These results are similar to another randomized trial of melatonin in children with ADHD.[30]

Long-term use of melatonin in children
A long-term trial of melatonin also reported that it is well tolerated.[33] A parental survey of children with ADHD and chronic sleep-onset insomnia treated on average for 3.7 years reported no serious adverse events or treatment-related comorbidities. Most children surveyed used melatonin daily. Parents also reported improved behavior and mood.[33]

Ramelteon

A potential medication to consider in the treatment of sleep-onset insomnia or delayed sleep phase syndrome in adolescents is ramelteon. Ramelteon is a selective melatonin type 1 and 2 receptor agonist that has been approved for sleep-onset insomnia in patients aged 18 years and older.[34] It lacks the potential for abuse commonly associated with hypnotics. Systematic trials in younger patients are not available. A case study did report efficacy in an 18-year-old patient and a 7-year-old patient with autism and insomnia.[35]

HYPERTENSIVES
Clonidine

Clonidine was originally marketed for the treatment of hypertension under the trade name Catapres, but its sedating properties have led to its use as a soporific. No randomized trials of clonidine specifically for children with insomnia were found. Clonidine is a central α2-adrenergic receptor agonist, with a half-life of 6 to 24 hours. Onset of action is within 1 hour, and its peak effects are at 2 to 4 hours. At least 50% is excreted unchanged in the urine. Side effects include hypotension, bradycardia, irritability, anticholinergic effects (eg, dry mouth), and REM suppression. With abrupt discontinuation, rebound hypertension and REM rebound can occur. There is no manufacturer-recommended hypnotic dose but, in practice, the starting dose is usually 25 μg.[4,36]

Benzodiazepines

Benzodiazepine hypnotics have been used extensively in adults with insomnia. Benzodiazepine hypnotics are less commonly used for children with insomnia, although, in theory, they should have similar effectiveness as in adults. The mechanism of action is based on activation of the γ-aminobutyric acid (GABA) receptor.[37] Benzodiazepines may have muscle-relaxing properties and should be avoided in anyone with suspected OSA syndrome. On a polysomnogram, benzodiazepines may alter normal sleep architecture. There can be drug-related artifacts such as atypical sleep spindles and suppression of slow wave sleep. An important exception is clonazepam, which is often an option for insomnia in children. Clonazepam is discussed in more detail later.[38]

Zolpidem, zaleplon, eszopiclone

There are 3 nonbenzodiazepine hypnotics currently available in the United States[39,40]: zolpidem (immediate release and extended release), eszopiclone, and zaleplon. Their use in children is considered off-label, and therefore no official dosing guidelines are available. None of these medications is available in liquid form, which makes them difficult to administer to small children. These newer medications preserve the overall sleep architecture. At the recommended doses, they do not typically have the insomnia rebound effects experienced with benzodiazepine hypnotics when they are abruptly stopped. Rebound insomnia refers to an exacerbation of insomnia on abrupt cessation of a hypnotic. The degree of resulting insomnia is more severe than the initial insomnia before starting hypnotics.

All of these hypnotics should be given as the child is being put to bed. Administering the medication much in advance of bedtime and waiting for it to take effect may result in an increase in paradoxic effects and greater risk of physical injury from ataxia.

Zolpidem and zaleplon dosage

The standard adult dose of immediate-release zolpidem and zaleplon is 10 mg. They both have a rapid onset of action and shorten sleep latency. Zolpidem has a half-life of 2.5 hours and zaleplon has a half-life of 1 hour. This difference in duration is clinically important. Zolpidem may help improve both sleep-onset and, to some degree, sleep maintenance insomnia symptoms. Zaleplon typically only improves the sleep-onset insomnia, and is not expected to significantly increase the total sleep time. Zaleplon's shorter half-life may allow it to be administered after sleep disruption in some situations to help the patient to return to sleep, but this practice has not been studied in children.[41]

Zolpidem, both in the immediate-release and extended-release form, are widely prescribed for adults with insomnia. Although its use in children is off-label, some limited data are available. Blummer and colleagues[7] studied the pharmacokinetic profile of zolpidem in children. In this study, the pharmacokinetics of zolpidem were assessed in an open-label protocol in children with insomnia. Twenty-one children were divided evenly into 3 groups: ages 2 to 6 years, ages 7 to 12 years, and ages 13 to 18 years. Overall, zolpidem was well tolerated, and a pediatric dose of 0.25 mg/kg was recommended for future efficacy studies, with a maximum dose of 20 mg.

The standard adult dose of immediate-release zolpidem is 10 mg, and the extended-release dose is 12.5 mg. The standard adult dose may be prescribed to older children who can swallow the pill. It is not necessary to lower the dose because these medications have short half-lives and minimal side effects. Clearance of zolpidem in children is 3 times higher than in young adults, and it is lower in elderly adults.[39] A 5-mg size pill of immediate-release zolpidem and a 6.25-mg pill of the extended-release form are available and intended for use in the elderly or patients with decreased hepatic clearance. In the authors' experience, giving a lower dosage to children may be either ineffective or result in frightening sleep epiphenomena such as hypnagogic hallucinations. To avoid these adverse events, a higher dose may be needed. The medication is most effective when taken on an empty stomach.

An 8-week, multicenter, double-blind, placebo-controlled study of zolpidem in children with ADHD was published, but it failed to find significant efficacy.[42]

Eszopiclone dosage
Eszopiclone is a nonbenzodiazepine hypnotic that was recently approved in the United States.[43–45] This medication has a longer half-life (6 hours) than zolpidem and zaleplon, and may, theoretically, be helpful in children because they typically sleep longer than adults. To date, there are no published studies in children.

OFF-LABEL USE OF PRESCRIPTION HYPNOTICS

Prescription hypnotics do not have an FDA indication for adolescents younger than 18 years. An off-label use as an adjunct to the behavioral modification of the circadian problem may be considered in certain clinical situations. Because these patients typically only have sleep-onset insomnia without significant nocturnal disruption, a short-acting hypnotic agent may be considered for a short period of time. Zaleplon, a nonbenzodiazepine hypnotic, may theoretically be used in adolescents with delayed sleep phase syndrome. Zaleplon has a short elimination half-life of approximately 1 hour. This short duration of action, unlike diphenhydramine, minimizes any next-day sedation or risk of rebound insomnia. Rebound insomnia is more typical of short-acting benzodiazepine hypnotics such as triazolam. Gradual tapering of the benzodiazepines dose may avoid a significant rebound insomnia effect.

OFF-LABEL USE OF NEUROLEPTICS

Neuroleptics such as risperidone, quetiapine, aripiprazole, and olanzapine are typically prescribed to treated psychiatric conditions. Their off-label use in children with psychiatric or developmental disorders has been reported.[46–49] Neuroleptics are also used off-label to treat insomnia in adults.[50–52] Given this situation, it is tempting to consider the use of neuroleptics in the treatment of sleep disorders such as insomnia in children. However, there are no published data on the use neuroleptics in the treatment of otherwise healthy children with insomnia. Although these medications may facilitate sleep and have effects on sleep architecture, such as increasing slow wave sleep, their routine use to treat sleep disorders in children is not recommended. In addition, excessive weight gain is a report side effect of some neuroleptics, which would exacerbate any sleep-disordered breathing present in the child.

NARCOLEPSY IN CHILDREN AND ADOLESCENTS

Narcolepsy is a neurologic syndrome characterized by excessive daytime sleepiness that is typically associated with cataplexy, sleep paralysis, and hypnagogic hallucinations. Patients often have disturbed nocturnal sleep and pathologic manifestations related to rapid REM sleep. Age at onset varies from childhood to the fifth decade, with a peak in adolescents and young adults.[53] The first symptoms often develop at approximately the time of puberty. Although the cause is not clear, narcolepsy has been shown to be caused by dysfunction of hypocretin/orexin activity in the hypothalamus, primarily through an autoimmune mechanism.[54–58]

Treatment of Narcolepsy in Children

Successful treatment of narcolepsy needs to include both behavioral and pharmacologic treatments. Behavioral treatment includes developing healthy sleep habits and avoiding sleep deprivation. A brief nap of 15 to 20 minutes once or twice daily should improve alertness and should be encouraged as a lifelong practice.

Drug therapy must take into account that narcolepsy is a lifelong illness, and patients have to receive medication for years. Tolerance or addiction may be seen with some compounds. Treatment of narcolepsy thus balances avoidance of side effects, including tolerance, with maintenance of an active life. Physicians need to monitor for the development of hypertension, abnormal liver function, depression, irritability, anorexia, insomnia, or psychosis associated with medications.[59]

Pharmacotherapies targeted to treating daytime sleepiness and cataplexy are the mainstays of narcolepsy treatment. Most studies on medications for narcolepsy have been performed in adults; no double-blind placebo-controlled trials of medication have been specifically conducted for children with narcolepsy.

Sodium oxybate (γ-hydroxybutyrate)

Sodium oxybate (γ-hydroxybutyrate; GHB) is indicated in the treatment of narcolepsy with cataplexy and is FDA approved for both the treatment of cataplexy and excessive daytime sleepiness (EDS). As a therapeutic agent in narcolepsy-cataplexy, its mechanisms of action are incompletely understood, but clinically it has been shown to greatly reduce cataplexy, as well as treat daytime sleepiness and improve sleep fragmentation/disturbed sleep typical of narcolepsy-cataplexy.[60–63] The improvement in cataplexy is more rapid than the effect on daytime sleepiness, which may take up to 6 to 8 weeks. GHB has powerful central nervous system depressant effects, and it has been shown to increase slow wave sleep.

Sodium oxybate/GHB dosing It has a short half-life (90–120 minutes), so the first dose is taken at bedtime, and a second dose is most commonly taken 2.5 to 4 hours later, although timing may vary between patients. The recommended starting dose in adults is 4.5 g/d divided into 2 equal doses of 2.25 g. Dosing may be increased gradually over 8 weeks or longer, with a typical adult dose goal of 6 to 9 g, which has been shown to be effective for improvements in EDS and nocturnal sleep.[64]

In a pediatric narcolepsy series reported from Stanford, 85% of children (similar rates for prepubertal, peripubertal, and postpubertal children) were treated with sodium oxybate with a reportedly high positive effect on daytime sleepiness, disturbed nighttime sleep, and cataplexy.[65] Irritability and nausea were commonly reported side effects, and the report found no impact of the use of sodium oxybate on the occurrence of subsequent puberty. The investigators also reported that sodium oxybate alone, or in association with 1 other drug, modafinil, was sufficient treatment in half of prepubertal cases of narcolepsy-cataplexy.[66]

Amphetamines for narcolepsy Central nervous system stimulants have been the drugs most widely used in the treatment of narcolepsy, and amphetamines were first proposed in 1935.[67] However, several side effects may arise, including irritability, anxiety, nervousness, headache, psychosis, tachycardia, hypertension, nocturnal sleep disturbances, tolerance, and drug dependence. The use of methylphenidate was later encouraged because of a shorter half-life and lower incidence of similar side effects.

Modafinil and armodafinil for narcolepsy

Modafinil is considered a first-line therapy for EDS associated with narcolepsy in adults. Modafinil has been reported in the treatment of EDS in narcoleptic children[68,69] and has also been reported to be effective in the treatment of excessive daytime sleepiness in Prader-Willi syndrome.[70]

The mechanism of this wake-promoting drug is unknown, but it is different from that of amphetamines and is hypothesized to work on hypothalamic wake-promoting circuits. The results of several multicenter trials in adults have shown improvements in objective measures of sleepiness and improved wakefulness in narcoleptic patients, and additive effects have been shown when used with GHB.[62,71,72]

Armodafinil is the R-enantiomer of modafinil with a longer duration of action, approved in 2007 for the treatment of EDS in narcolepsy. Armodafinil has been shown to improve EDS throughout the day in randomized, double-blind, placebo-controlled trials, and produced improvements in the multiple sleep latency test (MSLT) at doses of 150 to 250 mg. The use of armodafinil in children has not been recommended.[73]

Modafinil dosing Doses of 200 to 400 mg are typically used, with morning and noon-hour administration. Elimination half-life is 10 to 12 hours.

Modafinil side effects With modafinil there have been reports of significant drug reactions in children, including reports of skin rash and possible erythema multiforme/Stevens-Johnson syndrome.[74]

Modafinil can reduce the effectiveness of oral contraceptives, and therefore patients should be advised to use additional forms of contraception. Abuse potential for this medication is low and discontinuation of modafinil is not associated with rebound hypersomnolence, nor is there evidence of tolerance.

Modafinil toxicity The toxicity of modafinil has been reviewed.[75,76] An adolescent attempted to commit suicide by ingesting 5000 mg of modafinil. Approximately 2 hours following ingestion, the patient complained of headache, nausea, and abdominal pain. An electrocardiogram showed prolonged QTc interval. Observation for 72 hours revealed 24 hours of inability to sleep, tachycardia, and dyskinesia. There was no deterioration of kidney or liver functions, and no change in complete blood count or blood pressure. The youngest unintentional modafinil ingestion was in a 1-year-old child.[75]

Antidepressants for cataplexy Before the availability of sodium oxybate, the only FDA-approved medication for narcolepsy and cataplexy, antidepressants were the mainstay treatment of cataplexy. Tricyclic antidepressants such as imipramine and clomipramine, which block presynaptic reuptake of catecholamines, were commonly used. However anticholinergic side effects were also common. Selective serotonin reuptake inhibitors replaced tricyclics in popularity to treat cataplexy. Newer antidepressants with selective noradrenergic/serotonergic uptake inhibition remain good choices in adults, with respect to both side effect profile and efficacy for cataplexy. The most commonly used drug in this class is venlafaxine at typical doses of 75 to 150 mg once daily, but can be used as low as 37.5 mg in young patients with narcolepsy. Atomoxetine, a highly specific noradrenergic reuptake blocker, has also been effective for treatment of cataplexy as well as EDS in adults and children, and may be useful in resistance cataplexy at doses of 18 to 100 mg in 1 or 2 divided doses.[77] Atomoxetine has an FDA warning of potential suicidal ideations in children and adolescents.

Sleep-disordered Breathing in Children

Sleep-disordered breathing is a clinical syndrome ranging from simple snoring to potentially life-threatening OSA. This clinical spectrum can occur at any age. There is realization now that patients may be symptomatic in the absence of frank apneas.[78] This realization has led to use of the term sleep-disordered breathing to better describe the clinical spectrum, which includes snoring, upper airway resistance syndrome (UARS), and obstructive hypopnea syndrome. Symptoms of sleep-disordered breathing include nocturnal snoring, mouth breathing, and a palate that is narrow and high-arched.

Pharmacologic Treatment of OSA in Children

In the past, oxygen and protriptyline were advocated for OSA, but now are not considered mainline treatments.[79] Adenotonsillectomy and continuous positive airway pressure therapy (CPAP) have been the mainstays of treatment. Orthodontics are also playing a role in the treatment of OSA using rapid maxillary expansion.[80,81] Although most children with OSA respond to surgery, the possibility of residual symptoms or intolerance to the mainstream treatments requires additional management. Obese children and adolescents with OSA were reported to be more likely to remain symptomatic despite adenotonsillectomy.[82] Although the use of medication to avoid surgery or CPAP for OSA in children is appealing, there is insufficient clinical experience to recommend any medication as a long-term treatment. No randomized trials for this treatment have been reported in children with OSA. Reports of adverse psychiatric events have been reported in children using montelukast.[83] The possibility of medication adverse events must be weighed against the potential morbidity of surgery or difficulties with CPAP. Individual clinical decisions with close follow-up need to be made in children who are CPAP intolerant or have residual symptoms of OSA despite surgery.

RLS

RLS is a chronic familial neurologic disorder.[84] It is characterized by leg discomfort that makes the patients want to move their legs. The leg discomfort may be hard to describe, and in children may be characterized as growing pains.[85–87] The discomfort is more common in the evening and is relieved with movement. RLS is associated with poor-quality sleep. This effect on sleep may lead to daytime behavior that mimics ADHD.[88–92] Iron deficiency exacerbates RLS symptoms and monitoring of serum ferritin is recommended. Iron supplementation may be helpful in children with RLS.[93] Vitamin C may help improve iron absorption.

RLS Treatment in Children

Dopamine precursors and agonists have been effective in relieving both RLS and periodic leg movements syndrome (PLMS).[94]

Levodopa

Levodopa, the metabolic precursor of dopamine used to treat Parkinson disease, is also used to treat RLS during sleep in both adults and children.[95,96] The main complication of levodopa therapy for RLS is the development of worsening symptoms during the afternoon or early evening, despite adequate control later at night. This phenomenon, termed restless legs augmentation, may occur frequently, sometimes within months after initiating therapy. If augmentation occurs, the offending agent should be discontinued, and a different medication should be used. In addition to motor fluctuations and nausea, other adverse effects that may be observed with levodopa therapy include hallucinations, confusion, and orthostatic hypotension. These other side effects are more typically seen in adult patients with Parkinson disease using higher dosages than are used in the treatment of PLMS and RLS. The use of levodopa in RLS has greatly decreased as selective dopamine agonists have become more available.

Pramipexole and ropinirole

Selective dopamine agonists are potent treatments for periodic limb movements disorders and RLS. They tend to have fewer side effects than carbidopa/levodopa. Pramipexole and ropinirole are the most commonly used medications in this category.[94] Pramipexole and ropinirole are both FDA approved for the treatment of RLS in adults.[97–99] Selective dopaminergic agonists have similar side effects to carbidopa/levodopa but at a lower frequency. These agents are more potent and allow lower dosages than with carbidopa/levodopa. Montplaisir and colleagues[100] found pramipexole to be effective in a double-blind placebo-controlled study in adults. The starting dose in adults in this study was 0.375 mg. In children, the lowest dose available is an empiric starting dose. Pramipexole is available in a 0.125-mg tablet. This tablet is scored and can be halved if an even lower starting dosage is desired. If the medication is tolerated, then the dose can be gradually increased, as necessary, to optimize efficacy. There is a case report of an 11-year-old girl with RLS and depressive symptoms that improved with 0.5 mg of ropinirole.[101]

Dosage adjustments Regardless of which medication is used, it is important to make medication changes slowly, because the symptoms of RLS seem to fluctuate independently of the medication. In addition, if the dosage is too high, significant side effects may occur. We advise parents to only adjust the medication once a week at most when they first start the medication. Once an effective dose is found, it typically does not need to be adjusted except to allow for the child's growth. In adults, the dosage of dopamine agonists for RLS usually does not exceed 1.5 mg, and it is often effective at a much lower dose.

Rotigotine Rotigotine is a new dopamine agonist approved for RLS in adults.[102–104] This medication is delivered via a skin patch and could be an option for children who cannot take medication by mouth. However, there are no published data on its use in children. It cannot be recommended in children younger than 18 years at this time.

Gabapentin Gabapentin has been reported to be effective in the treatment of RLS in adults.[105,106] There are no published trials of the use of gabapentin in children with RLS; however, gabapentin is effective in children for the treatment of epilepsy.[107,108] Somnolence is one of the most common side effects. An extended-release form, gabapentin enacarbil, has been studied and approved for adults with RLS.[109–112]

Opiates have long been known to be an effective treatment of RLS in adults,[113,114] but their use in children is not recommended.

Parasomnias

According to the *International Classification of Sleep Disorders* (ICSD), parasomnias are groups of clinical disorders in which undesirable events or experiences occur during entry into sleep, within sleep, or during arousals from sleep.[84] The ICSD describes more than a dozen different parasomnias, most of which can occur in children. The phenomena of sleep paralysis, night terrors, and sleepwalking were once interpreted as supernatural events; family cultural beliefs need to be addressed when parasomnias arise in a child.

Among these disorders, parasomnias associated with arousals are common in children and include the clinical spectrum of confusional arousals, sleep terrors, and sleepwalking. Confusional arousals may be partial manifestations of sleep terrors and sleepwalking events. The individual is disoriented, speech and mentation are slow, and response to questioning is confused.[84] These behaviors usually last only a few minutes in children and can be precipitated by forced awakenings out of slow wave sleep. The condition is benign and tends to decrease over time. However, a child with a tendency to have these events may also be at risk for sleepwalking, and parents/caretakers should be warned of this possibility. The events can be minimized by avoiding situations that can increase slow wave sleep or result in sleep disruption.

Nocturnal seizures versus parasomnias
Parasomnias such as sleepwalking and sleep terrors need to be distinguished from nocturnal seizures. The timing of seizures is different from that of sleepwalking and sleep terrors. The timing of nocturnal seizures does not cluster during slow wave sleep in the first third of the night.

Seizures also do not usually arise from REM sleep. The motor activity of generalized tonic-clonic seizures is different from these parasomnias. Tongue biting and urinary incontinence are not characteristically seen in sleepwalking and night terrors. Patients with generalized nocturnal seizures have a low risk of daytime seizures.[115] The motor activity of a partial complex seizure may be more difficult to distinguish from parasomnias and may resemble a confusional arousal.[116] The overall clinical picture can usually help with the diagnosis. If a patient has been injured during an apparent parasomnia, a comprehensive neurologic evaluation should be considered, including a sleep-deprived electroencephalogram.

Epilepsy versus parasomnias
Some forms of epilepsy may be misidentified as benign parasomnia and as narcolepsy in children.[117] Frontal lobe epilepsy is poorly understood and often unrecognized by health care workers dealing with children and may be misdiagnosed as a sleep disorder or psychiatric problem. Age of onset of epilepsy varies from infancy to adolescence. Seizures are typically brief (30 seconds to 2 minutes), stereotypic, nocturnal, and can occur several times during the night. Seizures have an explosive onset, characterized by screaming, agitation, stiffening, kicking or bicycling of the legs, and incontinence. The movements are not symmetric. The interictal electroencephalogram is usually normal. Long-term video electroencephalographic monitoring is required to show the frontal epileptic discharges. Seizure control is difficult and may require epilepsy surgery.[118]

PARASOMNIA TREATMENT IN CHILDREN

There are no medications with an FDA indication in children for any of the different parasomnias listed in the ICSD.[84,119] This article discusses off-label use of pharmacotherapies for parasomnias in youth.

Benzodiazepines

Benzodiazepines, which have been used extensively in adults with insomnia, are the most commonly used agents for the off-label treatment of parasomnias. Benzodiazepines have been particularly useful for arousal parasomnias such as sleepwalking and REM sleep behavior disorder. The mechanism of action is based on activation of the GABA receptor complex.[37] Benzodiazepines may have muscle-relaxing properties and should be used with caution if comorbid sleep-disordered breathing is suspected. On a polysomnogram, benzodiazepines may alter the normal sleep stages referred to as sleep architecture. There can be drug-related artifacts such as atypical sleep spindles and suppression of slow wave sleep.

Clonazepam

Among the benzodiazepine class, clonazepam is the most common medication used in the treatment of parasomnias.[38,120,121] The clinical use of clonazepam in parasomnias may be popular because of familiarity with the drug along with the putative clinical efficacy.

Clonazepam's effectiveness may be caused by increasing the arousal threshold.

Clonazepam is rapidly and completely absorbed after oral administration. Onset of action is 20 to 60 minutes. The time to peak level is 1 to 3 hours. Duration of action is 6 to 8 hours in children and up to 12 hours in adults. The bioavailability is about 90%. Maximum plasma concentrations are reached within 1 to 4 hours after oral administration. The half-life of clonazepam is typically 30 to 40 hours. The half-life tends to be longer in adults than in children. The metabolism is extensively hepatic and it is excreted in urine. Clonazepam can be used to prevent parasomnias associated with partial arousals, such as sleep terrors or sleepwalking. When parasomnias are frequent and disturbing to the patient and family, a low dose of clonazepam at 0.25 to 0.5 mg may be helpful.[122] Clonazepam is available in thin wafers that dissolve on the tongue, so the child does not have to swallow a pill.

Clonazepam has been studied as pharmacotherapy for arousal parasomnias in the last 2 decades. It has predominantly been studied in adults and, specifically, in those who have had a sleep–related injury. Schenck and colleagues[123] in 1989 studied 100 patients with various parasomnias who presented to their sleep center with nocturnal injuries and who underwent polysomnography. Fifty-four of these patients were diagnosed with either sleep terrors or sleepwalking (age of onset ranging from 3 to 58 years). Clonazepam was prescribed for 28 of these patients. Most reportedly had significant improvement in sleep up to 6 years after starting treatment. Schenck and Mahowald[124] also reported a study of 170 adults with sleep-related injuries between 1982 and 1994, of whom 69 had either sleepwalking or sleep terrors; other sleep diagnoses. Eighty-six percent of these patients had complete or near-complete control of their symptoms. There have also been case reports of patients with behaviors such as driving and sleep violence who have been diagnosed with sleepwalking and have also responded to clonazepam.[124,125]

SUMMARY

There is a need for more information on the pharmacologic management of sleep disorders in children. Pharmacologic guidelines need to be developed specifically for sleep disorders in children. These guidelines should be FDA approved for the specific sleep disorder and pediatric age group. Easy-to-swallow, chewable, or liquid forms of these medications are needed. Integration of behavioral and pharmacologic treatments may yield better patient outcomes, and would require psychiatrists and other health care providers to have a comprehensive understanding of clinical sleep disorders in children. Training programs should enhance pediatricians' knowledge of the pharmacologic treatment of sleep disorders in children.

REFERENCES

1. Alonso Alvarez ML, Teran Santos J, Cordero Guevara JA, et al. Reliability of respiratory polygraphy for the diagnosis of sleep apnea-hypopnea syndrome in children. Arch Bronconeumol 2008;44:318–23 [in Spanish].

2. Pelayo R, Chen W, Monzon S, et al. Pediatric sleep pharmacology: you want to give my kid sleeping pills? Pediatr Clin North Am 2004;51:117–34.
3. Owens JA, Moturi S. Pharmacologic treatment of pediatric insomnia. Child Adolesc Psychiatr Clin North Am 2009;18:1001–16.
4. Schnoes CJ, Kuhn BR, Workman EF, et al. Pediatric prescribing practices for clonidine and other pharmacologic agents for children with sleep disturbance. Clin Pediatr (Phila) 2006;45:229–38.
5. Owens JA, Rosen, Mindell JA. Medication use in the treatment of pediatric insomnia: results of a survey of community-based pediatricians. Pediatrics 2003;111(5 Pt 1):e628–35.
6. Stojanovski SD, Rasu RS, Balkrishnan R, et al. Trends in medication prescribing for pediatric sleep difficulties in US outpatient settings. Sleep 2007;30:1013–7.
7. Blumer JL, Reed MD, Steinberg F, et al. Potential pharmacokinetic basis for zolpidem dosing in children with sleep difficulties. Clin Pharmacol Ther 2008;83(4):551–8.
8. Morgenthaler TI, Owens J, Alessi C, et al. Practice parameters for behavioral treatment of bedtime problems and night wakings in infants and young children. Sleep 2006;29:1277–81.
9. Haydon RC 3rd. Are second-generation antihistamines appropriate for most children and adults? Arch Otolaryngol Head Neck Surg 2001;127:1510–3.
10. Meltzer EO. Comparative safety of H1 antihistamines. Ann Allergy 1991;67:625–33.
11. Baker AM, Johnson DG, Levisky JA, et al. Fatal diphenhydramine intoxication in infants. J Forensic Sci 2003;48:425–8.
12. Corey JP, Houser SM, Ng BA. Nasal congestion: a review of its etiology, evaluation, and treatment. Ear Nose Throat J 2000;79:690–3, 6, 8 passim.
13. Gengo F, Gabos C, Miller JK. The pharmacodynamics of diphenhydramine-induced drowsiness and changes in mental performance. Clin Pharmacol Ther 1989;45:15–21.
14. Albert KS, Hallmark MR, Sakmar E, et al. Pharmacokinetics of diphenhydramine in man. J Pharmacokinet Biopharm 1975;3:159–70.
15. Simons KJ, Watson WT, Martin TJ, et al. Diphenhydramine: pharmacokinetics and pharmacodynamics in elderly adults, young adults, and children. J Clin Pharmacol 1990;30:665–71.
16. Merenstein D, Diener-West M, Halbower AC, et al. The Trial of Infant Response to Diphenhydramine: the TIRED study–a randomized, controlled, patient-oriented trial. Arch Pediatr Adolesc Med 2006;160:707–12.
17. Adam EK, Snell EK, Pendry P. Sleep timing and quantity in ecological and family context: a nationally representative time-diary study. J Fam Psychol 2007;21:4–19.
18. Dinndorf PA, McCabe MA, Frierdich S. Risk of abuse of diphenhydramine in children and adolescents with chronic illnesses. J Pediatr 1998;133:293–5.
19. Nigro N, Eandi M. Sleep: notes on pediatric pharmacotherapy (in the light of current knowledge of its principal characteristics). Minerva Pediatr 1975;27:1999–2007 [in Italian].
20. Pershad J, Palmisano P, Nichols M. Chloral hydrate: the good and the bad. Pediatr Emerg Care 1999;15:432–5.
21. Zee PC. Shedding light on the effectiveness of melatonin for circadian rhythm sleep disorders. Sleep 2010;33:1581–2.
22. van Geijlswijk IM, van der Heijden KB, Egberts AC, et al. Dose finding of melatonin for chronic idiopathic childhood sleep onset insomnia: an RCT. Psychopharmacology 2010;212:379–91.

23. van Geijlswijk IM, Korzilius HP, Smits MG. The use of exogenous melatonin in delayed sleep phase disorder: a meta-analysis. Sleep 2010;33:1605–14.
24. Wagner J, Wagner ML, Hening WA. Beyond benzodiazepines: alternative pharmacologic agents for the treatment of insomnia. Ann Pharmacother 1998;32: 680–91.
25. Touitou Y. Human aging and melatonin. Clinical relevance. Exp Gerontol 2001; 36:1083–100.
26. Buscemi N, Vandermeer B, Hooton N, et al. Efficacy and safety of exogenous melatonin for secondary sleep disorders and sleep disorders accompanying sleep restriction: meta-analysis. BMJ 2006;332:385–93.
27. Jan JE, Tai J, Hahn G, et al. Melatonin replacement therapy in a child with a pineal tumor. J Child Neurol 2001;16:139–40.
28. Smits MG, Nagtegaal EE, van der Heijden J, et al. Melatonin for chronic sleep onset insomnia in children: a randomized placebo-controlled trial. J Child Neurol 2001;16:86–92.
29. Weiss MD, Wasdell MB, Bomben MM, et al. Sleep hygiene and melatonin treatment for children and adolescents with ADHD and initial insomnia. J Am Acad Child Adolesc Psychiatry 2006;45:512–9.
30. Van der Heijden KB, Smits MG, Van Someren EJ, et al. Effect of melatonin on sleep, behavior, and cognition in ADHD and chronic sleep-onset insomnia. J Am Acad Child Adolesc Psychiatry 2007;46:233–41.
31. Wasdell MB, Jan JE, Bomben MM, et al. A randomized, placebo-controlled trial of controlled release melatonin treatment of delayed sleep phase syndrome and impaired sleep maintenance in children with neurodevelopmental disabilities. J Pineal Res 2008;44:57–64.
32. Wirojanan J, Jacquemont S, Diaz R, et al. The efficacy of melatonin for sleep problems in children with autism, fragile X syndrome, or autism and fragile X syndrome. J Clin Sleep Med 2009;5:145–50.
33. Hoebert M, van der Heijden KB, van Geijlswijk IM, et al. Long-term follow-up of melatonin treatment in children with ADHD and chronic sleep onset insomnia. J Pineal Res 2009;47:1–7.
34. Johnson MW, Suess PE, Griffiths RR. Ramelteon: a novel hypnotic lacking abuse liability and sedative adverse effects. Arch Gen Psychiatry 2006;63: 1149–57.
35. Stigler KA, Posey DJ, McDougle CJ. Ramelteon for insomnia in two youths with autistic disorder. J Child Adolesc Psychopharmacol 2006;16:631–6.
36. Ingrassia A, Turk J. The use of clonidine for severe and intractable sleep problems in children with neurodevelopmental disorders–a case series. Eur Child Adolesc Psychiatry 2005;14:34–40.
37. Ashton H. Guidelines for the rational use of benzodiazepines. When and what to use. Drugs 1994;48:25–40.
38. Wills L, Garcia J. Parasomnias: epidemiology and management. CNS Drugs 2002;16:803–10.
39. Salva P, Costa J. Clinical pharmacokinetics and pharmacodynamics of zolpidem. Therapeutic implications. Clin Pharmacokinet 1995;29:142–53.
40. Weitzel KW, Wickman JM, Augustin SG, et al. Zaleplon: a pyrazolopyrimidine sedative-hypnotic agent for the treatment of insomnia. Clin Ther 2000;22: 1254–67.
41. Zammit GK, Corser B, Doghramji K, et al. Sleep and residual sedation after administration of zaleplon, zolpidem, and placebo during experimental middle-of-the-night awakening. J Clin Sleep Med 2006;2:417–23.

42. Blumer JL, Findling RL, Shih WJ, et al. Controlled clinical trial of zolpidem for the treatment of insomnia associated with attention-deficit/hyperactivity disorder in children 6 to 17 years of age. Pediatrics 2009;123:e770–6.
43. Najib J. Eszopiclone, a nonbenzodiazepine sedative-hypnotic agent for the treatment of transient and chronic insomnia. Clin Ther 2006;28:491–516.
44. Roth T, Walsh JK, Krystal A, et al. An evaluation of the efficacy and safety of eszopiclone over 12 months in patients with chronic primary insomnia. Sleep Med 2005;6:487–95.
45. Walsh JK, Krystal AD, Amato DA, et al. Nightly treatment of primary insomnia with eszopiclone for six months: effect on sleep, quality of life, and work limitations. Sleep 2007;30:959–68.
46. Masi G, Cosenza A, Millepiedi S, et al. Aripiprazole monotherapy in children and young adolescents with pervasive developmental disorders: a retrospective study. CNS Drugs 2009;23:511–21.
47. Valicenti-McDermott MR, Demb H. Clinical effects and adverse reactions of off-label use of aripiprazole in children and adolescents with developmental disabilities. J Child Adolesc Psychopharmacol 2006;16:549–60.
48. Harrison-Woolrych M, Garcia-Quiroga J, Ashton J, et al. Safety and usage of atypical antipsychotic medicines in children: a nationwide prospective cohort study. Drug Saf 2007;30:569–79.
49. Capone GT, Goyal P, Grados M, et al. Risperidone use in children with Down syndrome, severe intellectual disability, and comorbid autistic spectrum disorders: a naturalistic study. J Dev Behav Pediatr 2008;29:106–16.
50. Sokolski KN, Brown BJ. Quetiapine for insomnia associated with refractory depression exacerbated by phenelzine. Ann Pharmacother 2006;40:567–70.
51. Juri C, Chana P, Tapia J, et al. Quetiapine for insomnia in Parkinson disease: results from an open-label trial. Clin Neuropharmacol 2005;28:185–7.
52. Doan RJ. Risperidone for insomnia in PDDs. Can J Psychiatry 1998;43:1050–1.
53. Guilleminault C, Pelayo R. Narcolepsy in prepubertal children. Ann Neurol 1998; 43:135–42.
54. Nishino S, Mignot E. Narcolepsy and cataplexy. Handb Clin Neurol 2011;99: 783–814.
55. Kornum BR, Faraco J, Mignot E. Narcolepsy with hypocretin/orexin deficiency, infections and autoimmunity of the brain. Curr Opin Neurobiol 2011; 21:897–903.
56. Kawashima M, Lin L, Tanaka S, et al. Anti-Tribbles homolog 2 (TRIB2) autoantibodies in narcolepsy are associated with recent onset of cataplexy. Sleep 2010; 33:869–74.
57. Dauvilliers Y, Montplaisir J, Cochen V, et al. Post-H1N1 narcolepsy-cataplexy. Sleep 2010;33:1428–30.
58. Aran A, Lin L, Nevsimalova S, et al. Elevated anti-streptococcal antibodies in patients with recent narcolepsy onset. Sleep 2009;32:979–83.
59. Guilleminault C, Pelayo R. Narcolepsy in children: a practical guide to its diagnosis, treatment and follow-up. Paediatr Drugs 2000;2:1–9.
60. Lammers GJ, Arends J, Declerck AC, et al. Gammahydroxybutyrate and narcolepsy: a double-blind placebo-controlled study. Sleep 1993;16:216–20.
61. US Xyrem Multicenter Study Group. Sodium oxybate demonstrates long-term efficacy for the treatment of cataplexy in patients with narcolepsy. Sleep Med 2004;5:119–23.
62. Black J, Houghton WC. Sodium oxybate improves excessive daytime sleepiness in narcolepsy. Sleep 2006;29:939–46.

63. A randomized, double blind, placebo-controlled multicenter trial comparing the effects of three doses of orally administered sodium oxybate with placebo for the treatment of narcolepsy. Sleep 2002;25:42–9.

64. Scharf MB, Lai AA, Branigan B, et al. Pharmacokinetics of gammahydroxybutyrate (GHB) in narcoleptic patients. Sleep 1998;21:507–14.

65. Aran A, Einen M, Lin L, et al. Clinical and therapeutic aspects of childhood narcolepsy-cataplexy: a retrospective study of 51 children. Sleep 2010;33: 1457–64.

66. Aran A, Einen M, Lin L. Clinical aspects and management issues in childhood narcolepsy-cataplexy. Sleep, in press.

67. Littner M, Johnson SF, McCall WV, et al. Practice parameters for the treatment of narcolepsy: an update for 2000. Sleep 2001;24:451–66.

68. Ivanenko A, Tauman R, Gozal D. Modafinil in the treatment of excessive daytime sleepiness in children. Sleep Med 2003;4:579–82.

69. Yeh SB, Schenck CH. Efficacy of modafinil in 10 Taiwanese patients with narcolepsy: findings using the multiple sleep latency test and Epworth Sleepiness Scale. Kaohsiung J Med Sci 2010;26:422–7.

70. De Cock VC, Diene G, Molinas C, et al. Efficacy of modafinil on excessive daytime sleepiness in Prader-Willi syndrome. Am J Med Genet A 2011;155: 1552–7.

71. Randomized trial of modafinil as a treatment for the excessive daytime somnolence of narcolepsy: US modafinil in narcolepsy multicenter study group. Neurology 2000;54:1166–75.

72. Broughton RJ, Fleming JA, George CF, et al. Randomized, double-blind, placebo-controlled crossover trial of modafinil in the treatment of excessive daytime sleepiness in narcolepsy. Neurology 1997;49:444–51.

73. Lankford DA. Armodafinil: a new treatment for excessive sleepiness. Expert Opin Investig Drugs 2008;17:565–73.

74. Rugino T. A review of modafinil film-coated tablets for attention-deficit/hyperactivity disorder in children and adolescents. Neuropsychiatr Dis Treat 2007;3:293–301.

75. Spiller HA, Borys D, Griffith JR, et al. Toxicity from modafinil ingestion. Clin Toxicol (Phila) 2009;47:153–6.

76. Neuman G, Shehadeh N, Pillar G. Unsuccessful suicide attempt of a 15 year old adolescent with ingestion of 5000 mg modafinil. J Clin Sleep Med 2009;5: 372–3.

77. Billiard M. Narcolepsy: current treatment options and future approaches. Neuropsychiatr Dis Treat 2008;4:557–66.

78. Carroll JL. Obstructive sleep-disordered breathing in children: new controversies, new directions. Clin Chest Med 2003;24:261–82.

79. Marcus CL, Ward SL, Mallory GB, et al. Use of nasal continuous positive airway pressure as treatment of childhood obstructive sleep apnea. J Pediatr 1995;127: 88–94.

80. Villa MP, Rizzoli A, Miano S, et al. Efficacy of rapid maxillary expansion in children with obstructive sleep apnea syndrome: 36 months of follow-up. Sleep Breath 2011;15:179–84.

81. Pirelli P, Saponara M, Guilleminault C. Rapid maxillary expansion in children with obstructive sleep apnea syndrome. Sleep 2004;27:761–6.

82. Bhattacharjee R, Kheirandish-Gozal L, Spruyt K, et al. Adenotonsillectomy outcomes in treatment of obstructive sleep apnea in children: a multicenter retrospective study. Am J Respir Crit Care Med 2010;182:676–83.

83. Wallerstedt SM, Brunlof G, Sundstrom A, et al. Montelukast and psychiatric disorders in children. Pharmacoepidemiol Drug Saf 2009;18:858–64.
84. International classification of sleep disorders. 2nd edition. Westchester (IL): American Academy of Sleep Medicine; 2005, http://www.aasmnet.org/store/product.aspx?pid=101.
85. Picchietti D, Allen RP, Walters AS, et al. Restless legs syndrome: prevalence and impact in children and adolescents–the Peds REST study. Pediatrics 2007;120: 253–66.
86. Picchietti DL, Stevens HE. Early manifestations of restless legs syndrome in childhood and adolescence. Sleep Med 2008;9(7):770–81.
87. Mohri I, Kato-Nishimura K, Tachibana N, et al. Restless legs syndrome (RLS): an unrecognized cause for bedtime problems and insomnia in children. Sleep Med 2008;9(6):701–2.
88. Picchietti DL, Walters AS. Moderate to severe periodic limb movement disorder in childhood and adolescence. Sleep 1999;22:297–300.
89. Hening W, Allen R, Earley C, et al. The treatment of restless legs syndrome and periodic limb movement disorder. An American Academy of Sleep Medicine review. Sleep 1999;22:970–99.
90. Picchietti D. Is iron deficiency an underlying cause of pediatric restless legs syndrome and of attention-deficit/hyperactivity disorder? Sleep Med 2007;8: 693–4.
91. Picchietti DL, Arbuckle RA, Abetz L, et al. Pediatric restless legs syndrome: analysis of symptom descriptions and drawings. J Child Neurol 2011;26: 1365–76.
92. England SJ, Picchietti DL, Couvadelli BV, et al. L-Dopa improves restless legs syndrome and periodic limb movements in sleep but not attention-deficit-hyperactivity disorder in a double-blind trial in children. Sleep Med 2011;12:471–7.
93. Patrick LR. Restless legs syndrome: pathophysiology and the role of iron and folate. Altern Med Rev 2007;12:101–12.
94. Littner MR, Kushida C, Anderson WM, et al. Practice parameters for the dopaminergic treatment of restless legs syndrome and periodic limb movement disorder. Sleep 2004;27:557–9.
95. Chesson AL Jr, Wise M, Davila D, et al. Practice parameters for the treatment of restless legs syndrome and periodic limb movement disorder. An American Academy of Sleep Medicine report. Standards of Practice Committee of the American Academy of Sleep Medicine. Sleep 1999;22:961–8.
96. Walters AS, Mandelbaum DE, Lewin DS, et al. Dopaminergic therapy in children with restless legs/periodic limb movements in sleep and ADHD. Dopaminergic Therapy Study Group. Pediatr Neurol 2000;22:182–6.
97. Oertel WH, Stiasny-Kolster K, Bergtholdt B, et al. Efficacy of pramipexole in restless legs syndrome: a six-week, multicenter, randomized, double-blind study (effect-RLS study). Mov Disord 2007;22:213–9.
98. Allen RP, Ritchie SY. Clinical efficacy of ropinirole for restless legs syndrome is not affected by age at symptom onset. Sleep Med 2008;9(8):899–902.
99. Quilici S, Abrams KR, Nicolas A, et al. Meta-analysis of the efficacy and tolerability of pramipexole versus ropinirole in the treatment of restless legs syndrome. Sleep Med 2008;9(7):715–26.
100. Montplaisir J, Nicolas A, Denesle R, et al. Restless legs syndrome improved by pramipexole: a double-blind randomized trial. Neurology 1999;52:938–43.
101. Cortese S, Konofal E, Lecendreux M. Effectiveness of ropinirole for RLS and depressive symptoms in an 11-year-old girl. Sleep Med 2009;10:259–61.

102. Schreglmann SR, Gantenbein AR, Eisele G, et al. Transdermal rotigotine causes impulse control disorders in patients with restless legs syndrome. Parkinsonism Relat Disord 2012;18:207–9.

103. Oertel W, Trenkwalder C, Benes H, et al. Long-term safety and efficacy of rotigotine transdermal patch for moderate-to-severe idiopathic restless legs syndrome: a 5-year open-label extension study. Lancet Neurol 2011;10:710–20.

104. Oertel WH, Benes H, Garcia-Borreguero D, et al. Rotigotine transdermal patch in moderate to severe idiopathic restless legs syndrome: a randomized, placebo-controlled polysomnographic study. Sleep Med 2010;11:848–56.

105. Saletu M, Anderer P, Saletu-Zyhlarz GM, et al. Comparative placebo-controlled polysomnographic and psychometric studies on the acute effects of gabapentin versus ropinirole in restless legs syndrome. J Neural Transm 2010;117:463–73.

106. Garcia-Borreguero D, Larrosa O, de la Llave Y, et al. Treatment of restless legs syndrome with gabapentin: a double-blind, cross-over study. Neurology 2002;59:1573–9.

107. Mills JK, Ruslan NE, Lewis TG, et al. Retention rate of gabapentin in children with intractable epilepsies at 1 year. Seizure 2012;21:28–31.

108. Haig GM, Bockbrader HN, Wesche DL, et al. Single-dose gabapentin pharmacokinetics and safety in healthy infants and children. J Clin Pharmacol 2001;41:507–14.

109. Hayes WJ, Lemon MD, Farver DK. Gabapentin enacarbil for treatment of restless legs syndrome in adults. Ann Pharmacother 2012;46:229–39.

110. Lee DO, Ziman RB, Perkins AT, et al. A randomized, double-blind, placebo-controlled study to assess the efficacy and tolerability of gabapentin enacarbil in subjects with restless legs syndrome. J Clin Sleep Med 2011;7:282–92.

111. Ellenbogen AL, Thein SG, Winslow DH, et al. A 52-week study of gabapentin enacarbil in restless legs syndrome. Clin Neuropharmacol 2011;34:8–16.

112. Gabapentin encarbil (Horizant) for restless leg syndrome. Med Lett Drugs Ther 2011;53:70–1.

113. Silver N, Allen RP, Senerth J, et al. A 10-year, longitudinal assessment of dopamine agonists and methadone in the treatment of restless legs syndrome. Sleep Med 2011;12:440–4.

114. Trzepacz PT, Violette EJ, Sateia MJ. Response to opioids in three patients with restless legs syndrome. Am J Psychiatry 1984;141:993–5.

115. D'Alessandro R, Guarino M, Greco G, et al. Risk of seizures while awake in pure sleep epilepsies: a prospective study. Neurology 2004;62:254–7.

116. Lahorgue Nunes M, Ferri R, Arzimanoglou A, et al. Sleep organization in children with partial refractory epilepsy. J Child Neurol 2003;18:763–6.

117. Kotagal P. The relationship between sleep and epilepsy. Semin Pediatr Neurol 2001;8:241–50.

118. Sinclair DB, Wheatley M, Snyder T. Frontal lobe epilepsy in childhood. Pediatr Neurol 2004;30:169–76.

119. Attarian H. Treatment options for parasomnias. Neurol Clin 2010;28:1089–106.

120. Mahowald MW, Schenck CH, Bornemann MA. Pathophysiologic mechanisms in REM sleep behavior disorder. Curr Neurol Neurosci Rep 2007;7:167–72.

121. Schenck CH, Arnulf I, Mahowald MW. Sleep and sex: what can go wrong? A review of the literature on sleep related disorders and abnormal sexual behaviors and experiences. Sleep 2007;30:683–702.

122. Pelayo R, Dubik M. Pediatric sleep pharmacology. Semin Pediatr Neurol 2008;15:79–90.

123. Schenck CH, Milner DM, Hurwitz TD, et al. A polysomnographic and clinical report on sleep-related injury in 100 adult patients. Am J Psychiatry 1989;146: 1166–73.

124. Schenck CH, Mahowald MW. Long-term, nightly benzodiazepine treatment of injurious parasomnias and other disorders of disrupted nocturnal sleep in 170 adults. Am J Med 1996;100:333–7.

125. Schenck CH, Mahowald MW. A polysomnographically documented case of adult somnambulism with long-distance automobile driving and frequent nocturnal violence: parasomnia with continuing danger as a noninsane automatism? Sleep 1995;18:765–72.

Empirical Evidence for Psychopharmacologic Treatment in Early-Onset Psychosis and Schizophrenia

Ann E. Maloney, MD*, Lauren J. Yakutis, BA, Jean A. Frazier, MD

KEYWORDS

- Psychopharmacologic treatment • Psychosis • Early-onset schizophrenia

KEY POINTS

- Youth affected by psychosis are often impaired.
- Psychosis in youth is likely to be chronic and intermittent and interferes with learning and relationships.
- Youth may not reveal much about their symptoms unless they are directly asked about them.
- Results of several studies indicate that antipsychotics are helpful in treating psychotic symptoms. However, a federally funded study called Treatment of Early Onset Schizophrenia Spectrum Disorders (TEOSS) revealed no differences between first-generation and second-generation antipsychotics in terms of efficacy and few differences in side effect profiles.
- Monitoring response to treatment and adverse effects resulting from antipsychotics is essential. Monitoring can be performed in collaboration with colleagues in primary care and by engaging families in this process.
- Future treatments for psychotic youth may include nonpharmacologic along with pharmacologic approaches. Drug discovery efforts are focusing on finding new agents with fewer side effects for youth.
- Neurocognition is an important target for these youth.

Disclosures: Dr Maloney has received software for research from Posit Sciences, software and dance mats for research from Konami Digital Entertainment, and research funding from the National Institutes of Health (NIH) and the US Department of Agriculture. Ms Yakutis has no conflicts to report. Dr Frazier has received grant support from NIH, Roche Seaside Therapeutics, Pfizer, and Glaxo Smith Kline.
Department of Psychiatry, Child and Adolescent NeuroDevelopment Initiative (CANDI), University of Massachusetts Memorial Health Care, University of Massachusetts Medical School, Worcester, MA, USA
* Corresponding author. Department of Psychiatry, Child and Adolescent NeuroDevelopment Initiative (CANDI), Biotech One–Suite 100, 365 Plantation Street, Worcester, MA 01605.
E-mail address: Ann.Maloney@umassmed.edu

Child Adolesc Psychiatric Clin N Am 21 (2012) 885–909
http://dx.doi.org/10.1016/j.chc.2012.07.011
1056-4993/12/$ – see front matter © 2012 Elsevier Inc. All rights reserved.
childpsych.theclinics.com

OVERVIEW OF DISEASE

Psychosis may initially present during childhood or adolescence. Because half of all major mental illnesses start early in life,[1] child and adolescent mental health providers need to ask directly about psychotic symptoms when conducting mental status examinations. Psychotic symptoms, such as hallucinations and delusions, may be present in several disorders, including the primary psychotic disorders (schizophrenia and schizoaffective and schizophreniform disorders). Affective disorders with psychotic features are more common in youth than primary psychotic disorders. Approximately 40% to 60% of youth with bipolar disorder have psychotic features[2,3] and studies have shown that 15% to 35% of depressed youth have psychosis.[4–6] Psychotic mania presents with marked energy, obvious insomnia, and paranoid thought processes.[7] On the other hand, psychotic depression is more often accompanied by delusions and bizarre thinking.[8] Primary psychotic disorders tend to present with significant functional impairments.[9,10] Even before the diagnosis of schizophrenia is made, aggression and school problems are cited by parents as significant.[11] Psychosis is not so rare as many clinicians in child psychiatry might think.[12] Estimates of schizophrenia before age 18 years vary, but between ages 13 and 19 years, the prevalence is believed to be about 0.5%.[13]

Diagnostic criteria used for early-onset schizophrenia (EOS) are the same as those used in the adult-onset disorder, except that psychotic symptoms are present before age 18 years in EOS. The terms very early-onset schizophrenia or childhood-onset schizophrenia (COS) are reserved to describe those youth who have illness onset before the age of 13 years.[14] There are some developmental differences in the characteristics of symptoms that are associated with age on presentation. Specifically, youth are more likely to have multimodal hallucinations (eg, visual and auditory phenomena) than adults. For example, most of the National Institute of Mental Health (NIMH) COS cohort reported visual hallucinations.[15] In addition, these youngsters have more difficulty recognizing their symptoms as abnormal, and may not complain spontaneously about hallucinations.[16]

Youth who experience EOS and COS frequently show greater premorbid problems with attention, learning, and socialization when compared with those with adult-onset schizophrenia.[10,17,18] Communication deviance is a predictor of outcome in youth at clinical high risk for psychosis, and attention should be focused on poverty of speech and subtle communication disturbances during interviews with these youngsters.[19] Youth with schizophrenia spectrum disorders often have impaired cognition and social withdrawal.[20,21] Cognitive symptoms include impaired memory, attention, verbal processing, and executive function, and these deficits are highly correlated with loss of function in school, community, and social relationships.[18,22]

The incidence of EOS is not well established. However, at least 5% of adults with schizophrenia became ill before 14 years of age and up to 20% became ill before 18 years of age.[23–27] Negative symptoms are closely related to age of onset, as are measures of executive functioning and sustained attention.[28]

More males than females experience COS (2:1), and more males experience EOS than females.[14] In a small sample of 28 youth with childhood-onset illness (mean age 14.5 ± 2.3 years), indices of pubertal development showed no relationship to onset of psychosis.[29]

Financial costs associated with schizophrenia are high, when evaluated over a lifetime, according to the President's New Freedom Commission on Mental Heath Report.[30] There is also evidence of a shortened life span for those with schizophrenia because of increased risk for cardiovascular disease.[31] This article focuses on how to mitigate risks associated with this illness.

In clinical trials, lengthy but validated instruments are used to make a diagnosis (such as K-SADS-PL [Schedule for Affective Disorders and Schizophrenia for School-Age Children-Present and Lifetime Version]).[32] However, mental health providers in practice have time constraints, which limit the usefulness of these research instruments in the clinical arena. Clinicians need to keep in mind psychotic illness in their differential diagnoses and closely question youth about psychotic symptoms, because they are often hidden in presentation and may not be the chief complaint of the child, the referring clinician, or the parents.[10] It is important to directly question youth and parents about psychotic symptoms. Child psychiatrists are often the first to ask about these symptoms.[11]

WORKUP OF EOS

When assessing a child with new-onset psychosis, it is important to rule out medical/neurologic conditions that can manifest in psychotic signs and symptoms by completing a thorough workup.[14] There is no agreed standard for the initial medical workup across the American, Canadian, and New Zealand practice guidelines.[33] Nonetheless, across these practice guidelines, the following are consistently recommended:

- Careful physical examination, with attention to the neurologic examination
- Vital signs and measurements of body mass index (BMI, calculated as weight in kilograms divided by the square of height in meters)
- Laboratory tests with consideration of the complete blood count
- Electrolytes, glucose, calcium, blood urea nitrogen/creatinine, liver function tests
- Erythrocyte sedimentation rate
- Syphilis test
- Antinuclear antibody
- Ceruloplasmin
- Vitamin B_{12}
- Pregnancy test (women)
- Thyroid functions
- Prolactin
- Hepatitis C
- Human immunodeficiency virus
- Toxicology
- Heavy metal screening
- If clinically indicated, consideration can be given to neuroimaging, electrocardiography, fluorescent in situ hybridization (for 22q11 deletion syndrome), and electroencephalography.

In studies from the adult literature, about 3% of first-episode cases can be attributed to a medical condition, which mimics psychosis. Particular attention should be paid to the possibility of substance-induced thought disorder and the role of cannabis in the duration and the onset of symptoms.[34–36] Cannabis use can change the long-term course of the psychosis, depending on discontinued or continued use. For example, in 1 study, ongoing cannabis use had a deleterious effect on functional outcomes, but stopping use after the first psychotic episode contributed to a clear improvement over the study period, which was on average 7.67 ± 0.94 years.[37] An Australian research group found that cannabis use started before psychosis onset in 87.6% of individuals (n = 625, age range: 14–29 years).[38] In addition, the earlier age at onset of cannabis use has been associated with an earlier age of onset of psychosis.[39,40]

Before starting treatment, it is essential to obtain a good patient history, asking about personal and family history of diabetes dyslipidemia, hypertension, or cardiovascular disease. A child presenting with a family history for metabolic disorders may prompt the prescriber to collaborate with the primary care provider and possibly a specialist during the course of treatment.[41]

EMPIRICAL EVIDENCE FOR INTERVENTIONS FOR EARLY-ONSET PSYCHOSIS/SCHIZOPHRENIA

There have been about 3 times as many trials conducted using second-generation antipsychotics in youth compared with trials using first-generation medications. Six studies were published between the 1960s and 1990s using first-generation agents (FGAs). Although only a few trials were published in the 1990s using the second-generation medications, more than 20 studies have been completed since then. Some studies were conducted with 1 medication, some were placebo controlled, and some were head-to-head designs. Most of the published trials have reported a decrease in psychotic symptoms with active medications.[42] **Table 1** contains information about antipsychotic medications, including US Food and Drug Administration (FDA) indications and typical dose ranges used in pediatric clinical trials.

Table 1		
Antipsychotic doses and FDA indications for the treatment of schizophrenia in youth		
Medication (Brand Name)	**Dose Range**	**FDA Approval for Ages**
Second-Generation Medications		
Risperidone (Risperdal)	0.5–3 mg/d by mouth divided into twice a day or 3 times a day (maximum 6 mg/d)	≥13 y for schizophrenia
Olanzapine (Zyprexa)	2.5–10 mg/d by mouth divided into twice a day or 3 times a day (maximum 20 mg/d)	13–17 y as second-line treatment of schizophrenia
Quetiapine (Seroquel)	25–800 mg/d by mouth divided into twice a day or 3 times a day	≥13 y for schizophrenia
Aripiprazole (Abilify)	2–30 mg/d by mouth divided into twice a day or 3 times a day	13–17 y for schizophrenia
First-Generation Medications		
Fluphenazine (Prolixin)	2.5–10 mg by mouth divided into twice a day or three times a day (maximum 40 mg/d)	>12 y for schizophrenia
Loxapine (Loxatine)	60–100 mg by mouth divided into twice a day to four times a day dosing (maximum 250 mg/d)	≥16 y for schizophrenia
Trifluoperazine (Stelazine)	1–2 mg by mouth twice a day (maximum 40 mg/d)	Adults and children (6–12 y) for schizophrenia
Thioridazine (Mellaril)	50–100 mg/d divided into twice a day to 4 times a day (maximum 800 mg/d)	Adults and children for schizophrenia

When reviewing these studies, it is important to understand the rating scales that were used to evaluate effectiveness. Many investigators used the reduction of positive or negative symptoms on the Positive and Negative Syndrome Scale (PANSS)[43] or the Scale for the Assessment of Positive Symptoms[44] in combination with the Scale for the Assessment of Negative Symptoms (SANS).[45] Others selected the change scores on the Clinical Global Impression-Severity (CGI-S) or the Clinical Global Impression-Improvement (CGI-I).[46] Scores on the CGI-S of 3 or lower (mildly ill) at end point or scores on the CGI-I of 1 or 2, or a combination of measures, may be chosen to determine response.[47]

EVIDENCE BASIS FOR THE FGAS

One team of investigators studied loxapine (mean dose: 87.5 mg/d), haloperidol (mean dose: 9.8 mg/d), and placebo in adolescents with EOS.[48] Both active medications were effective in reducing psychotic symptoms, and loxapine, a congener of clozapine, was superior to haloperidol. In a study of haloperidol versus placebo using a crossover design, children with schizophrenia were randomly assigned to either 4 weeks of haloperidol or 4 weeks of placebo, or alternatively, 4 weeks of placebo and 4 weeks of haloperidol.[49] Haloperidol was superior to placebo for reduction of target symptoms and optimal dose was 0.5 to 3.5 mg/d (0.02–0.12 mg/kg/d).

In another study, 2 older agents were compared with each other (thiothixene, mean dose 16.2 mg, range: 4.8–42.6 mg, and thioridazine, mean dose: 178 mg, range: 91–228 mg). There were no differences in the rapidity of symptom abatement or the extent of the improvement at the study end.[50] Side effects for both medications included drowsiness (n = 7 on thiothixene; n = 6 on thioridazine). Some patients taking thiothixene experienced extrapyramidal symptoms (n = 7) and some taking thioridazine experienced dizziness (n = 2) and orthostatic hypotension (n = 1).[50]

EVIDENCE BASIS FOR THE SECOND-GENERATION AGENTS

These agents, also called atypical antipsychotics, have become more frequently used than FGAs, partially because of a lower risk for tardive dyskinesia.[51] Approvals for the second-generation medications from the FDA have occurred only recently. For example, risperidone and aripiprazole were approved in 2007 for youth with schizophrenia (ages 13–17 years). In 2009, olanzapine and quetiapine were approved for the treatment of youths (ages 13–17 years) with that disorder.

Clozapine

The first second-generation agent (SGA) that was systematically studied in youth was clozapine. Clozapine was initially studied in an open-label trial,[52] and then in a 6-week double-blind randomized trial at the NIMH in a group of 21 treatment-refractory youth.[53] In the double-blind study, the efficacy and adverse effects of clozapine and haloperidol were compared in the treatment of youth with COS (mean age: 14.0 ± 2.3 years). Final doses were 176 ± 149 mg/d for clozapine and 16 ± 8 mg/d for haloperidol. Clozapine was superior to haloperidol on all measures of psychosis (P = .04–.002). Both positive and negative symptoms of schizophrenia improved. However, neutropenia and seizures were concerns, such that one-third of the group had to discontinue using clozapine.

Therapeutically, clozapine has shown superiority in terms of efficacy in several head-to-head comparisons with other agents.[53–55] For example, in 1 study, clozapine-treated youth had a 66% improvement on the Brief Psychiatric Rating Scale (BPRS),[56] whereas the olanzapine group had 33% improvement (n = 39).[57]

In a retrospective study of Korean youth with treatment-refractory EOS, those treated with clozapine had a significant reduction in number of hospital days, and although neutropenia (a lowered absolute neutrophil count [ANC, measured in cells/mm³ of blood; 1000–1500 = mild; 500–1000 = moderate; <500 = severe]) developed in 27%, none developed agranulocytosis (severe and dangerous ANC count <100).[58] Clozapine dosing varies in studies from an average of 176 mg/d[53] to an average of 403.1 mg/d.[57] Many child and adolescent clinicians are concerned about the adverse effects and the burden of monitoring blood work on this agent. Agranulocytosis occurs in about 0.6% of youth treated with clozapine, but concurrent treatment with lithium can help to increase the white blood cell count.[59] The risk for this hematologic side effect is highest during the first 3 months of treatment, with a cumulative risk of 0.80% after 1 year.[60] This medication is associated with hypersalivation and increased seizure risk, so obtaining a careful history about epilepsy is warranted before starting clozapine. There have been reports of pancreatitis on this medication as well.[61] Despite its side effect profile, clozapine may be an important option for treatment-refractory cases. In clinical practice, it is generally accepted that when antipsychotic treatment with 2 different agents has either failed to yield improvement in EOS/COS or resulted in intolerable side effects, a clozapine trial is warranted.[62]

Olanzapine

Olanzapine is generally not considered a first-line treatment predominantly because of its metabolic side effect profile, although the FDA approved its use in EOS.[63] In 1 study, olanzapine was compared with placebo over 6 weeks in 107 adolescents with schizophrenia. There was significant improvement on the Brief Psychiatric Rating Scale-Child (BPRS-C)[64] ($P = .003$) and the CGI-S ($P = .004$), as well as the PANSS total ($P = .005$) and the PANSS positive ($P = .002$) scores in those on olanzapine. The treatment response rate, as defined a priori as a 30% reduction or greater on the BPRS-C total and a CGI-S of 3 or lower, did not differ significantly between olanzapine and placebo (37.5% and 25.7%, $P = .278$).[47] In general, olanzapine is associated with more metabolic side effects and significant weight gain when compared with other agents; however, it is overall better tolerated than other agents, when considering all causes for discontinuation.[65,66] The mean effective dose in 1 study of psychotic youth was 12.3 ± 3.5 mg mg/d.[65]

In a study of psychotic youth comparing olanzapine with risperidone and haloperidol in the treatment of psychosis in adolescents, 88% of patients treated with olanzapine, 74% treated with risperidone, and 53% treated with haloperidol met response criteria, defined by a change in scores on the BPRS-C total.[65] In a study of 96 adolescents with EOS treated with doses of 5 to 15 mg/d of olanzapine, 62.5% met response criteria at week 6.[67] Across studies, the mean dose at end point ranged from 11.1 to 26.2 mg/d.[47,57] A recent study indicated that younger patients may experience higher plasma levels at a given dose of olanzapine because of greater body water and less adipose tissue in childhood.[68] Olanzapine also comes in an orally disintegrating tablet (ODT) and can be helpful for reduction of acute agitation symptoms by the sublingual route, although no studies have been conducted using this preparation in youth.

Risperidone

Open-label studies with risperidone commenced in 1997 with a 3-week trial in a group of 10 youth. All had positive responses on the PANSS (20% reduction) and on other measures of response over 6 weeks.[69] One multisite study involved a 6-week double-blind randomized trial of risperidone in 160 youths with schizophrenia.[70] Patients were randomized to either placebo or to risperidone 1 to 3 mg/d or risperidone 4 to 6 mg/d and then titrated from the minimum dose by either 1 mg/d or 4 mg/d, respectively. Both active treatment groups showed significant improvement on the PANSS compared with placebo, although patients given the higher dose of risperidone (4–6 mg/d) had a higher incidence of extrapyramidal symptoms, dizziness, and hypertonia than patients given the lower dose of the agent (1–3 mg).[70] Risperidone has strong dopaminergic-blocking properties and therefore potent prolactin-increasing effects. In a series of adolescents treated openly with risperidone, galactorrhea was noted in 3 male patients and also in 2 female patients.[71] Mean end point dose range across studies was 1 to 6 mg/d.[70] Risperidone now also comes in a longer-acting formulation (injectable microspheres of 25, 37.5, or 50 mg every 14 days), yet no data have been published in youth with this formulation. In addition, risperidone also comes in an ODT, which can be useful in select patients, although there are no data on its use in youth.

Quetiapine

Quetiapine has been studied in an open-label, 12-week study conducted in 56 youth, aged 12 to 17 years, who were diagnosed with schizophrenia spectrum disorders.[72] In all, 27 youth completed the study; 17 terminated early because of lack of effectiveness. Only 35% fulfilled the response criterion at end point. Somnolence (21.4%) and fatigue (17.9%) were the most frequent side effects. Another research group assessed the safety and tolerability of this medication during an open-label extension study in 10 adolescents, 7 of whom had schizoaffective disorder.[73] There were no reports of tardive dyskinesia or extrapyramidal symptoms. However, there was nonsignificant weight gain at week 64. These investigators also performed a 23-day intensive pharmacokinetic study in 10 youth (ages 12.3–15.9 years), and found that quetiapine was well tolerated. Doses of quetiapine were given twice a day starting at 25 mg and ending at 800 mg/d. These investigators reported that 9 youth had postural tachycardia and that 6 of 10 had an average weight gain of 1.5 kg, with a range of 0.5 kg to 5.5 kg.[74] This agent has also been studied in a multisite double-blind placebo-controlled trial, which resulted in approval of the agent by the FDA for the treatment of adolescents with schizophrenia.[75]

Ziprasidone

Ziprasidone has been studied in an 8-week open-label flexible dose study with adolescents aged 9 to 18 years with schizophrenia spectrum disorders. The mean dose was 117 ± 49.2 mg/d. Sedation and weight gain were the most common side effects. Of the 40 subjects treated in the study, 10 showed symptoms of activation and 9 developed either mania or hypomania.[76] In that group of 40 youth, QT_c interval prolongation was 3.61 ± 17.55 milliseconds. Ziprasidone was also examined in another open-label study because of early concerns about the potential for Qtc interval prolongation.[77] That group studied 8 males and 5 females, aged 13 to 18 years, and 1 patient had an increase (19 milliseconds) in the QT_c interval prolongation. The most common side effects in that case series were akathisia and agitation.

Aripiprazole

The safety and efficacy of aripiprazole were evaluated in a double-blind randomized placebo-controlled study of high and low doses in adolescents with schizophrenia.[78] Patients were assigned to placebo or to a 10 mg or 30 mg dose of aripiprazole for 6 weeks. Of the 302 patients enrolled, 258 completed the trial. Both the high and low dose of aripiprazole were found to be well tolerated, and patients taking either dose showed a significant reduction in their PANSS scores compared with placebo.[78]

Aripiprazole was used in combination with clozapine in a study of 15 transition-age youth with schizophrenia (8 male; mean age: 19.3 ± 1.2 years). The combination was used because monotherapy with clozapine did not sufficiently reduce symptoms in these youth. Patients were described as receiving augmentation with aripiprazole over 11.1 ± 9.7 months. At end point, the mean daily aripiprazole dose was 8.2 ± 3.6 mg (range 5–15 mg). This strategy also had the effect of lowering the mean daily dosages of clozapine from 260 ± 84 mg (range 1250–400 mg) to 181 ± 93 mg (range 25–400). Mean CGI-S scores improved significantly from 5.3 (baseline) to 4.5 (P = .003, d = 0.76), and end point CGI-I decreased from 3.7 (at 1 month) to 3.3 (end point) (P = .212, d = 0.45).[79]

Paliperidone

A multisite 6-week double-blind parallel group study of paliperidone extended-release (ER) treatment was conducted for adolescents, ages 12 to 17 years, with a diagnosis of schizophrenia.[80] Of 201 patients randomized, 138 completed the study. Patients were randomly assigned to either placebo or a low, medium, or high fixed paliperidone ER dose based on weight (patients weighing 29–51 kg at baseline received 1.5 mg [low], 3 mg [medium], or 6 mg [high] and patients weighing 51 kg at baseline received 1.5 mg [low], 6 mg [medium], or 12 mg [high]). Results, determined by a change in PANSS score from baseline to end point, were significant for the adolescents receiving the medium dose of paliperidone ER but not for those receiving the high or low dose compared with placebo. There was also a significant difference between patients taking a dose of 3, 6, or 12 mg compared with placebo. Paliperidone was well tolerated and the most common side effects were somnolence, insomnia, tremor, headache, and akathisia.

TREATMENT OF EARLY ONSET SCHIZOPHRENIA SPECTRUM DISORDERS STUDY

Until 2008, most antipsychotic studies were conducted for FDA registration. Before the publication of the results of the Treatment of Early Onset Schizophrenia Spectrum Disorders (TEOSS) study, many clinicians believed in the superiority of second-generation medications and used them more than FGAs. TEOSS was designed to rigorously study the treatment of youth with EOS between the ages 8 and 19 years and was launched at about the same time as a similarly designed study in adults.[10,81] The adult study, called Clinical Antipsychotic Trials of Intervention Effectiveness (CATIE), was a nationwide public health-focused clinical trial designed to compare the first-generation medications with the SGAs.[82] Results from that adult study supplied important information to clinicians and showed that first-generation and second-generation antipsychotics were comparably effective but were associated with high rates of discontinuation, side effects, or failure to control symptoms. Similarly, TEOSS set out to compare the efficacy and safety of 2 second-generation antipsychotics (olanzapine and risperidone) with a first-generation antipsychotic (molindone). TEOSS was a double-blind multisite trial that randomly assigned youth to olanzapine (2.5–20 mg/d), risperidone (0.5–6 mg/d), or molindone (10–140 mg/d, plus 1 mg/d of benztropine). The primary outcome was response to treatment, defined as a CGI-I score of 1 or 2 and 20% or greater reduction in PANSS total score after 8 weeks of treatment. A total of 116 children were dosed with a medication in this study. No significant differences in efficacy were found among treatment groups (molindone: 50%; olanzapine: 34%; risperidone: 46%).[83] There also were no significant differences in the magnitude of symptom reduction between treatment arms, so all 3 medications were essentially equal. Perhaps one of the most enduring results of TEOSS was that the investigators noted safety findings were what differentiated the treatments and that weight gain was a concern, particularly in the olanzapine arm. This pivotal study highlights the differential metabolic effects of antipsychotics in youth, and, coupled with the CATIE results, suggests that the first-generation antipsychotics are just as likely to work well clinically as the SGAs in youth with schizophrenia.

TEOSS was also designed to be more than an acute trial; it had an extension phase, which lasted up to 44 weeks. Only youth who were responders (with 20% reduction in PANSS scores plus a CGI-I ≤2) after acute treatment were allowed to continue in the extension period. Fifty-four youth began the extension phase, but only 14 completed the study protocol.[84] The most common reasons for discontinuation were adverse effects or inadequate efficacy. Similar to the acute trial, there were no differences among the 3 treatment arms in terms of symptom reduction on the PANSS or the CGI-I. In addition, all treatment groups in the 44-week extension study showed statistically significant weight gain, with no between-group differences in the magnitude of weight gain.[84] Extrapyramidal side effects (EPS), such as pacing and restlessness, were more commonly seen in the molindone-treated patients. Only about 12% of those originally enrolled in TEOSS completed 12 months of treatment with their original medication. Considering these results, better and safer treatments for youth with EOS are critically needed.

Studies before TEOSS showed that youth with EOS had more pronounced neurocognitive deficits than adults.[85] In TEOSS, investigators conducted neurocognitive testing to understand possible medication effects on neurocognitive outcomes.[18,21] The investigators hypothesized that the SGAs would address both the negative symptoms and cognitive deficits in EOS. Seventy-seven of 116 TEOSS participants (66%) had extensive prebaseline and postbaseline neurocognitive data. No significant differences emerged in the neurocognitive outcomes between the 3 medication groups. Across all 3 arms, youth experienced only modest improvement in neurocognitive function, and these improvements were largely unrelated to baseline symptoms or symptom change.[18] The modest treatment effect sizes seen in this study could easily be accounted for by practice effects.[86] This study highlights the critical need for the development of more efficacious interventions for the cognitive dysfunction seen in these youth. A summary of clinical trials using antipsychotic agents is included in **Table 2**.

There are no studies that have been designed to treat youth with EOS who have another comorbid condition according to the criteria of the *Diagnostic and Statistical Manual of Mental Disorders*. There are studies that have included youth with mood disorders, such as those with schizoaffective disorder, and many of these youth have been treated with thymoleptics. For example, stable doses of thymoleptics for 30 days before enrollment were acceptable in the TEOSS study. About 20% of the 116 individuals in TEOSS were on concomitant medications (eg, selective serotonin reuptake inhibitors, mood stabilizers, and other agents).[83]

LONG-TERM EVIDENCE

There are few studies regarding the long-term course of EOS. Child-onset and adult-onset schizophrenia spectrum illnesses usually stabilize over time.[87] In 1 study of functional outcomes of 110 youth during their first episode of psychosis (ages 9–17 years), using a case-control design, cases had lower scores of both adolescence adjustment and global functioning.[88] One promising finding is that the longer the treatment, the better the outcomes, according to the epidemiologic literature.[89]

Table 2
Summaries for pediatric schizophrenia spectrum medication trials

Reference	N (Number of Patients)	Age Range (y)	Diagnosis	Length of Study (wk)	Study Design	Medication(s) Studied	Main Finding/Outcome Measure
Wolpert et al, 1967[104]	16	8–15	Childhood schizophrenia	8	Double-blind randomized	Thiothixene vs trifluoperazine	Thiothixene worked well; few side effects; comparable with trifluoperizine
Waizer et al, 1972[105]	18	5–13	Childhood schizophrenia	12	Single-blind	Thiothixene	All improved on thiothixene as noted by psychiatrist Global Impression
Engelhardt et al, 1973[106]	30	6–12	Childhood schizophrenia	12	Double-blind	Fluphenazine vs haloperidol	Both effective; few side effects
Pool et al, 1976[48]	75	13–18	Acute schizophrenia or exacerbation	4	Double-blind	Loxapine vs haloperidol vs placebo	Side effects minimal but extrapyramidal phenomena and somnolence; both loxapine and haloperidol > placebo
Realmuto et al, 1984[50]	21	11–18	Met DSM-III criteria for schizophrenia	4-6	Randomized; blinded rating	Thioridazine vs thiothixene	No differences; slightly different side effects; drowsiness for both; optimal dose for thiothixene: 30 mg/kg/d; for thioridazine: 3.3 mg/kg/d; overall not much improvement
Spencer et al, 1992[49]	16	5–11	Met DSM-III-R criteria for schizophrenia	10-wk crossover design	Double-blind, placebo-controlled	Haloperidol vs placebo	Haloperidol > placebo in children
Frazier et al, 1994[52]	11	12–17	DSM-III-R criteria for schizophrenia	6	Open-label	Clozapine	More than half showed improvement on BPRS

Study	N	Age	Diagnosis		Design	Comparison	Results
Kumra et al, 1996[53]	21	16–18	DSM-III-R criteria for schizophrenia	6	Double-blind parallel	Clozapine v haloperidol	Clozapine > haloperidol (BPRS-C, PANSS, CGI)
Armenteros et al, 1997[69]	10	11–18	DSM-IV criteria for schizophrenia	8	Open pilot	Risperidone	Risperidone significant improvement on positive and negative symptoms
Turetz et al, 1997[107]	11	9–13	DSM-III-R criteria COS	16	Open-label	Clozapine	Overall clinically significant reduction in parameters, especially positive symptoms; most improvement in first 6–8 wk
Kumra et al, 1998[108]	23 (with comparison studies) 8 open-label olanzapine	6–18	DSM-III-R criteria for schizophrenia	8	Open-label	Olanzapine	Open-label data then compared with similar 6-wk trial with clozapine; olanzapine proved effective for some of the 8 patients
Sholevar et al, 2000[109]	16	6–13	DSM-IV criteria for schizophrenia	Average 11.3 d	Open-label	Olanzapine	Most patients improved
Ratzoni et al, 2002[93]	50	13–20	46 patients had schizophrenia, 2 had schizoaffective disorder, and 2 conduct disorder all determined by DSM-IV	12	Measuring weight gain	Olanzapine vs risperidone, vs haloperidol	Olanzapine and risperidone groups experienced significant weight gain between baseline and end point ($P<.01$), whereas the average weight of the haloperidol group did not change
Findling et al, 2003[110]	16	12–17	DSM-IV criteria for schizophrenia, schizoaffective disorder, or schizophreniform disorder	8	Open-label	Olanzapine	Improvements in PANSS, CGI, and CGAS

(continued on next page)

Table 2
(continued)

Reference	N (Number of Patients)	Age Range (y)	Diagnosis	Length of Study (wk)	Study Design	Medication(s) Studied	Main Finding/ Outcome Measure
Woods et al, 2003[111]	60	12–45	Prodromal (preschizophrenia)	8	Double-blind randomized placebo-controlled	Olanzapine vs placebo	Olanzapine > placebo; olanzapine group significant weight gain
Sikich et al, 2004[65]	50	8–19	Permitted primary diagnoses were psychosis NOS, schizophreniform disorder, schizophrenia, schizoaffective disorder, delusional disorder, major depression with psychotic features, and bipolar affective disorder with psychotic features	8	Double-blind randomized	Risperidone haloperidol olanzapine	Olanzapine best tolerated, no difference efficacy of 3 groups BPRS-C
Schimmelmann et al, 2007[72]	56	12–17	DSM-IV criteria for schizophrenia, schizoaffective, or schizophreniform disorder, with a PANSS total score of ≥60 points	12	Open-label	Quetiapine	Significant reductions in PANSS total and positive scores were detected; significant weight gain occurred
Shaw et al, 2006[54]	25	7–16	DSM-IV criteria for schizophrenia	8	Double-blind randomized	Clozapine vs olanzapine	Clozapine > olanzapine (SANS, CGI)
Mozes et al, 2006[112]	25	9–14	Unmodified DSM-IV criteria for schizophrenia	12	Open-label	Risperidone vs olanzapine	Both successful; no significant difference

Study						Outcome
Quintana et al, 2007[113]	16	8–17	DSM-IV criteria for schizophrenia	10	Open-label	Olanzapine	12 patients showed significant improvement; males improved more but gained more weight; weight gain significant
Fleischhaker et al, 2007[114]	45	9–21	45 inpatients without weight-related diseases. 28 patients had a diagnosis of schizophrenia, 5 pervasive developmental disorders, 3 cannabis-related disorders, 2 schizoaffective disorder, 2 anxiety disorders, 2 disruptive behavior disorders, 1 obsessive-compulsive disorder, 1 histrionic personality disorder, and 1 Tourette disorder	6	Measuring weight gain	Olanzapine vs risperidone vs clozapine	Weight gain was significantly higher for the olanzapine group (mean = 4.6 kg, SD = 1.9) than for the risperidone (mean = 2.8 kg, SD = 1.3) and clozapine (mean = 2.5 kg ± 2.9) groups. Olanzapine and risperidone, but not clozapine, caused a disproportionately higher weight gain in children and adolescents compared with adults
Kumra et al, 2008[57]	39	10–18	DSM-IV criteria for schizophrenia	12	Randomized and double-blind design	Clozapine vs high-dose olanzapine	Clozapine > olanzapine

(continued on next page)

Table 2
(continued)

Reference	N (Number of Patients)	Age Range (y)	Diagnosis	Length of Study (wk)	Study Design	Medication(s) Studied	Main Finding/ Outcome Measure
Findling et al, 2008[78]	302	13–17	DSM-IV diagnosis of schizophrenia	6	Randomized double-blind placebo-controlled	Aripiprazole high (30 mg/d) vs low (10 mg/d)	EPS, somnolence. tremor for high > low
Sikich et al, 2008[83]	119	8–19	DSM-IV diagnosis of schizophrenia	8	Double-blind randomized placebo-controlled	Risperidone olanzapine (olanzapine arm of study prematurely ended in TEOSS because of weight gain) molindone	No difference in drug, 50% responded but olanzapine treatment also led to significant increases in fasting cholesterol, low-density lipoprotein, insulin and liver transaminases plus rapid weight gain
Berger et al, 2008[115]	141	15–25	Drug-naive first-episode psychosis patients	4-wk double-blind; followed by 8-wk flexible dose	Double-blind randomized	200 mg/d vs 400 mg/d quetiapine	Safe; well tolerated; suggested dose of 250–300 mg
DelBello et al, 2008[116]	63	10–17	23 children total, 17 of whom had schizophrenia spectrum disorders	27	Open-label flexible dosing	Ziprasidone	Starting dose of 20 mg/d titrated to between 80 and 160 mg/d over 1–2 wk seems optimal for most patients

Study	N	Age	Diagnosis	Duration	Design	Treatment	Results
Dittmann et al, 2008[67]	96	12–19	DSM-IV criteria for schizophrenia, schizoaffective, or schizophreniform disorders	24	Open-label	Olanzapine	Mean BPRS total scores decreased significantly from baseline; the rate of patients considered markedly ill or worse (CGI-S) decreased from 83.3% (baseline) to 37.5% (week 6, LOCF). The most common reported adverse event was weight gain
Jensen et al, 2008[117]	30	10–18	DSM-IV criteria for a schizophrenia-spectrum disorder (schizophrenia, schizoaffective, schizophreniform, psychotic disorder not otherwise specified)	12	Open-label; flexible dose	Risperidone vs olanzapine vs quetiapine	No differences
Haas et al, 2009[118]	160	13–17	DSM-IV diagnosis of schizophrenia	6	Randomized double-blind placebo-controlled	Risperidone low (1–3 mg) and risperidone high (4–6 mg)	Both better than placebo
Haas et al, 2009[119]	257	13–17	DSM-IV diagnosis of schizophrenia	8	Double-blind	Risperidone low and risperidone high (1.5–6 mg)	High better than low dose
Kryzhanovskaya et al, 2009[120]	107	13–17	DSM-IV diagnosis of schizophrenia	6	Randomized double-blind placebo-controlled	Olanzapine vs placebo	Better than placebo (BPRS-C; PANSS; CGI-S)

(continued on next page)

Table 2
(continued)

Reference	N (Number of Patients)	Age Range (y)	Diagnosis	Length of Study (wk)	Study Design	Medication(s) Studied	Main Finding/ Outcome Measure
Arango et al, 2009[121]	50	12–18	Diagnosis of psychosis (ie, schizophrenia or any other psychotic disorder according to DSM-IV criteria)	72	Open-label; randomized quetiapine or olanzapine	Quetiapine vs olanzapine	No difference besides side effect of weight gain
Findling et al, 2010[84]	54 of the 116 dosed were eligible to enter maintenance trial	8–19	Diagnostic criteria for schizophrenia, schizophreniform disorder, or schizoaffective disorder	44-wk maintenance treatment	Double-blind maintenance	Risperidone olanzapine molindone	No differences noted
Singh et al, 2011[80]	201	12–17	DSM-IV diagnosis of schizophrenia	6	Randomized double-blind	Paliperidone vs placebo	With weight-based treatment, only paliperidone ER medium treatment (3–6 mg) resulted in significant improvement in symptoms of schizophrenia in adolescents, as did 3, 6, and 12 mg by dose strengths

Abbreviations: CGAS, Children's Global Assessment Scale; DSM-III, Diagnostic and Statistical Manual of Mental Disorders, Third Edition; DSM-III-R, Diagnostic and Statistical Manual of Mental Disorders, Third Edition, Revised; DSM-IV, Diagnostic and Statistical Manual of Mental Disorders, Fourth Edition; SD, standard deviation; NOS, not otherwise specified; LOCF, last observation carried forward.

MONITORING OF ANTIPSYCHOTIC TREATMENTS

For the clinician starting an antipsychotic or accepting a patient into care taking this class of medication, it is advisable to obtain a thorough history and document the baseline comprehensive metabolic profile. Monitoring should proceed systematically and in partnership with primary care.[90] Monitoring metabolic parameters is essential, including glucose, insulin, liver function tests, cardiovascular, and hematologic changes.[42,66] When starting ziprasidone, obtaining a 12-lead electrocardiogram is suggested. Obtaining prolactin levels is indicated for a child who is treated with an antipsychotic and clinically has changes in the menstrual cycle or who develops

---

CLINICAL VIGNETTE

Fourteen-year-old JT was seen in the emergency department after she told her school counselor that she was seeing things that were not there and was very scared. Her teachers recently noted that she looked as if she had not showered in a while. She was evaluated by a crisis worker, who discovered that she had been having a difficult time for about 6 months. Although an honor student in past years, this school year was not going well for her. Her mother noted that she was isolating and not seeing her lacrosse friends, preferring to spend more time on her computer. When pressed, there were some concerns about bizarre behaviors: JT felt she "had to do what the voices told her to do," like putting certain items of food in the freezer "so we can check them later for poison." On mental status examination, there was thought blocking, distraction, clear ambivalence when asked questions, and attention to internal stimuli. She was disheveled and mumbled to herself quietly. After an extensive negative medical workup, performed in collaboration with her primary care provider, the child psychiatrist made a diagnosis of a primary psychotic disorder and began treatment. At first, JT did well on risperidone, which began at 0.5 mg by mouth twice a day and was gradually increased to 4 mg/d in divided doses, but she was upset about gaining weight (6.35 kg [14 pounds], which boosted her from a BMI of 83% to 96% in a few weeks). After a time, her medication was switched to aripiprazole, but this medication made her feel anxious and the voices returned. She started with 2 mg by mouth twice a day and was all the way up to 30 mg/ day when she decided that this was not working for her, and her clinician and family concurred. The family read on the Internet that older medications could also be tried, and found out that an aunt who had schizophrenia had taken perphenazine with good results. JT was not as lucky as her aunt; she had akathisia on this FGA when they titrated up to 32 mg/d in divided doses. The side effects were unresponsive to benzatropine and to diphenhydramine and she became frustrated with her lack of progress. The clinician spent time with the family over several sessions discussing the risks and benefits of clozapine and they decided to initiate this agent.

Four months later, JT emerged from her final examinations and told her mother "I feel like my old self again." She had passed her courses (with extra tutoring) and she appeared much like she had the year before, because she was more engaged, was paying more attention to her self-care, and she became interested in being the team manager in lacrosse. Together, they also decided to try metformin to alleviate the weight gain she had experienced on this agent.[96] Metformin (gradually increased to 100 mg by mouth twice a day) made her feel better and she was not gaining more weight on her final effective dose of 250 mg by mouth twice a day of clozapine. While on metformin, she also began improving her level of activity and incorporating more fresh fruits and vegetables in her daily diet. Her BMI decreased from the 96th percentile to the 85th, and she was able to accept this new weight and said that her jeans fit "well enough." When another teen in her town, a family friend, had a similar first episode, JT's parents spoke to the family at a Family-to-Family National Alliance on Mental Illness meeting. Over time, the 2 friends became closer and the families learned to help their daughters to lower stress and to pay careful attention to self-care and sleep. Both had positive outcomes, but struggled to handle their symptoms as they aged.

gynecomastia.[91] In addition to being a potential medical issue, weight gain during treatment can be upsetting to youth. In a study of 20 adolescents with antipsychotic treatment, one-third perceived the side effect of weight gain as distressing as early as 2 weeks after initiation of the treatment regimen.[92] Given that many youth in antipsychotic trials experience greater than 7% body weight gain,[55,60,61,63,65,93] asking about this side effect is warranted. Because child psychiatrists have noted for decades that weight gain accompanies treatment with SGAs, some have investigated the use of adjunctive agents, such as metformin, to minimize the weight gain. These studies have shown safety as well as some efficacy.[94–96] Tracking growth is now easier with downloadable free forms (http://www.cdc.gov/growthcharts and accompanying BMI calculators). Blood pressure norms can also be tracked with tables provided by the National High Blood Pressure Education Program Working Group.[97] Parents can be taught to look for EPS in their children, and clinicians can examine periodically for EPS. We can also track tardive dyskinesia symptoms using the Abnormal Involuntary Movement Scale.[98]

Because SGA prescribing in children increased 6-fold in a short period (between 1993 and 2002),[99] many regulators introduced measures to monitor this growth in prescriptive practice. Some states have imposed rules and have even required petitions to courts before starting youth in state custody on antipsychotic medications. States have also gradually moved to controlling formularies and try to make psychiatrists aware of the rising costs of second-generation antipsychotics.

SUMMARY/FUTURE DIRECTIONS

The literature from the past 2 decades has informed the field that our current psychopharmacologic treatments for youth with psychosis have benefits but highlight that drug development efforts to discover safer and more effective interventions are warranted. Longer-term data on our current agents are needed regarding efficacy and the long-term metabolic consequences of these agents, such as impact on fertility, bone growth, and cardiovascular effects. Future trials ideally should be of longer duration because this would increase our understanding of both the long-term benefits and adverse effects of these agents. In addition, the field would benefit from studies focused on nonpharmacologic adjunctive treatments, particularly on cognitive remediation and neuroplasticity-based treatments.[100–103] New approaches are clearly needed for children suffering with EOS.

REFERENCES

1. Kessler RC, Berglund P, Demler O, et al. Lifetime prevalence and age-of-onset distributions of DSM-IV disorders in the National Comorbidity Survey Replication. Arch Gen Psychiatry 2005;62(6):593–602.
2. McGlashan TH. Adolescent versus adult onset of mania. Am J Psychiatry 1988; 145(2):221–3.
3. Loranger AW, Levine PM. Age at onset of bipolar affective illness. Arch Gen Psychiatry 1978;35(11):1345–8.
4. Carlson GA, Kashani JH. Manic symptoms in a non-referred adolescent population. J Affect Disord 1988;15(3):219–26.
5. Chambers WJ. Psychotic symptoms in prepubertal major depressive disorder. Arch Gen Psychiatry 1982;39:921–7.
6. Ryan ND, Puig-Antich J. Pharmacological treatment of adolescent psychiatric disorders. J Adolesc Health Care 1987;8(1):137–42.

7. Kafantaris V, Coletti DJ, Dicker R, et al. Adjunctive antipsychotic treatment of adolescents with bipolar psychosis. J Am Acad Child Adolesc Psychiatry 2001;40(12):1448–56.
8. Schultz SK, Miller DD, Oliver SE, et al. The life course of schizophrenia: age and symptom dimensions. Schizophr Res 1997;23(1):15–23.
9. Buckley PF, Correll CU, Miller AL. First-episode psychosis: a window of opportunity for best practices. CNS Spectr 2007;12(9 Suppl 15):1–12 [discussion: 13–4]; [quiz: 15–6].
10. Frazier JA, McClellan J, Findling RL, et al. Treatment of early-onset schizophrenia spectrum disorders (TEOSS): demographic and clinical characteristics. J Am Acad Child Adolesc Psychiatry 2007;46(8):979–88.
11. Schaeffer JL, Ross RG. Childhood-onset schizophrenia: premorbid and prodromal diagnostic and treatment histories. J Am Acad Child Adolesc Psychiatry 2002;41(5):538–45.
12. Sikich L. Efficacy of atypical antipsychotics in early-onset schizophrenia and other psychotic disorders. J Clin Psychiatry 2008;69(Suppl 4):21–5.
13. Werry JS. Child and adolescent (early onset) schizophrenia: a review in light of DSM-III-R. J Autism Dev Disord 1992;22(4):601–24.
14. American Academy of Child and Adolescent Psychiatry. AACAP official action. Summary of the practice parameters for the assessment and treatment of children and adolescents with schizophrenia. J Am Acad Child Adolesc Psychiatry 2000;39(12):1580–2.
15. David CN, Greenstein D, Clasen L, et al. Childhood onset schizophrenia: high rate of visual hallucinations. J Am Acad Child Adolesc Psychiatry 2011;50(7):681–686. e3.
16. Russell AT. The clinical presentation of childhood-onset schizophrenia. Schizophr Bull 1994;20(4):631–46.
17. Rapoport JL, Addington A, Frangou S. The neurodevelopmental model of schizophrenia: what can very early onset cases tell us? Curr Psychiatry Rep 2005;7(2):81–2.
18. Frazier JA, Giuliano AJ, Johnson JL, et al. Neurocognitive outcomes in the treatment of early-onset schizophrenia spectrum disorders study. J Am Acad Child Adolesc Psychiatry 2012;51(5):496–505.
19. Bearden CE, Wu KN, Caplan R, et al. Thought disorder and communication deviance as predictors of outcome in youth at clinical high risk for psychosis. J Am Acad Child Adolesc Psychiatry 2011;50(7):669–80.
20. Asarnow JR, Tompson MC, McGrath EP. Annotation: childhood-onset schizophrenia: clinical and treatment issues. J Child Psychol Psychiatry 2004;45(2):180–94.
21. Hooper SR, Giuliano AJ, Youngstrom EA, et al. Neurocognition in early-onset schizophrenia and schizoaffective disorders. J Am Acad Child Adolesc Psychiatry 2010;49(1):52–60.
22. Oie MR, Rund BR. Neuropsychological deficits in adolescent-onset schizophrenia compared with attention deficit hyperactivity disorder. Am J Psychiatry 1999;156:1216–22.
23. Hafner H, Nowotny B. Epidemiology of early-onset schizophrenia. Eur Arch Psychiatry Clin Neurosci 1995;245:80–92.
24. Maziade M, Bouchard S, Gingras N, et al. Long-term stability of diagnosis and symptom dimensions in a systematic sample of patients with onset of schizophrenia in childhood and early adolescence. II: postnegative distinction and childhood predictors of adult outcome. Br J Psychiatry 1996;169(3):371–8.

25. Thomsen PH. Schizophrenia with childhood and adolescent onset-a nationwide register-based study. Acta Psychiatr Scand 1996;94(3):187–93.
26. Schimmelmann BG, Conus P, Cotton S, et al. Pre-treatment, baseline, and outcome differences between early-onset and adult-onset psychosis in an epidemiological cohort of 636 first-episode patients. Schizophr Res 2007;95(1–3):1–8.
27. Luoma S, Hakko H, Ollinen T, et al. Association between age at onset and clinical features of schizophrenia: the Northern Finland 1966 birth cohort study. Eur Psychiatry 2008;23(5):331–5.
28. Bellino S, Rocca P, Patria L, et al. Relationships of age at onset with clinical features and cognitive functions in a sample of schizophrenia patients. J Clin Psychiatry 2004;65(7):908–14.
29. Frazier JA, Alaghband-Rad J, Jacobsen L, et al. Pubertal development and onset of psychosis in childhood onset schizophrenia. Psychiatry Res 1997;70(1):1–7.
30. Hogan M, Adams J, Arrendonodo R, et al. Achieving the promise: transforming mental health care in America. Rockville (MD): Government Printing Press; 2003.
31. Newcomer JW, Hennekens CH. Severe mental illness and risk of cardiovascular disease. JAMA 2007;298(15):1794–6.
32. Kaufman J, Birmaher B, Brent D, et al. Schedule for affective disorders and schizophrenia for school-age children-present and lifetime version (K-SADS-PL): initial reliability and validity data. J Am Acad Child Adolesc Psychiatry 1997;36(7):980–8.
33. Freudenreich O, Charles Schulz S, Goff DC. Initial medical work-up of first-episode psychosis: a conceptual review. Early Interv Psychiatry 2009;3(1):10–8.
34. Compton MT, Kelley ME, Ramsay CE, et al. Association of pre-onset cannabis, alcohol, and tobacco use with age at onset of prodrome and age at onset of psychosis in first-episode patients. Am J Psychiatry 2009;166(11):1251–7.
35. Arendt M, Rosenberg R, Foldager L, et al. Cannabis-induced psychosis and subsequent schizophrenia-spectrum disorders: follow-up study of 535 incident cases. Br J Psychiatry 2005;187(6):510–5.
36. Amar M, Potvin S. Cannabis and psychosis: what is the link? J Psychoactive Drugs 2007;39:131–42.
37. Gonzalez-Pinto A, Alberich S, Barbeito S, et al. Cannabis and first-episode psychosis: different long-term outcomes depending on continued or discontinued use. Schizophr Bull 2011;37(3):631–9.
38. Schimmelmann BG, Conus P, Cotton S, et al. Prevalence and impact of cannabis use disorders in adolescents with early onset first episode psychosis. Eur Psychiatry 2012;27(6):463–9.
39. Schimmelmann BG, Conus P, Cotton SM, et al. Cannabis use disorder and age at onset of psychosis-a study in first-episode patients. Schizophr Res 2011; 129(1):52–6.
40. Kumra S. Schizophrenia and cannabis use. Minn Med 2007;90(1):36–8.
41. Lehman AF, Lieberman JA, Dixon LB, et al. Practice guideline for the treatment of patients with schizophrenia, second edition. Am J Psychiatry 2004;161(Suppl 2): 1–56.
42. Masi G, Liboni F. Management of schizophrenia in children and adolescents: focus on pharmacotherapy. Drugs 2011;71(2):179–208.
43. Kay SR, Fiszbein A, Opler LA. The Positive and Negative Syndrome Scale (PANSS) for schizophrenia. Schizophr Bull 1987;13:262–76.
44. Andreasen N. The scale for the Assessment of Positive Symptoms (SAPS). Iowa (IA): The University of Iowa Press; 1984.
45. Andreasen N. Scale for the Assessment of Negative Symptoms (SANS). Iowa (IA): The University of Iowa Press; 1983.

46. Rush J. Psychiatric measures. In: Guy W, editor. Clinical Global Impressions (CGI) Scale. Washington, DC: APA; 2000.
47. Kryzhanovskaya L, Schulz SC, McDougle C, et al. Olanzapine versus placebo in adolescents with schizophrenia: a 6-week, randomized, double-blind, placebo-controlled trial. J Am Acad Child Adolesc Psychiatry 2009;48(1):60–70.
48. Pool D, Bloom W, Mielke DH, et al. A controlled evaluation of loxitane in seventy-five adolescent schizophrenic patients. Curr Ther Res Clin Exp 1976;19(1):99–104.
49. Spencer EK, Kafantaris V, Padron-Gayol M, et al. Haloperidol in schizophrenic children: early findings from a study in progress. Psychopharmacol Bull 1992; 28:183–6.
50. Realmuto GM, Erickson WD, Yellin AM, et al. Clinical comparison of thiothixene and thioridazine in schizophrenic adolescents. Am J Psychiatry 1984;141:440–2.
51. Correll CU, Leucht S, Kane JM. Lower risk for tardive dyskinesia associated with second-generation antipsychotics: a systematic review of 1-year studies. Am J Psychiatry 2004;161(3):414–25.
52. Frazier JA, Gordon CT, McKenna K, et al. An open trial of clozapine in 11 adolescents with childhood-onset schizophrenia. J Am Acad Child Adolesc Psychiatry 1994;33(5):658–63.
53. Kumra S, Frazier JA, Jacobsen L, et al. Childhood-onset schizophrenia: a double-blind clozapine-haloperidol comparison. Arch Gen Psychiatry 1996;53:1090–7.
54. Shaw P, Sporn A, Gogtay N, et al. Childhood-onset schizophrenia: a double-blind, randomized clozapine-olanzapine comparison. Arch Gen Psychiatry 2006;63(7):721–30.
55. Kumra S, Kranzler H, Gerbino-Rosen G, et al. Clozapine versus "high-dose" olanzapine in refractory early-onset schizophrenia: an open-label extension study. J Child Adolesc Psychopharmacol 2008;18(4):307–16.
56. Overall JE, Gorham DR. The Brief Psychiatric Rating Scale (BPRS): recent developments in ascertainment and scaling. Psychopharmacol Bull 1988;24: 97–9.
57. Kumra S, Kranzler H, Gerbino-Rosen G, et al. Clozapine and "high-dose" olanzapine in refractory early-onset schizophrenia: a 12-week randomized and double-blind comparison. Biol Psychiatry 2008;63(5):524–9.
58. Kim Y, Kim BN, Cho SC, et al. Long-term sustained benefits of clozapine treatment in refractory early onset schizophrenia: a retrospective study in Korean children and adolescents. Hum Psychopharmacol 2008;23(8):715–22.
59. Sporn A, Gogtay N, Ortiz-Aguayo R, et al. Clozapine-induced neutropenia in children: management with lithium carbonate. J Child Adolesc Psychopharmacol 2003;13(3):401–4.
60. Alvir JM, Lieberman JA. Agranulocytosis: incidence and risk factors. J Clin Psychiatry 1994;55(Suppl B):137–8.
61. Wehmeier PM, Heiser P, Remschmidt H. Pancreatitis followed by pericardial effusion in an adolescent treated with clozapine. J Clin Psychopharmacol 2003;23(1):102–3.
62. Findling RL, Frazier JA, Gerbino-Rosen G, et al. Is there a role for clozapine in the treatment of children and adolescents? J Am Acad Child Adolesc Psychiatry 2007;46(3):423–8.
63. Maloney AE, Sikich L. Olanzapine approved for the acute treatment of schizophrenia or manic/mixed episodes associated with bipolar I disorder in adolescent patients. Neuropsychiatr Dis Treat 2010;6:749–66.
64. Overall J, Pfefferbaum B. The brief psychiatric rating scale for children. Psychol Bull 1982;18(2):10–6.

65. Sikich L, Hamer RM, Bashford RA, et al. A pilot study of risperidone, olanzapine, and haloperidol in psychotic youth: a double-blind, randomized, 8-week trial. Neuropsychopharmacology 2004;29(1):133–45.
66. Correll CU, Manu P, Olshanskiy V, et al. Cardiometabolic risk of second-generation antipsychotic medications during first-time use in children and adolescents. JAMA 2009;302(16):1765–73.
67. Dittmann RW, Meyer E, Freisleder FJ, et al. Effectiveness and tolerability of olanzapine in the treatment of adolescents with schizophrenia and related psychotic disorders: results from a large, prospective, open-label study. J Child Adolesc Psychopharmacol 2008;18:54–69.
68. Aichhorn W, Marksteiner J, Walch T, et al. Age and gender effects on olanzapine and risperidone plasma concentrations in children and adolescents. J Child Adolesc Psychopharmacol 2007;17(5):665–74.
69. Armenteros JL, Whitaker AH, Welikson M, et al. Risperidone in adolescents with schizophrenia: an open pilot study. J Am Acad Child Adolesc Psychiatry 1997; 36(5):694–700.
70. Pandina G, Kushner S, Karcher K, et al. An open-label, multicenter evaluation of the long-term safety and efficacy of risperidone in adolescents with schizophrenia. Child Adolesc Psychiatry Ment Health 2012;6(1):23.
71. Holzer L, Eap CB. Risperidone-induced symptomatic hyperprolactinaemia in adolescents. J Clin Psychopharmacol 2006;26(2):167–71.
72. Schimmelmann BG, Mehler-Wex C, Lambert M, et al. A prospective 12-week study of quetiapine in adolescents with schizophrenia spectrum disorders. J Child Adolesc Psychopharmacol 2007;17(6):768–78.
73. McConville B, Carrero L, Sweitzer D, et al. Long-term safety, tolerability, and clinical efficacy of quetiapine in adolescents: an open-label extension trial. J Child Adolesc Psychopharmacol 2003;13(1):75–82.
74. McConville BJ, Arvanitis LA, Thyrum PT, et al. Pharmacokinetics, tolerability, and clinical effectiveness of quetiapine fumarate: an open-label trial in adolescents with psychotic disorders. J Clin Psychiatry 2000;61(4):252–60.
75. AstraZeneca. Quetiapine fumarate (SEROQUEL) compared to placebo in the treatment of adolescent patients with schizophrenia (ANCHOR 112). In: Clinical-Trials.gov [Internet]. Bethesda (MD): National Library of Medicine (US); 2000. Accessed July 12, 2012. Available at: http://clinicaltrials.gov/ct2/show/NCT00090324. NLM Identifier: NCT00090324.
76. Ambler D, Maloney A, Hunt-Harrison T, et al. Ziprasidone in early onset schizophrenia and schizoaffective disorder. Biol Psychiatry 2006;59(Suppl 8):1s–264s.
77. Patel NC, Sierk P, Dorson PG, et al. Experience with ziprasidone. J Am Acad Child Adolesc Psychiatry 2002;41(5):495.
78. Findling RL, Robb A, Nyilas M, et al. A multiple-center, randomized, double-blind, placebo-controlled study of oral aripiprazole for treatment of adolescents with schizophrenia. Am J Psychiatry 2008;165(11):1432–41.
79. Bachmann CJ, Lehr D, Theisen FM, et al. Aripiprazole as an adjunct to clozapine therapy in adolescents with early-onset schizophrenia: a retrospective chart review. Pharmacopsychiatry 2009;42(4):153–7.
80. Singh J, Robb A, Vijapurkar U, et al. A randomized, double-blind study of paliperidone extended-release in treatment of acute schizophrenia in adolescents. Biol Psychiatry 2011;70(12):1179–87.
81. McClellan J, Sikich L, Findling RL, et al. Treatment of early-onset schizophrenia spectrum disorders (TEOSS): rationale, design, and methods. J Am Acad Child Adolesc Psychiatry 2007;46(8):969–78.

82. Stroup TS, Lieberman JA, McEvoy JP, et al. Effectiveness of olanzapine, quetiapine, risperidone, and ziprasidone in patients with chronic schizophrenia following discontinuation of a previous atypical antipsychotic. Am J Psychiatry 2006;163(4):611–22.

83. Sikich L, Frazier JA, McClellan J, et al. Double-blind comparison of first- and second-generation antipsychotics in early-onset schizophrenia and schizo-affective disorder: findings from the treatment of early-onset schizophrenia spectrum disorders (TEOSS) study. Am J Psychiatry 2008;165(11): 1420–31.

84. Findling RL, Johnson JL, McClellan J, et al. Double-blind maintenance safety and effectiveness findings from the treatment of early-onset schizophrenia spectrum (TEOSS) study. J Am Acad Child Adolesc Psychiatry 2010;49(6):583–94.

85. White T, Ho BC, Ward J, et al. Neuropsychological performance in first-episode adolescents with schizophrenia: a comparison with first-episode adults and adolescent control subjects. Biol Psychiatry 2006;60(5):463–71.

86. Goldberg TE, Keefe RS, Goldman RS, et al. Circumstances under which practice does not make perfect: a review of the practice effect literature in schizophrenia and its relevance to clinical treatment studies. Neuropsychopharmacology 2010;35(5):1053–62.

87. Remschmidt H, Martin M, Fleischhaker C, et al. Forty-two-years later: the outcome of childhood-onset schizophrenia. J Neural Transm 2007;114(4):505–12.

88. Castro-Fornieles J, Parellada M, Gonzalez-Pinto A, et al. The child and adolescent first-episode psychosis study (CAFEPS): design and baseline results. Schizophr Res 2007;91(1–3):226–37.

89. Rani F, Murray ML, Byrne PJ, et al. Epidemiologic features of antipsychotic prescribing to children and adolescents in primary care in the United Kingdom. Pediatrics 2008;121(5):1002–9.

90. Correll CU, Penzner JB, Parikh UH, et al. Recognizing and monitoring adverse events of second-generation antipsychotics in children and adolescents. Child Adolesc Psychiatr Clin North Am 2006;15(1):177–206.

91. Correll CU, Carlson HE. Endocrine and metabolic adverse effects of psychotropic medications in children and adolescents. J Am Acad Child Adolesc Psychiatry 2006;45(7):771–91.

92. Schimmelmann BG, Paulus S, Schacht M, et al. Subjective distress related to side effects and subjective well-being in first admitted adolescents with early-onset psychosis treated with atypical antipsychotics. J Child Adolesc Psychopharmacol 2005;15(2):249–58.

93. Ratzoni G, Gothelf D, Brand-Gothelf A, et al. Weight gain associated with olanzapine and risperidone in adolescent patients: a comparative prospective study. J Am Acad Child Adolesc Psychiatry 2002;41(3):337–43.

94. Klein DJ, Cottingham EM, Sorter M, et al. A randomized, double-blind, placebo-controlled trial of metformin treatment of weight gain associated with initiation of atypical antipsychotic therapy in children and adolescents. Am J Psychiatry 2006;163(12):2072–9.

95. Klein DJ, Cottingham EM, Sorter M, et al. A randomized, double-blind, placebo-controlled trial of metformin treatment of weight gain associated with initiation of atypical antipsychotic therapy in children and adolescents. Am J Psychiatry 2006;163(12):2072–9.

96. Shin L, Bregman H, Breeze JL, et al. Metformin for weight control in pediatric patients on atypical antipsychotic medication. J Child Adolesc Psychopharmacol 2009;19(3):275–9.

97. National High Blood Pressure Education Program Working Group on High Blood Pressure in C, Adolescents. The fourth report on the diagnosis, evaluation, and treatment of high blood pressure in children and adolescents. Pediatrics 2004; 114(2 Suppl 4th Report):555–76.

98. Abnormal involuntary movement scale (AIMS). Psychopharmacol Bull 1988; 24(4):781–3.

99. Olfson M, Blanco C, Liu L, et al. National trends in the outpatient treatment of children and adolescents with antipsychotic drugs. Arch Gen Psychiatry 2006;63(6):679–85.

100. Fisher M, Holland C, Merzenich MM, et al. Using neuroplasticity-based auditory training to improve verbal memory in schizophrenia. Am J Psychiatry 2009; 166(7):805–11.

101. Gard DE, Fisher M, Garrett C, et al. Motivation and its relationship to neurocognition, social cognition, and functional outcome in schizophrenia. Schizophr Res 2009;115(1):74–81.

102. Subramaniam K, Luks Tracy L, Fisher M, et al. Computerized cognitive training restores neural activity within the reality monitoring network in schizophrenia. Neuron 2012;73(4):842–53.

103. Wykes T, Huddy V, Cellard C, et al. A meta-analysis of cognitive remediation for schizophrenia: methodology and effect sizes. Am J Psychiatry 2011;168(5): 472–85.

104. Wolpert A, Hagamen MB, Merlis S. A comparative study of thiothixene and trifluoperazine in childhood schizophrenia. Curr Ther Res Clin Exp 1967;9(9): 482–5.

105. Waizer J, Polizos P, Hoffman SP, et al. A single-blind evaluation of thiothixene with outpatient schizophrenic children. J Autism Child Schizophr 1972;2(4):378–86.

106. Engelhardt DM, Polizos P, Waizer J, et al. A double-blind comparison of fluphenazine and haloperidol in outpatient schizophrenic children. J Autism Child Schizophr 1973;3(2):128–37.

107. Turetz M, Mozes T, Toren P, et al. An open trial of clozapine in neuroleptic-resistant childhood-onset schizophrenia. Br J Psychiatry 1997;170:507–10.

108. Kumra S, Jacobsen L, Lenane M, et al. Childhood-onset schizophrenia: an open-label study of olanzapine in adolescents. J Am Acad Child Adolesc Psychiatry 1998;37(4):377–85.

109. Sholevar EH, Baron DA, Hardie TL. Treatment of childhood-onset schizophrenia with olanzapine. J Child Adolesc Psychopharmacol 2000;10(2):69–78.

110. Findling R, McNamara J, Youngstrom E, et al. A prospective, open-label trial of olanzapine in adolescents with schizophrenia. J Am Acad Child Adolesc Psychiatry 2003;42(2):170–5.

111. Woods SW, Breier A, Zipursky RB, et al. Randomized trial of olanzapine versus placebo in the symptomatic acute treatment of the schizophrenic prodrome. Biol Psychiatry 2003;54(4):453–64.

112. Mozes T, Ebert T, Michal SE, et al. An open-label randomized comparison of olanzapine versus risperidone in the treatment of childhood-onset schizophrenia. J Child Adolesc Psychopharmacol 2006;16(4):393–403.

113. Quintana H, Wilson MS 2nd, Purnell W, et al. An open-label study of olanzapine in children and adolescents with schizophrenia. J Psychiatr Pract 2007;13(2): 86–96.

114. Fleischhaker C, Heiser P, Hennighausen K, et al. Weight gain associated with clozapine, olanzapine and risperidone in children and adolescents. J Neural Transm 2007;114(2):273–80.

115. Berger GE, Proffitt TM, McConchie M, et al. Dosing quetiapine in drug-naive first-episode psychosis: a controlled, double-blind, randomized, single-center study investigating efficacy, tolerability, and safety of 200 mg/day vs. 400 mg/day of quetiapine fumarate in 141 patients aged 15 to 25 years. J Clin Psychiatry 2008;69(11):1702–14.
116. DelBello MP, Versavel M, Ice K, et al. Tolerability of oral ziprasidone in children and adolescents with bipolar mania, schizophrenia, or schizoaffective disorder. J Child Adolesc Psychopharmacol 2008;18(5):491–9.
117. Jensen JB, Kumra S, Leitten W, et al. A comparative pilot study of second-generation antipsychotics in children and adolescents with schizophrenia-spectrum disorders. J Child Adolesc Psychopharmacol 2008;18(4):317–26.
118. Haas M, Unis AS, Armenteros J, et al. A 6-week, randomized, double-blind, placebo-controlled study of the efficacy and safety of risperidone in adolescents with schizophrenia. J Child Adolesc Psychopharmacol 2009;19(6):611–21.
119. Haas M, Eerdekens M, Kushner S, et al. Efficacy, safety and tolerability of two dosing regimens in adolescent schizophrenia: double-blind study. Br J Psychiatry 2009;194(2):158–64.
120. Kryzhanovskaya LA, Robertson-Plouch CK, Xu W, et al. The safety of olanzapine in adolescents with schizophrenia or bipolar I disorder: a pooled analysis of 4 clinical trials. J Clin Psychiatry 2009;70(2):247–58.
121. Arango C, Robles O, Parellada M, et al. Olanzapine compared to quetiapine in adolescents with a first psychotic episode. Eur Child Adolesc Psychiatry 2009; 18(7):418–28.

Pharmacologic Treatment of Bipolar Disorder in Children and Adolescents

Benjamin I. Goldstein, MD, PhD[a],*, Roberto Sassi, MD, PhD[b], Rasim S. Diler, MD[c]

KEYWORDS

- Bipolar • Manic • Psychopharmacotherapy • Antipsychotics • Mood stabiliziers
- Comorbidities

KEY POINTS

- There is a substantial rigorous evidence base regarding treatment of mania among youth, whereas less is known regarding the treatment of youth with bipolar depression, mainenance treatment, and treatment in the presence of certain comorbidities.
- Response rates in studies of treatments of acute manic and mixed episodes among children and adolescents are comparable to those among adults.
- Youth seem highly responsive to second-generation antipsychotics (SGAs) and especially sensitive to their metabolic side effects.
- Combination treatment and continuation treatment are common clinical scenarios, but there is limited evidence to guide this treatment.
- Provided that mood is first stabilized with a first-line antimanic medication, stimulant treatment of comorbid attention-deficit/hyperactivity disorder (ADHD) seems safe and effective.

OVERVIEW

Bipolar disorder (BD) is a recurrent and severe illness characterized by substantial symptomatic burden, comorbidity, functional impairment, and suicide risk.[1–5] Child-onset and adolescent-onset BD may be even more severe and may have an even worse prognosis than adult-onset BD.[4,6–8] Although case descriptions of mania in children have been available for almost a century,[9,10] it is only within approximately the past 15 to 20 years that rigorous research on this topic has been conducted.[a]

---

[a] Departments of Psychiatry and Pharmacology, Sunnybrook Health Sciences Centre, University of Toronto Faculty of Medicine, Toronto, ON, Canada; [b] Department of Psychiatry and Behavioural Neurosciences, McMaster University Faculty of Health Sciences, Hamilton, ON, Canada; [c] Western Psychiatric Institute and Clinic, University of Pittsburgh School of Medicine, Pittsburgh, PA, USA
* Corresponding author. Department of Psychiatry, Sunnybrook Health Sciences Centre, 2075 Bayview Avenue, Room FG-53, Toronto, Ontario M4N-3M5, Canada.
E-mail address: benjamin.goldstein@sunnybrook.ca

[a] For the purpose of this review, unless otherwise indicated, the term, *BP*, encompasses all subtypes (I, II, cyclothymia, and NOS), and the term, *pediatric*, refers to children and/or adolescents ≤19 years of age.

Child Adolesc Psychiatric Clin N Am 21 (2012) 911–939
http://dx.doi.org/10.1016/j.chc.2012.07.004
1056-4493/12/$ – see front matter © 2012 Elsevier Inc. All rights reserved.

Recently, compelling international data from the World Health Organization indicate that BD is the fourth leading cause of disability among adolescents ages 15 to 19 years worldwide, accounting for fully 5% of total disability in this age range.[11] There is still an active debate in the scientific literature on whether the dramatic increase in rates of pediatric BD (PBD) diagnoses in clinical settings over the past decades[12,13] is mostly related to better awareness of this problem, an interpretation of the definition of bipolarity in children that is too broad, and/or upcoding in settings where health insurance reimbursement is diagnosis dependent.[9,14–16] It is also possible that rates are actually increasing, although epidemiologic data to date suggest otherwise.[17] Although prescriptions for mood-stabilizing medications for children have increased dramatically,[18] unfortunately it seems that the majority of youth with BD may not access treatment for their illness.[19] Similarly, despite controversies regarding overdiagnosis, the number of youth who receive diagnoses of BD in clinical settings is much less than expected based on the population prevalence of BD.[20]

Despite these controversies, the validity of the *Diagnostic and Statistical Manual of Mental Disorders* (Fourth Edition) criteria as applied in youth has been supported by substantial evidence.[1,16,21] Recent findings from the Course and Outcome of Bipolar Youth study indicate that the longitudinal course of PBD is in many ways comparable to that of adults: 90% experience pathologic elation, most experience recovery and recurrences, depression is the prevailing polarity; and subsyndromal symptoms predominate.[1] Compared with adults with BD, however, youth with BD spend more time with syndromal and clinically significant subsyndromal symptoms, in particular mixed states, and have far more changes in symptomatic status.[22] Younger children have even fewer typical presentations than adolescents.[23]

The frequency of symptomatic recurrences in BD in general,[24,25] specifically in child and adolescent BD,[1,26,27] underscores the importance of mood stabilizing medications. Over the past decade there has been tremendous progress in the evidence regarding the pharmacologic treatment of PBD. By virtue of the tremendous growth of research in the area of PBD, this review cannot address all of the important topics that are salient to the treatment of PBD. Previous publications have addressed treatment algorithms and guidelines for PBD,[28,29] and other recent reviews have comprehensively examined the existing literature on the pharmacologic treatment of PBD.[30–33] There is limited literature regarding the treatment of PBD among preschoolers[34–36] and regarding alternative treatments of PBD,[37] which are topics not specifically addressed in this review. The issue of treatment-emergent mania associated with antidepressants and psychostimulants has been recently comprehensively examined and is not reviewed here,[38] and the same is true of metabolic tolerability.[39,40]

This review focuses mainly on published articles regarding the treatment of school-aged children and adolescents with PBD. In light of the systematic reviews, large randomized controlled trial (RCT) data are emphasized wherever possible. This review addresses the treatment of acute manic/mixed episodes, including combination treatment, the preliminary literature regarding bipolar depression among youth, treatment in the face of comorbid conditions, and maintenance treatment. Finally, suggestions regarding future directions are offered.

EMPIRIC EVIDENCE
Acute Manic and Mixed Episodes

Lithium
Lithium was the first drug approved by the Food and Drug Administration for the treatment of mania in children 12 years and older, a decision largely owed to lithium's long

history of use in adults (**Table 1**).[b,41] Open-label studies of lithium in pediatric mania have shown significant improvement in both manic and depressive symptoms after 4 to 6 weeks of treatment, with a response rate between 38% and 55%.[42–44] These studies allowed the use of adjunctive medications, however, including antipsychotics, limiting conclusions about lithium monotherapy. In an open-label study, children with manic or mixed episodes were randomized to receive lithium, divalproex sodium (DVPX), or carbamazepine for 6 weeks.[43] Their results suggest that DVPX is more effective, with response rates of 53%, whereas lithium and carbamazepine had an equally lower response of 38%. Although all agents showed large effect sizes (ESs), these differences among the treatments were not statistically significant. Moreover, no placebo group was included, limiting efficacy conclusions. Preliminary data from the multisite Collaborative Lithium Trials (N = 61) found a 58% response rate to open-label lithium.[45] A randomized, double-blind, placebo-controlled study evaluating the efficacy of lithium in acute mania has been presented but not yet published.[46] In an 8-week trial with 153 manic/mixed patients with PBD, response rates did not differ significantly for lithium (41%) and placebo (30%) whereas DVPX (56%) did yield significantly greater response than placebo. A previous study examining lithium for adolescents with comorbid PBD and substance use disorders[47] and findings from the multisite Treatment of Early Age Mania study are described later.[48] A randomized double-blind placebo-controlled lithium discontinuation study has also been reported.[49] After 4 weeks on open-label lithium treatment, 40 patients ages 12 to 18 years with PBD-I and in a manic episode who responded to lithium monotherapy, defined as 33% decline in the total Young Mania Rating Scale (YMRS), enrolled in the double-blind arm of the study, in which they either continued with lithium for another 2 weeks or received placebo after a quick taper period. No significant differences in exacerbation rates were found between the subjects who continued lithium treatment and those who were switched to placebo. Important limitations of this preliminary study include a small sample size, discontinuation before recovery, and rapid discontinuation.

Anticonvulsants

Divalproex
Small, open-label trials of DVPX in acute pediatric mania have reported response rates ranging from 53% to 75%.[50–52] A large (N = 150; 10–17 years old) 4-week industry-sponsored multicenter study found a similar response rate for DVPX (24%) and placebo (23%).[53] Controlled trials comparing DVPX with SGAs are discussed.

Lamotrigine
There are no double-blind placebo-controlled studies of lamotrigine for mania/hypomania in PBD; however, open-label data show promise. In a prospective 12-week trial of 39 children (6–17 years) with PBD and manic symptoms, there was a significant reduction in manic symptoms and 54% responded to ($\geq$50% reduction in symptoms) lamotrigine.[54] Fifteen subjects developed some form of skin rash, and of those only 6 discontinued the trial due to a rash deemed related to lamotrigine, all of which resolved after treatment discontinuation. None developed Stevens-Johnson syndrome.

---

[b] For the purpose of this review, response and remission rates are reported as indicated in the original publications. Definitions for response and remission vary across different studies, however, and differ based on the scale used and/or the cut-off used (eg, percentage change and absolute score).

Table 1
Dosing and effectiveness of bipolar disorder medications

Medication	Dosing	Effectiveness/Efficacy	Side Effects	Black Box Warnings, Contraindications	Comment
Antipsychotics					
Aripiprazole	5–30 mg	2 Positive RCTs for acute mania, 1 positive RCT for maintenance	Sedation, stomach discomfort, extrapyramidal side effects	Class black box warnings regarding suicidality; contraindication if previous hypersensitivity to drug (applied to all medications)	Doses in the higher range (20–30 mg/d) may be needed in acute mania, but maintenance treatment can be achieved with lower doses (5–10 mg/d), minimizing side effects.
Olanzapine	5–20 mg	1 Positive RCT for acute mania	Increased appetite, somnolence, sedation, weight gain, dyslipidemia, dysglycemia		Very efficacious in acute mania, but metabolic side effects are noticeable even after 3 of weeks of treatment. Combining topiramate with olanzapine may mitigate the treatment-emergent weight gain.

Quetiapine	150–600 mg	1 Positive unpublished RCT for acute mania, 1 negative RCT for bipolar depression, 1 positive RCT as augmentation to DVPX in acute mania, 1 RCT (no placebo arm) comparing favorably to DVPX in acute mania	Sedation, dizziness, gastrointestinal upset, weight gain, dyslipidemia, dysglycemia	Treatment of acute mania required doses around 400 mg/d in most studies. The 600-mg/d regimen did not seem more effective than 400 mg/d. In bipolar depression, doses up to 600 mg/d were not effective among adolescents, in contrast to the positive results in adults.
Risperidone	0.5–6 mg	1 Positive RCT for acute mania, 2 RCTs (no placebo arm) comparing risperidone favorably to lithium and DVPX in acute mania	Fatigue, extrapyramidal side effects, elevated prolactin levels, weight gain, elevations in cholesterol levels. Elevated prolactin may cause intolerable side effects in few cases.	Small doses (0.5–2.5 g/d) were as effective as high doses (3–6 mg/d) to treat acute mania, with fewer side effects.

(continued on next page)

Table 1
(continued)

Medication	Dosing	Effectiveness/Efficacy	Side Effects	Black Box Warnings, Contraindications	Comment
Ziprasidone	80–160 mg	1 Positive unpublished RCT for acute mania.	Sedation, headaches, gastrointestinal upset. QTc and weight changes were not observed in the few available studies	Contraindicated in patients with a known history of QT prolongation or arrhythmia history, in patients with recent acute myocardial infarction and in patients with uncompensated heart failure hypokalemia or hypomagnesemia. Ziprasidone should not be given with other drugs that cause QTc prolongation.	Very few data currently available on its efficacy in PBD. Risk-benefit may be optimized in patients at risk of metabolic syndrome.
Mood stabilizers					
Carbamazepine	400–2000 mg in Divided doses, blood levels 4–10 mEq/L	Modest response rates in open studies	Dizziness, drowsiness, vision changes, double vision, upset GI, loss of appetite, dry mouth, weight gain, potential for severe dermatologic reactions	Black box warning regarding serious dermatologic reactions, and suggestion to screen Asian patients for HLA-B*1502 (generally not used if positive). Black box warning regarding aplastic anemia,	Paucity of data precludes specific recommendations at present.

agranulocytosis. Contraindicated if hypersensitivity to carbamazepine, TCAs, HLA-B*1502 allele, history of hepatic porphyria, bone marrow depression, MAOI within 14 d.

Significant teratogenic potential, use with caution in females, ensuring 2 reliable means of contraception.

	Dose	RCTs	Side effects	Warnings/Contraindications	Notes
DVPX	500–2000 mg, blood levels 50–150mEq/L	Three negative RCTs but one unpublished RCT was better than placebo. Head-to-head trials show that SGAs have better ESs and are overall better tolerated than DVPX.	Weight gain, tremor, nausea, diarrhea, cognitive dulling, sedation, fatigue, ataxia, dizziness; also, hepatic failure, thrombocytopenia, pancreatitis, potential for severe dermatologic reactions, polycyctic ovarian disease	Black box warning for hepatoxicity, teratogenicity, pancreatitis. Contraindications if hypersensitivity, hepatic disease or impairment, urea cycle disorders.	
Lamotrigine	25–400 mg in Divided doses during titration. Blood levels available, but link with outcomes not yet established.	No RCTs. Open-label studies are promising	Abdominal symptoms, dizziness, ataxia, headache, tremor, blurred vision, diplopia, potential for severe dermatologic reactions	Black box warning for serious rash (Stevens-Johnson, toxic epidermal necrolysis). Younger age is only clear predictive risk factor. Rapid dose titration, high starting dose, or concomitant DVPX are other potential risk factors.	May help with symptoms of hypomania, may be preferred in depressive phase. Requires low initiation dose and slow titration. Lack of significant weight gain is a benefit.

(continued on next page)

Table 1
(continued)

Medication	Dosing	Effectiveness/Efficacy	Side Effects	Black Box Warnings, Contraindications	Comment
Lithium	300–1800 mg, Blood levels 0.6–1.2 mEq/L	The first medication approved by FDA but grandfathered. One unpublished study was negative and the other RCT that included prepubertal children showed poorer response rate than risperidone. Maintenance studies negative but had few subjects and short duration.	Lithium toxicity (dizziness, clumsiness, unsteady gait, slurred speech, coarse tremors, abdominal pain, vomiting, sedation, confusion and blurry vision), polyuria, polydipsia, tremor, weight gain, nausea, diarrhea, cognitive dulling, sedation, leukocytosis, possible ECG T-wave changes Possible renal failure and hypothyroidism.	Black box warning for lithium toxicity. Narrow therapeutic index. Potentially lethal in overdose.	May consider preferentially if a parent has lithium-responsive BD. Interactions with common medications, including anti-inflammatories.
Oxcarbazepine	300- mg bid to 2400 mg/d in Adults	Case reports were promising, but the only RCT was negative.	Less concern about hepatic enzyme induction, and does not require blood monitoring, but otherwise similar to carbamazepine (eg, dizziness, drowsiness, vision changes, double vision, upset GI, loss of appetite, dry mouth, weight gain, skin reaction)	Hypersensitivity	In RCT, 19% on oxcarbazepine discontinued, vs 4% in placebo group. Six patients on oxcarbazepine and none on placebo required hospitalization. Negative RCT combined with tolerability concerns reduce enthusiasm for this option.

Topiramate	50–400 mg in Divided doses	One RCT was terminated and available result is negative.	Flushing skin, upset GI, dizziness, memory impairment, decreased concentration, tiredness, decreased appetite	Hypersensitivity	May be combined with SGA for weight concerns; a study is now in progress for using it in comorbid substance use.
Stimulants and NRIs for comorbid ADHD					
Atomoxetine	Target 0.8–1.2 mg/kg	1 Open trial, large ES	No manic/mixed episodes, but 2/12 subjects discontinued due to worsening mood symptoms.	Black box warning regarding suicidality. Contraindicated if hypersensitivity, MAOI within 14 d, angle-closure glaucoma, cardiac structural abnormalities, cardiomyopathy, severe arrhythmias, pheochromocytoma	Promising signal from open trial
Methylphenidate	5–15 mg bid	1 positive RCT	Most side effects in RCT were similar to placebo. Potential side effects for stimulants include irritability, insomnia, tics, rebound effects, anorexia.	Black box warning regarding use in patients with substance use disorders. Similar contraindications to atomoxetine, also contraindicated if agitation present, age <6 y, history of tics.	May require lower than usual stimulant doses. Treatment-associated psychiatric adverse events (ie, hypo/mania, suicidality) in 2.5%–10%.

(continued on next page)

Table 1
(continued)

Medication	Dosing	Effectiveness/Efficacy	Side Effects	Black Box Warnings, Contraindications	Comment
Mixed amphetamine salts	5 mg bid	1 Positive RCT	1 in 30 Subjects became manic, but no systematic change in manic symptoms. Side effects as for methylphenidate.	Black box warning for high abuse potential and dependency. Similar contraindications to atomoxetine, also contraindicated if moderate-severe hypertension, hyperthyroidism, substance abuse history.	As for methylphenidate

Abbreviations: FDA, Food and Drug Administration; GI, gastrointestinal; MAOI, monoamine oxidase inhibitors.
Note: for a summary of other information, including half-life, cytochrome P-450 metabolism, excretion, pregnancy category, and FDA indications, see Hamrin V, Iennaco JD. Psychopharmacology of pediatric bipolar disorder. Expert Rev Neurother 2011;10:1053; and Pfeifer JC, Kowatch RA, DelBello MP. Pharmacotherapy of bipolar disorder in children and adolescents: recent progress. CNS Drugs 2010;24:575.

Carbamazepine

Despite promising observational findings,[55–58] few treatment studies have examined carbamazepine. In a comparative study, the ES for carbamazepine was similar to that of lithium.[43] In an 8-week prospective open-label trial of extended-release carbamazepine monotherapy for 27 manic/mixed/hypomanic children ages 6 to 12, 52% experienced at least 30% reduction in manic symptoms and 34% achieved remission (YMRS <12).[59]

Oxcarbazepine

Oxcarbazepine, an analog of carbamazepine with fewer side effects and better pharmacokinetic properties, had shown some promise as a treatment of acute mania in adults.[60] Despite promising case reports in youth,[61,62] however, oxcarbazepine did not show a statistically significant difference from placebo in any of the outcome measures in a large, double-blind, placebo-controlled trial when examining the whole sample of 116 subjects.[63] When separating children (7–12 years) from adolescents (13–18 years), however, 41% percent of the children in the oxcarbazepine group and 17% of those in the placebo group achieved at least a 50% reduction in YMRS scores. Among adolescents, the results on this measure were similar for oxcarbazepine and placebo (43% and 40%, respectively). Although the overall differences were not statistically significant, it is possible that this study was underpowered to detect efficacy differences in the younger subsample.

Topiramate

One retrospective study suggested that adjunctive topiramate reduces the severity of bipolar mania in pediatric patients.[64] A 4-week, double-blind, placebo-controlled trial of topiramate in pediatric mania, however, was prematurely terminated by the industry sponsor due to negative findings in adults, after recruiting 56 of a planned 230 subjects.[65] Although reduction of mean manic symptom scores was 2-fold greater in the topiramate group, this difference was not significant. A significant steeper slope of improvement in the topiramate group tentatively suggests that improvement may have been more rapid.

Second-Generation Antipsychotics

Risperidone

Confirming previous findings from open-label trials and chart reviews,[66,67] a 3-week study of 169 children ages 10 to 17 years demonstrated the efficacy of risperidone for mania. Subjects were randomly assigned to placebo, low-dose risperidone (0.5–2.5 mg/d), or high-dose risperidone (3–6 mg/d). Significant clinical improvement was observed with both risperidone treatment groups within the first week. Response rates in the low-dose (59%) and high-dose (63%) groups were superior to placebo (26%). There was a dose-dependent increase in the frequency of side effects in the active group.

Olanzapine

Confirming previous findings from open-label trials and chart reviews,[68–70] olanzapine's efficacy in treating acute mania was supported by a 3-week, double-blind, placebo-controlled, multisite study of 161 adolescents ages 13 to 17 years.[71] Olanzapine was superior to placebo within the first week. Response (48.6% vs 22.2%) and remission (35.2% vs 11.1%) were also superior for olanzapine at week 3.

Quetiapine

Chart reviews have suggested that quetiapine is effective and safe in PBD both as monotherapy augmentation.[72] There is only 1 double-blind placebo-controlled monotherapy trial of quetiapine in acute pediatric mania, which has not yet been published. Data from this study were presented in meetings,[73] however, and results are available online.[74] Subjects (N = 284) ages 10 to 17 years were randomized to receive either fixed-dose quetiapine (400 mg/d), quetiapine (600 mg/d), or placebo in this multisite, 3-week study. Response rates were 64%, 58%, and 37% for quetiapine (400 mg), quetiapine (600 mg), and placebo respectively.

Aripiprazole

Chart reviews and open-label studies provided preliminary evidence for aripiprazole in acute PBD mania.[75–78] In a large (N = 413), 4-week, double-blind, placebo-controlled randomized trial of aripiprazole monotherapy, subjects were randomly assigned to placebo or target doses of aripiprazole of either 10 mg/d or 30 mg/d.[79] Superiority of aripiprazole over placebo was evident by the end of 1 week for both doses. At study endpoint, response rates were 44.8%, 63.6%, and 26.1% for aripiprazole (10 mg), aripiprazole (30 mg), and placebo, respectively. Another randomized, double-blind, placebo-controlled monotherapy trial examined the efficacy of aripiprazole in treating youth with PBD and comorbid ADHD during a manic or mixed episode.[80] In this 6-week trial (N = 43), patients weighing less than 50 kg received a starting dose of 2 mg/d, whereas the other patients started on 5 mg/d. Doses were increased by 5 mg weekly as needed and tolerated, up to 20 mg/d. YMRS scores decreased significantly at endpoint when compared with baseline, and patients on aripiprazole presented with better response (88.9% vs 52%) and remission (72% vs 32%) rates when compared with placebo, respectively. No significant reductions in ADHD or depressive symptoms were observed, however.

Ziprasidone

To date there are limited published data on efficacy and safety of ziprasidone for PBD.[81–83] An open-label 8-week study examined ziprasidone monotherapy for 21 PBD patients 6 to 17 years with significant manic symptoms and reported a 33% response rate.[82] Findings from a 4-week, double-blind, placebo-controlled study of ziprasidone in pediatric mania (N = 237) have not been published yet but were presented in international meetings[84] and are currently available on Food and Drug Administration Web site.[74] Ziprasidone was titrated up to 120 to 160 mg/d in divided doses over the first 1 to 2 weeks depending on body weight (80–160 mg/d for subjects weighing at least 45 kg; 60–80 mg/d for subjects less than 45 kg) and then flexibly dosed. Ziprasidone was efficacious only for the subjects weighing 45 kg or more, and the active and placebo groups separated as early as week 1. The number of children on the under–45 kg group was small, and findings may have been constrained by low dosing. Response rate for ziprasidone (62%) was significantly greater than for placebo (35%). There was only minimal QTc prolongation, and no significant weight or metabolic changes. A subsequent placebo-controlled adjunctive methylphenidate study from this sample is discussed later.

COMPARATIVE EFFICACY OF SECOND-GENERATION ANTIPSYCHOTICS VERSUS TRADITIONAL MOOD STABILIZERS

A recent comparative analysis examined all double-blind, placebo-controlled trials of acute treatment of mania for both adults (23 trials) and youth (9 trials) available to that date.[39] After pooling the trials and excluding the failed topiramate studies, the study found a significant difference in ESs favoring the SGAs when compared with classical mood stabilizers among youth but not among adults (ES = 0.65 vs 0.20, respectively). Carbamazepine was included as a mood stabilizer among adults whereas oxcarbazepine was included among youth. Nonetheless, a recent large meta-analysis also found that antipsychotics were overall more effective than mood stabilizers in treating mania in adults.[85]

Similar results were observed in a smaller (N = 37), randomized, double-blind, 6-week study comparing risperidone and DVPX in pediatric mania.[86] Risperidone was superior to DVPX in terms of response (78.1% vs 45.5%) and remission (62.5% vs 33%) rates. A double-blind randomized pilot study (N = 50) compared quetiapine to DVPX in acute adolescent manic or mixed episodes[87] and found significantly greater response and remission in the quetiapine group compared with the DVPX group (84% vs 56% and 60% vs 28%, respectively). Subgroup analyses suggested this advantage was restricted to patients with psychosis.

The Treatment of Early Age Mania study, a recent double-blind controlled trial, examined the antimanic efficacy of lithium, DVPX, and risperidone for PBD-I, manic/mixed episode, in patients age 6 to 15 years.[48] After screening 5671 children and adolescents, this multisite 8-week study enrolled 279 antimanic-naive subjects. The primary outcome measure was the Clinical Global Impression (CGI) for Bipolar Illness Improvement–Mania, with ratings of 1 or 2 (very much or much improved, respectively) counting as response to treatment. Subjects treated with risperidone had a significantly higher response rate (68%) than those treated with lithium (35.6%) or DVPX (24.0%). Differences between lithium and DVPX were not statistically significant.

Overall, the data currently available suggest that SGAs have better efficacy for treating acute mania in PBD than the classical mood stabilizers, lithium included. Whether these findings stand the tests of time and replication is not yet clear. Still, the treatment of acute mania is a brief intervention when contrasted to the treatment of bipolar depression or long-term maintenance, and pharmacologic decisions for all stages of illness should take into account tolerability and side-effect profiles of different medications.

COMBINATION TREATMENT

A substantial proportion of children with PBD require combination treatment.[57,88–90] Few rigorous studies have examined combination treatment in PBD, however, and they comprise a mixture of acute mania studies and continuation/maintenance treatment studies.

In 1 study, 30 subjects ages 12 to 18 years were randomized to receive DVPX plus placebo or DVPX plus quetiapine for 6 weeks.[91] Both groups had statistically significant reductions in YMRS scores, but the response rate in the DVPX plus quetiapine group (87%) was significantly greater than in the DVPX plus placebo group (53%). Increased sedation was the only side effect significantly more common in the group taking quetiapine. Although subjects in the DVPX plus quetiapine group gained more weight than on DVPX alone (4.2 ± 3.2 kg and 2.5 ± 2.1 kg, respectively), this difference was not statistically significant.

In a 1-year open-label trial, 21 children with manic or mixed episode who failed to adequately respond to an 8-week lithium monotherapy trial were treated adjunctively with risperidone, yielding a response rate of 85.7%.[92] Risperidone adjunctive to lithium or DVPX was also examined in an open-label, 6-month trial of 37 subjects ages 5 to 18 years during acute manic or mixed episode.[93] Both treatment strategies were well tolerated and produced similar significant improvements in manic symptoms.

An 8-week study compared the results of 2 partially concurrent trials of olanzapine plus topiramate and olanzapine monotherapy for PBD youth with current manic/mixed/hypomanic episodes. Combination treatment with topiramate was associated with significantly less weight gain but was not associated with greater manic symptom reduction.[94]

The combination of lithium and DVPX was also examined in an open-label trial (N = 90, up to 20 weeks) of lithium and DVPX in youth with PBD and a manic or hypomanic episode within the 3 months preceding enrollment.[95] Most subjects (81%) were in mixed or manic episodes at baseline. Antidepressants, antipsychotics, and stimulants were also allowed, as needed. Subjects who had experienced a manic episode while on therapeutic lithium or DVPX levels were excluded, likely enriching the sample for treatment-responsiveness. There was a significant reduction in manic and depressive symptoms at week 8 and end of study (mean 11.3 weeks), and 47% met criteria for clinical remission. This study was followed by a discontinuation monotherapy study (described later). A third study of 38 subjects who relapsed during monotherapy found that 90% were successfully restabilized during 8 weeks of open combination treatment with lithium and DVPX.[96]

BIPOLAR DEPRESSION

Similar to adults, depression is the primary source of symptomatic burden among youth with BP, who spend nearly 40% of the time with impairing depression symptoms (approximately half in the context of pure depressive states and half in the context of mixed states).[1] Depressive episodes are the most common manifestation (eg, more frequent, longer in duration) of BP in youth.[22,97] Followed prospectively, major depressive episodes are the most common form of syndromal recurrence (59.5% vs 20.9% hypomanic, 14.8% manic, and 4.8% mixed) among youth who had achieved recovery.[1] Nonetheless, depression is commonly undiagnosed in youth with BP.[98,99] Clinicians who do identify depression among youth with BP face the substantial challenge of how best to treat these youth. There is a paucity of controlled studies of pharmacotherapy for depression among youth with BP, and competing concerns about the risk for suicide and exacerbating or inducing mania with antidepressant treatment presents a dilemma.[100–103]

There have been few controlled studies of treatment of bipolar depression in adults[104]; however, guidelines are available to support clinical decision making.[105–108] Only 3 open studies and 1 placebo-controlled study are available in adolescents, and extant treatment guidelines for PBD do not explicitly address depression due to insufficient evidence.[109]

Lithium

The only available prospective study of lithium in bipolar youth with depression was an open-label 6-week acute treatment study of PBD-I depression in 22 inpatient adolescents ages 12 to 18 years, and this study reported a large ES of 1.7 with lithium monotherapy.[110] The Children's Depression Rating Scale–Revised (CDRS-R) scores decreased significantly from 64 ± 12.1 to 38.5 ± 17.6 (39.8% change) at the end of the sixth week and response (50% reduction in the CDRS-R score from baseline to endpoint) and remission (CDRS-R score ≤28 and a CGI–Bipolar Disorder Improvement score of 1 or 2, respectively) rates were 48% and 30%, respectively. Lithium was titrated to 1.0 mEq/L to 1.2 mEq/L and tolerated well.

Lamotrigine

Several case reports describe successful use of adjunctive lamotrigine for more than 6 months in youth with bipolar depression.[111,112] Similarly, a study of 46 youth with PBD I or PBD II reported that lamotrigine treatment (started in combination with an SGA for

8 weeks for acute mania/mixed mania or hypomania and then monotherapy [mean 200 mg/d] for the maintenance phase for 6 weeks) was effective in improving depressive symptoms during maintenance treatment.[113] Lamotrigine was well tolerated and slow titration resulted in a benign rash in 6.4% of patients that resolved with discontinuation of the medication or treatment with prednisone.

There is 1 lamotrigine study conducted in depressed bipolar adolescents ages 12 to 17 years. In this open-label 8-week acute treatment study of PBD-I, PBD-II, or BD not otherwise specified (NOS) depression, 20 outpatient adolescents reported an ES of 2.47 with lamotrigine monotherapy (65% of the subjects) or adjunctive therapy.[114] This study included mixed episodes and allowed concurrent medications. The CDRS-R scores decreased significantly from 58 ± 12.7 to 28 ± 11.6 (51.7% change) at the end of the eighth week and response (defined by a CGI-Improvement score of 1 or 2) and remission (a CDRS-R score ≤28 and a CGI-Improvement score of 1 or 2) rates were 84% and 58%, respectively. The symptomatic response rate (≥50% reduction in CDRS-R) was 63%. The mean lamotrigine dose was 131.6 ±31 mg/d and the medication was well tolerated without any significant skin reaction. It is difficult to compare open-label lithium and lamotrigine studies because of varying time frames (6 weeks lithium vs 8 weeks lamotrigine), modes of delivery (lithium monotherapy vs lamotrigine monotherapy or add-on), and sample characteristics (PBD-I depressed inpatients in lithium study vs PBD-I, PBD-II, and PBD-NOS depressed or mixed outpatients in lamotrigine study).

Quetiapine

The only double-blind randomized study of BP depression in youth (N = 32, ages 12–18 years, for 8 weeks) did not find differences between quetiapine (300–600 mg/d, endpoint quetiapine doses 403 ± 133 mg) and placebo.[115] Change in the primary measure, CDRS-R, was similar and the response rate was 71% in the quetiapine group and 67% in the placebo group. This study suggests the need for more and larger BP depression studies in youth considering the contrast between this study and the robust positive response to quetiapine in adults with BP I and BP II. Also, this study highlights the limitations of applying findings from studies of adults in treatment of BP youth. Alternatively, the findings may not be generalizable to all depressed BD youth with a more severe illness or other clinical characteristics. The investigators emphasized the high placebo response rate at the end of the study and the absence of placebo lead-in phase for the first week when discussing the possible reasons for negative results.

Antidepressants

The issue of whether to use antidepressants in BD has been debated, but few long-term, well-controlled studies have been done. A meta-analysis of 12 RCTs of bipolar depression in adults reported that antidepressants were more effective than placebo and did not induce more switching into mania[116]; however, a recent meta-analysis concluded otherwise, that antidepressants were not statistically superior to placebo or other current standard treatment of bipolar depression, but they were not associated with an increased risk of switch either.[117]

There are abundant data regarding the safety and efficacy of antidepressants among children and adolescents with anxiety disorder or major depressive disorder or unipolar depression.[118,119] Data on antidepressants in PBD are, however, limited. A retrospective chart review reported that depressed children with BD improved with antidepressant medications, but they were 3 times more likely to experience a subsequent manic episode.[103] Not all children in that study, however, were taking mood-stabilizing medication. Treatment guidelines for BD in children and adolescents were recently developed and, similar to adults, the panel discouraged antidepressant monotherapy trials in bipolar children, suggesting that selective serotonin reuptake inhibitors (SSRIs) or bupropion may be considered after mood stabilization.[109] The limited evidence regarding mania-inducing effects of antidepressants (and stimulants) in PBD has been thoroughly reviewed elsewhere.[38] Although there is no clear evidence that SSRIs (or stimulants) accelerate or exacerbate the natural course of BD, extra caution is warranted when considering these medications for youth who are at high risk for developing BD (eg, previous treatment-emergent hypo/manic episodes, history of psychosis, or family history of BD).[38] In addition to questions about precipitating the onset of BD and/or mood cycle acceleration, other important questions remain, such as, What are the predictors of treatment-emergent mania? Should these patients be rechallenged? and Do mood-stabilizing medications adequately mitigate this risk? Pending the prospective studies needed to answer these questions, increased caution is indicated when considering the use of antidepressants in PBD.

TREATMENT OF BIPOLAR DISORDER IN THE PRESENCE OF COMORBID CONDITIONS
ADHD

ADHD is among the most common comorbidities in BP[120] and presents unique treatment considerations. First, comorbid ADHD has been associated with decreased response to treatment of acute mania.[121–124] A recent meta-analysis, including 273 children and adolescents with BP, of whom approximately half had comorbid ADHD, found that the probability of response was significantly reduced (relative risk 0.88; 95% CI, 0.69–0.97; $P = .021$) among subjects with comorbid ADHD and that this association may be stronger among adolescents and among youth with BP-I.[123] Second, there have been concerns about the risk of treatment-emergent mania or destabilization in the context of treating youth with comorbid BP and ADHD with stimulants.[38] With regard to risks, recent studies suggest that 2.5% to 10% of patients treated with stimulants or atomoxetine (adjunctive to mood-stabilizing medication) experience psychiatric adverse events (ie, hypo/mania and/or suicidality) and that there was improvement with discontinuation of the stimulant. In those studies, however, participants had been stabilized with regard to their mood for at least 3 weeks while taking a first-line antimanic (aripiprazole, DVPX, or lithium).[125–128] American Academy of Child and Adolescent Psychiatry treatment guidelines advise that symptoms of BP should be stabilized first, and if impairing symptoms of ADHD persists, they may be judiciously treated, with stimulants as first-line treatment.[109]

Recent studies provide support for the efficacy of this approach. In a trial of 40 youth with BP and ADHD, 80% responded to antimanic treatment with valproate; however, in only 3 of 40 subjects did ADHD remit. Subjects were randomized to mixed amphetamine salts (MAS) (5 mg twice daily) or placebo in a 2-week crossover design. ADHD symptom reduction was significantly greater for MAS than for placebo.[127] Moreover, there was no carryover effect, meaning the benefits were observed only within the 2-week block of active treatment. One subject became manic after 4 weeks of MAS; however, there were no overall changes in manic symptoms and tolerability was good overall. A subsequent 4-week RCT of adjunctive methylphenidate versus placebo demonstrated a large ES for methylphenidate.[126] There were no systematic differences in manic or depressive symptoms or in adverse events. Irritability was common across both treatment conditions. Rebound phenomena were more common during methylphenidate treatment. In a third similar RCT of adjunctive methylphenidate or placebo added to aripiprazole, no significant between-group differences in ADHD symptoms were observed, although self-reported depressive symptoms improved significantly more with methylphenidate treatment.[125] A chart review and an open-treatment study of atomoxetine suggest that this medication may also be effective for comorbid ADHD.[128,129] Whereas tricyclic antidepressants may improve comorbid ADHD symptoms, they are also associated with significantly increased risk of relapse of manic symptoms.[130] Previously discussed limitations of the extant literature regarding pharmacologic treatment of comorbid ADHD among youth with BP include small sample sizes, short duration of follow-up, and use of rescue medications (eg, clonidine).[38]

Anxiety

Comorbid anxiety is highly prevalent in PBD,[120,131] and is associated with more severe depressive symptoms, lower likelihood of syndromic recovery, and increased risk of treatment-emergent mania/hypomania.[27,102,132,133] The impact of anxiety on treatment response in PBD is uncertain. A recent secondary analysis of 3 open-label olanzapine studies in PBD found that comorbid obsessive-compulsive disorder was associated with significantly poorer antimanic response (25% vs 63%).[134] Another recent study found that the absence of glutamate decarboxylase was significantly associated with nonresponse to mood stabilizers.[124] To date, no treatment studies have explicitly targeted comorbid anxiety in PBD. Both SSRIs and cognitive behavior therapy (CBT) are efficacious for pediatric anxiety in the absence of BD.[135] Taken together with the concerns (discussed previously) regarding the potential for treatment-emergent mania/hypomania, the absence of data regarding SSRIs for comorbid anxiety in PBD suggest that psychosocial treatment should be considered first. Pharmacologic and psychosocial treatment studies for comorbid anxiety in PBD are greatly needed.

Substance Use Disorders

Substance use disorders are common among adolescents with BD and are associated with significant morbidity.[136,137] The first randomized placebo-controlled study of lithium for PBD examined 25 adolescents with BP (N = 17) or major depressive disorder with predictors of future bipolarity (N = 8) and secondary substance dependence.[47] After 6 weeks, subjects in the lithium group were significantly less likely to have positive urine drug assays (approximately 10%) compared with subjects receiving placebo (approximately 35%) and had significantly greater improvement on the Children's Global Assessment Scale; however, impact on mood symptoms was not reported. A recently presented 16-week, randomized, double-blind, placebo-controlled study examined the efficacy of topiramate (average dose 175 mg/d) versus placebo, adjunctive to quetiapine, in 75 manic adolescents with co-occurring cannabis use disorders.[138] There was a significantly greater reduction in cannabis use in the topiramate group versus the placebo group. There was also significantly less weight gain, greater reduction in appetite, and greater rate of excitement as side effects of topiramate versus placebo.

Other Psychiatric Comorbidity

Other psychiatric comorbidities that have treatment implications include autism spectrum disorders (ASDs) and disruptive behavior disorders (DBDs). ASDs present challenges with regard to discerning treatment response of target symptoms, because in some cases the communication difficulties inherent in ASDs can make it difficult to parse the symptoms of BP from those of ASDs.[139] A recent secondary analysis of open-label SGA monotherapy studies examined 151 youth with BP, of whom 23 met criteria for comorbid ASDs. No significant differences in antimanic response or tolerability were observed.[140] Few data are available regarding the treatment of comorbid DBD among youth with BP. A case report suggested that topiramate may be effective for this comorbidity.[141] A double-blind study compared quetiapine and DVPX for the treatment of impulsivity and reactive aggression among adolescents with BP and comorbid DBD.[142] Both groups improved significantly over 4 weeks of treatment, and there were no significant between-group differences in effectiveness of speed of response.

LONG-TERM EVIDENCE OF TREATMENT OF BIPOLAR DISORDER

In comparison with data regarding acute manic/mixed episodes, few studies have examined continuation and/or maintenance treatment of PBD, and the data regarding treatment beyond 12-months' duration are sparse.

Mood Stabilizers

In addition to the 2-week randomized lithium discontinuation study (described previously), an 18-month observational study (N = 37) examined the role of lithium in continuation treatment after hospital discharge for acute mania.[143] The relapse rate among patients who discontinued lithium (N = 13) was 3 times greater compared with those who remained adherent with lithium throughout the 18 months (N = 24; 92.3% vs 37.5%, respectively). This small study did not, however, examine for potential confounding variables. Another study randomized 60 youth with PBD-I or PBD-II who had previously remitted on combination treatment with lithium and DVPX to monotherapy with either medication.[144] Treatment proceeded in double-blind fashion for up to 76 weeks. Time to median survival (50% relapse) did not differ significantly between the lithium (114 ± 57 days) and DVPX (112 ± 56 days) groups, both of which relapsed quickly. Finally, in a prospective, naturalistic, 8-year follow-up of children with first manic/mixed episodes, a greater number of weeks on lithium was associated with earlier recovery, controlling for demographic variables and exposure to other treatments.[145]

In a small chart review of 15 PBD youth treated with DVPX naturalistically for 1.4 ± 1.5 years, 53% were responders based on CGI-Improvement ratings, and one-third discontinued due to side effect (primarily weight gain).[146] A subsequent large study of 226 PBD youth examined effectiveness and safety of DVPX over 6 months of continuation treatment after a manic or mixed episode[147]; 99 subjects (44%) took DVPX for at least 180 days, and the mean duration of exposure was 124.4 days. Approximately two-thirds of subjects remained at least 70% compliant throughout the study. Effectiveness data were examined in the intent-to-treat sample (N = 199). Based on last-observation-carried-forward analyses, there was a mean decrease of 12.4 in YMRS scores. These data suggest that DVPX maintenance treatment seems well tolerated and may be associated with further symptomatic improvement. The effect of time cannot be parsed, however, from the effect of DVPX in this study, and RCT data are needed to determine how DVPX compares to placebo and/or other active treatments.

An open-label study of 46 youth with PBD examined the effect of 6 weeks of continuation treatment with lamotrigine (target dose 150 mg if ≤30 kg or 200 mg if >30 kg).[113] SGAs were tapered over 2 to 4 weeks so that by 8 weeks, treatment proceeded with lamotrigine monotherapy. Among subjects who were in remission at 8 weeks, 3 (23%) relapsed by the end of 14 weeks. Among subjects who were not in remission at 8 weeks, depressive symptoms continued to decrease with ongoing lamotrigine treatment. These findings, together with findings from adults, suggest the need for rigorous maintenance studies of lamotrigine in PBD. At present, there is insufficient data from which to draw conclusions about the potential benefits of maintenance lamotrigine for PBD.

Second-Generation Antipsychotics

A small study of 21 adolescents with PBD (67% PBD-NOS) retained 18 subjects throughout 48 weeks of follow-up.[148] Subjects were enrolled only after achieving 4 consecutive weeks of stability, and either continued on quetiapine or treated with quetiapine while tapering other medications. Thirteen subjects (72% of completers) were successfully maintained in remission on quetiapine monotherapy, with the remaining 5 subjects requiring adjunctive treatment targeting depressive and/or anxious symptoms.

A recent placebo-controlled study examined continuation treatment (phase II) for up to 72 weeks among 60 children ages 4 to 9 years with bipolar spectrum disorders

---

CLINICAL VIGNETTE: BIPOLAR DISORDER

Alexis is a 15-year-old white girl who lives with her mother and her 2 brothers, ages 9 and 12. Parents are divorced and have joint custody. Family psychiatric history is significant for major depressive disorder in her mother and maternal aunt, BD in maternal grandfather, and alcohol abuse and ADHD in her father. In addition, her youngest brother has been treated for anxiety.

Alexis is medically healthy and physically active. She has tried alcohol and cannabis on a few occasions but has not had any excessive use or related problems. She first presented for psychiatric treatment at the age of 8 for separation anxiety and school refusal. Her anxiety responded to psychosocial treatment and from ages 9 through 12 she was doing well academically, socially, and within the family. At age 12 her best friend moved to a different city, and what at first seemed a developmentally appropriate sadness evolved into a major depressive episode lasting 6 months.

She responded partially to CBT and eventually recovered completely with combination treatment with fluoxetine (20 mg) that was well tolerated with the exception of mild activation and insomnia. The following year she experienced another major depressive episode in the absence of any major stressors, which was effectively treated with another course of CBT.

Within the past school year she went on a school trip during which she experienced her first manic episode, necessitating hospitalization. She stabilized quickly on a medium dose of an SGA and was discharged to the care of her community psychiatrist. After gaining 12 pounds within the first few months of treatment, she became increasingly nonadherent with the SGA and had a second hospitalization, this time for a mixed manic episode. Her manic symptoms were again quickly improved with reinstitution of the SGA; however, her depressive symptoms became more prominent and persisted beyond discharge. Her outpatient psychiatrist titrated her dose somewhat and symptoms gradually improved to the point that she was functioning at approximately 70% of her healthy baseline. She continued to experience brief 2-day to 3-day intervals of hypomania, however, alternating with similar intervals of depression.

She also developed unprovoked panic attacks that she had 3 to 4 times per week. Her psychiatrist initiated adjunctive treatment with lithium. Within 4 weeks her symptoms had improved substantially, and by 16 weeks she had achieved recovery from depressive and hypo/manic symptoms.

At present, she continues to struggle with anxiety despite ongoing CBT. This has led to increased use of alcohol and cannabis in social settings, which she finds effective in reducing her social anxiety but also has led to some arguments with peers and her parents and which has resulted in some impulsive sexual behavior. She voices concern about the long-term effects of her combination pharmacologic treatment on her brain and body but elects to continue with treatment and defer discussion about discontinuing one or more of her medications until she reaches 12 months of sustained recovery.

(PBD-I, PBD-II, PBD-NOS, or cyclothymia) who had responded to open-label treatment with aripiprazole (phase I, N = 96).[34] However, 50% of subjects in the aripiprazole group and 90% of subjects in the placebo group discontinued within the first 4 weeks. The huge discrepancy in mean retention duration, 25.9 weeks for aripiprazole and 3 weeks for placebo, led the investigators to invoke the possibility of a nocebo effect (compromised blind leading to early discontinuation in the placebo group owing to expectations of lack of efficacy). In contrast to the robust evidence for SGAs in acute PBD manic/mixed episodes, there are limited maintenance data from which to draw conclusions. Studies are needed to determine whether SGAs are efficacious and tolerable for maintenance treatment of PBD, and the latter consideration is especially salient among youth.

CONCLUSIONS AND FUTURE DIRECTIONS FOR BIPOLAR DISORDER IN YOUTH

In summary, the literature to date supports several conclusions regarding the treatment of PBD. SGAs are highly efficacious for the treatment of acute manic/mixed episodes, although tolerability remains a major concern. The evidence regarding the traditional mood stabilizers lithium and DVPX suggest that they may be less efficacious than SGAs among youth; however, this conclusion remains tentative pending additional placebo-controlled trials. This impression comes from 2 different lines of evidence:

1. Head-to-head trials comparing SGAs to DVPX or lithium
2. Comparisons of the ESs of available placebo-controlled studies of SGAs and mood stabilizers

Remarkably, there are no published studies to date regarding lithium for the treatment of acute mania (or depression) in PBD, and this is an important future undertaking. Similarly, there is a lack of evidence that DVPX is an efficacious antimanic among youth. The existing evidence, however, is not sufficient to conclude that DVPX is ineffective. Existing data nonetheless draw into question what conclusion may be drawn regarding combination treatment. Preliminary open data suggest that combination treatment may be effective in terms of stabilizing PBD and subsequently restabilizing PBD after destabilization on monotherapy. Most data regarding combination treatment in randomized studies, however, involve the addition of an SGA to lithium or DVPX. Clinically, in the authors' view, it not clear whether it was the combination that was necessary or whether the SGAs are doing the heavy lifting in terms of antimanic benefit. As such, combination treatment studies should also examine the converse scenario, that is, adding lithium or DVPX to an SGA and comparing this to the addition of placebo. Expanding the evidence base regarding bipolar depression among youth is crucial. As with adults, depression is the most burdensome mood polarity in PBD. The failure of quetiapine to show even a modest signal versus placebo among depressed adolescents with BD is concerning. Although the response rate to quetiapine among youth was substantial (71%, vs 58% among adults), the placebo response rate among youth was far higher than among adults (67% vs 36.1%) invoking a possible ceiling effect.[149] Larger replication studies that address the limitations of the single RCT are warranted in light of the overwhelming evidence that quetiapine is efficacious for bipolar depression among adults. In addition, RCTs of lamotrigine, lithium, and SSRIs for bipolar depression in youth are warranted.

It is widely acknowledged that acute response and recovery are only the first steps of optimal treatment of BD. As such, long-term studies are needed to examine which medications best maintain recovery and prevent or at least prolong time to recurrence. The same studies should examine tolerability, because the cost-benefit in terms of metabolic side effects versus antimanic effect during the treatment of acute mania may differ from the cost-benefit of maintenance treatments. That is, there may be a larger role for traditional mood stabilizers in the maintenance treatment of PBD, whereas SGAs may be especially indicated for acute mania. Studies are needed, however, to determine whether this is the case. There are clinically relevant differences in metabolic side effects among SGAs, with some demonstrating more substantial and more ongoing weight gain than others.[150] With regard to comorbidities, similar to those of adults, studies examining comorbid anxiety are of paramount importance, because anxiety is a major source of symptomatic burden and functional impairment throughout the developmental progression of BD.

Because it is unlikely that any given medication will be effective for all youth with BD, improved ability to expeditiously provide individualized treatment is needed. Family history of treatment responsiveness is one such strategy but has yet to be rigorously examined in relation to clinical treatment decisions in youth.[151] Similarly, symptom clusters may be useful in informing treatment decisions. Few studies have compared the effects of different medications on different symptom clusters, and none to the authors' knowledge have assigned treatment on this basis. Finally, clinically relevant biomarkers will be central to progress in the treatment of PBD. Is there a role for pharmacogenetics in PBD? Can peripheral biomarkers be used to select treatments and/or monitor and predict treatment response? Do different neuroimaging biosignatures suggest the need for different treatments? Vigorous and concerted efforts to address these and other questions will ensure that the momentum of progress in the treatment of PBD is sustained over the coming years.

REFERENCES

1. Birmaher B, Axelson D, Goldstein B, et al. Four-year longitudinal course of children and adolescents with bipolar spectrum disorders: the Course and Outcome of Bipolar Youth (COBY) Study. Am J Psychiatry 2009;166(7):795–804.
2. Dennehy EB, Marangell LB, Allen MH, et al. Suicide and suicide attempts in the Systematic Treatment Enhancement Program for Bipolar Disorder (STEP-BD). J Affect Disord 2011;133(3):423–7.
3. Kupfer DJ. The increasing medical burden in bipolar disorder. JAMA 2005; 293(20):2528–30.
4. Leverich GS, Post RM, Keck JP, et al. The poor prognosis of childhood-onset bipolar disorder. J Pediatr 2007;150(5):485–90.
5. Soreca I, Fagiolini A, Frank E, et al. Relationship of general medical burden, duration of illness and age in patients with bipolar I disorder. J Psychiatr Res 2008;42:956–61.
6. Perlis RH, Dennehy EB, Miklowitz DJ, et al. Retrospective age at onset of bipolar disorder and outcome during two-year follow-up: results from the STEP-BD study. Bipolar Disord 2009;11(4):391–400.
7. Goldstein BI, Levitt AJ. Further evidence for a developmental subtype of bipolar disorder defined by age at onset: results from the national epidemiologic survey on alcohol and related conditions. Am J Psychiatry 2006;163(9):1633–6.
8. Perlis RH, Miyahara S, Marangell LB, et al. Long-term implications of early onset in bipolar disorder: data from the first 1000 participants in the systematic treatment enhancement program for bipolar disorder (STEP-BD). Biol Psychiatry 2004;55(9):875–81.
9. Carlson GA, Glovinsky I. The concept of bipolar disorder in children: a history of the bipolar controversy. Child Adolesc Psychiatr Clin N Am 2009;18(2):257–71.

10. Kraepelin E. Manic-depressive insanity and paranoia. Edinburgh (United Kingdom): E. S. Livingstone; 1921.
11. Gore FM, Bloem PJ, Patton GC, et al. Global burden of disease in young people aged 10-24 years: a systematic analysis. Lancet 2011;377(9783):2093–102.
12. Blader JC, Carlson GA. Increased rates of bipolar disorder diagnoses among U.S. child, adolescent, and adult inpatients, 1996-2004. Biol Psychiatry 2007; 62(2):107–14.
13. Moreno C, Laje G, Blanco C, et al. National trends in the outpatient diagnosis and treatment of bipolar disorder in youth. Arch Gen Psychiatry 2007;64(9): 1032–9.
14. Leibenluft E, Charney DS, Towbin KE, et al. Defining clinical phenotypes of juvenile mania. Am J Psychiatry 2003;160(3):430–7.
15. Wozniak J, Biederman J, Kiely K, et al. Mania-like symptoms suggestive of childhood-onset bipolar disorder in clinically referred children. J Am Acad Child Adolesc Psychiatry 1995;34(7):867–76.
16. Youngstrom EA, Birmaher B, Findling RL. Pediatric bipolar disorder: validity, phenomenology, and recommendations for diagnosis. Bipolar Disord 2008; 10(1 Pt 2):194–214.
17. Van Meter AR, Moreira AL, Youngstrom EA. Meta-analysis of epidemiological studies of bipolar disorder. J Clin Psychiatry 2011;72:1250–6.
18. Zito JM, Safer DJ, dosReis S, et al. Psychotropic practice patterns for youth: a 10-year perspective. Arch Pediatr Adolesc Med 2003;157(1):17–25.
19. Merikangas KR, He JP, Burstein M, et al. Service utilization for lifetime mental disorders in U.S. adolescents: results of the national comorbidity survey-adolescent supplement (NCS-A). J Am Acad Child Adolesc Psychiatry 2011; 50(1):32–45.
20. Merikangas KR, He JP, Burstein M, et al. Lifetime prevalence of mental disorders in U.S. adolescents: results from the National Comorbidity Survey Replication-Adolescent Supplement (NCS-A). J Am Acad Child Adolesc Psychiatry 2010; 49(10):980–9.
21. Stringaris A, Baroni A, Haimm C, et al. Pediatric bipolar disorder versus severe mood dysregulation: risk for manic episodes on follow-up. J Am Acad Child Adolesc Psychiatry 2010;49(4):397–405.
22. Birmaher B, Axelson D, Strober M, et al. Clinical course of children and adolescents with bipolar spectrum disorders. Arch Gen Psychiatry 2006;63(2):175–83.
23. Birmaher B, Axelson D, Strober M, et al. Comparison of manic and depressive symptoms between children and adolescents with bipolar spectrum disorders. Bipolar Disord 2009;11(1):52–62.
24. Judd LL, Akiskal HS, Schettler PJ, et al. The long-term natural history of the weekly symptomatic status of bipolar I disorder. Arch Gen Psychiatry 2002;59(6):530–7.
25. Judd LL, Akiskal HS, Schettler PJ, et al. A prospective investigation of the natural history of the long-term weekly symptomatic status of bipolar II disorder. Arch Gen Psychiatry 2003;60(3):261–9.
26. Geller B, Tillman R, Bolhofner K, et al. Child bipolar I disorder: prospective continuity with adult bipolar I disorder; characteristics of second and third episodes; predictors of 8-year outcome. Arch Gen Psychiatry 2008;65(10):1125–33.
27. DelBello MP, Hanseman D, Adler CM, et al. Twelve-month outcome of adolescents with bipolar disorder following first hospitalization for a manic or mixed episode. Am J Psychiatry 2007;164(4):582–90.
28. Dawson R, Lavori PW, Luby JL, et al. Adaptive strategies for treating childhood mania. Biol Psychiatry 2007;61(6):758–64.

29. McClellan J, Kowatch R, Findling RL, et al. Practice parameter for the assessment and treatment of children and adolescents with bipolar disorder. J Am Acad Child Adolesc Psychiatry 2007;46(1):107–25.
30. Hamrin V, Iennaco JD. Psychopharmacology of pediatric bipolar disorder. Expert Rev Neurother 2011;10(7):1053–88.
31. Liu HY, Potter MP, Woodworth KY, et al. Pharmacologic treatments for pediatric bipolar disorder: a review and meta-analysis. J Am Acad Child Adolesc Psychiatry 2012;50(8):749–62.
32. Thomas T, Stansifer L, Findling RL. Psychopharmacology of pediatric bipolar disorders in children and adolescents. Pediatr Clin North Am 2011;58(1):173–87.
33. Pfeifer JC, Kowatch RA, DelBello MP. Pharmacotherapy of bipolar disorder in children and adolescents: recent progress. CNS Drugs 2010;24(7):575–93.
34. Findling RL, Youngstrom EA, McNamara NK, et al. Double-blind, randomized, placebo-controlled long-term maintenance study of aripiprazole in children with bipolar disorder. J Clin Psychiatry 2012;73(1):57–63.
35. Kowatch R, Scheffer R, Delgado S, et al. Placebo controlled trial of valproate versus risperidone in preschool children with bipolar disorder. Presented at the Annual Meeting of the American Academy of Child and Adolescent Psychiatry. Toronto, Canada. 2011.
36. Biederman J, Mick E, Hammerness P, et al. Open-label, 8-week trial of olanzapine and risperidone for the treatment of bipolar disorder in preschool-age children. Biol Psychiatry 2005;58(7):589–94.
37. Potter M, Moses A, Wozniak J. Alternative treatments in pediatric bipolar disorder. Child Adolesc Psychiatr Clin N Am 2009;18(2):483–514, xi.
38. Goldsmith M, Singh M, Chang K. Antidepressants and psychostimulants in pediatric populations: is there an association with mania? Paediatr Drugs 2011;13(4):225–43.
39. Correll CU, Sheridan EM, DelBello MP. Antipsychotic and mood stabilizer efficacy and tolerability in pediatric and adult patients with bipolar I mania: a comparative analysis of acute, randomized, placebo-controlled trials. Bipolar Disord 2010;12(2):116–41.
40. Correll CU. Weight gain and metabolic effects of mood stabilizers and antipsychotics in pediatric bipolar disorder: a systematic review and pooled analysis of short-term trials. J Am Acad Child Adolesc Psychiatry 2007;46(6):687–700.
41. Thase ME, Denko T. Pharmacotherapy of mood disorders. Annu Rev Clin Psychol 2008;4:53–91.
42. Kafantaris V, Coletti DJ, Dicker R, et al. Lithium treatment of acute mania in adolescents: a large open trial. J Am Acad Child Adolesc Psychiatry 2003;42(9):1038–45.
43. Kowatch RA, Suppes T, Carmody TJ, et al. Effect size of lithium, divalproex sodium, and carbamazepine in children and adolescents with bipolar disorder. J Am Acad Child Adolesc Psychiatry 2000;39(6):713–20.
44. Strober M, Morrell W, Burroughs J, et al. A family study of bipolar I disorder in adolescence. Early onset of symptoms linked to increased familial loading and lithium resistance. J Affect Disord 1988;15(3):255–68.
45. Findling RL, Frazier JA, Kafantaris V, et al. The Collaborative Lithium Trials (CoLT): specific aims, methods, and implementation. Child Adolesc Psychiatry Ment Health 2008;2(1):21.
46. Kowatch R, Findling R, Scheffer R, et al. Placebo controlled trial of divalproex versus lithium for bipolar disorder. Presented at the Annual Meeting of the American Academy of Child and Adolescent Psychiatry. Boston, October 23–28, 2007.

47. Geller B, Williams M, Zimerman B, et al. Prepubertal and early adolescent bipolarity differentiate from ADHD by manic symptoms, grandiose delusions, ultrarapid or ultradian cycling. J Affect Disord 1998;51(2):81–91.

48. Geller B, Luby JL, Joshi P, et al. A randomized controlled trial of risperidone, lithium, or divalproex sodium for initial treatment of bipolar I disorder, manic or mixed phase, in children and adolescents. Arch Gen Psychiatry 2012;69(5): 515–28 [Epub 2012 Jan 2].

49. Kafantaris V, Coletti DJ, Dicker R, et al. Lithium treatment of acute mania in adolescents: a placebo-controlled discontinuation study. J Am Acad Child Adolesc Psychiatry 2004;43(8):984–93.

50. Papatheodorou G, Kutcher SP, Katic M, et al. The efficacy and safety of divalproex sodium in the treatment of acute mania in adolescents and young adults: an open clinical trial. J Clin Psychopharmacol 1995;15(2):110–6.

51. Pavuluri MN, Henry DB, Carbray JA, et al. Divalproex sodium for pediatric mixed mania: a 6-month prospective trial. Bipolar Disord 2005;7(3):266–73.

52. Wagner KD, Weller EB, Carlson GA, et al. An open-label trial of divalproex in children and adolescents with bipolar disorder. J Am Acad Child Adolesc Psychiatry 2002;41(10):1224–30.

53. Wagner KD, Redden L, Kowatch RA, et al. A double-blind, randomized, placebo-controlled trial of divalproex extended-release in the treatment of bipolar disorder in children and adolescents. J Am Acad Child Adolesc Psychiatry 2009;48(5):519–32.

54. Biederman J, Joshi G, Mick E, et al. A prospective open-label trial of lamotrigine monotherapy in children and adolescents with bipolar disorder. CNS Neurosci Ther 2010;16(2):91–102.

55. Davanzo P, Gunderson B, Belin T, et al. Mood stabilizers in hospitalized children with bipolar disorder: a retrospective review. Psychiatry Clin Neurosci 2003; 57(5):504–10.

56. Evans RW, Clay TH, Gualtieri CT. Carbamazepine in pediatric psychiatry. J Am Acad Child Adolesc Psychiatry 1987;26(1):2–8.

57. Kowatch RA, Sethuraman G, Hume JH, et al. Combination pharmacotherapy in children and adolescents with bipolar disorder. Biol Psychiatry 2003;53(11):978–84.

58. Woolston JL. Case study: carbamazepine treatment of juvenile-onset bipolar disorder. J Am Acad Child Adolesc Psychiatry 1999;38(3):335–8.

59. Joshi G, Wozniak J, Mick E, et al. A prospective open-label trial of extended-release carbamazepine monotherapy in children with bipolar disorder. J Child Adolesc Psychopharmacol 2010;20(1):7–14.

60. Hirschfeld RM, Kasper S. A review of the evidence for carbamazepine and oxcarbazepine in the treatment of bipolar disorder. Int J Neuropsychopharmacol 2004;7(4):507–22.

61. Davanzo P, Nikore V, Yehya N, et al. Oxcarbazepine treatment of juvenile-onset bipolar disorder. J Child Adolesc Psychopharmacol 2004;14(3):344–5.

62. Teitelbaum M. Oxcarbazepine in bipolar disorder. J Am Acad Child Adolesc Psychiatry 2001;40(9):993–4.

63. Wagner KD, Kowatch RA, Emslie GJ, et al. A double-blind, randomized, placebo-controlled trial of oxcarbazepine in the treatment of bipolar disorder in children and adolescents [see comment erratum appears in Am J Psychiatry 2006 Oct;163(10):1843]. Am J Psychiatry 2006;163(7):1179–86.

64. DelBello MP, Kowatch RA, Warner J, et al. Adjunctive topiramate treatment for pediatric bipolar disorder: a retrospective chart review. J Child Adolesc Psychopharmacol 2002;12(4):323–30.

65. Delbello MP, Findling RL, Kushner S, et al. A pilot controlled trial of topiramate for mania in children and adolescents with bipolar disorder. J Am Acad Child Adolesc Psychiatry 2005;44(6):539–47.
66. Biederman J, Mick E, Wozniak J, et al. An open-label trial of risperidone in children and adolescents with bipolar disorder. J Child Adolesc Psychopharmacol 2005;15(2):311–7.
67. Frazier JA, Meyer MC, Biederman J, et al. Risperidone treatment for juvenile bipolar disorder: a retrospective chart review. J Am Acad Child Adolesc Psychiatry 1999;38(8):960–5.
68. Chang KD, Ketter TA. Mood stabilizer augmentation with olanzapine in acutely manic children. J Child Adolesc Psychopharmacol 2000;10(1):45–9.
69. Soutullo CA, Sorter MT, Foster KD, et al. Olanzapine in the treatment of adolescent acute mania: a report of seven cases. J Affect Disord 1999;53(3):279–83.
70. Frazier JA, Biederman J, Tohen M, et al. A prospective open-label treatment trial of olanzapine monotherapy in children and adolescents with bipolar disorder. J Child Adolesc Psychopharmacol 2001;11(3):239–50.
71. Tohen M, Kryzhanovskaya L, Carlson G, et al. Olanzapine versus placebo in the treatment of adolescents with bipolar mania. Am J Psychiatry 2007;164(10):1547–56.
72. Marchand WR, Wirth L, Simon C. Quetiapine adjunctive and monotherapy for pediatric bipolar disorder: a retrospective chart review. J Child Adolesc Psychopharmacol 2004;14(3):405–11.
73. Delbello M, Findling R, Earley W, et al. Efficacy of quetiapine in children and adolescents with bipolar mania: a 3-week double-blind, randomized, placebo-controlled trial> Presented at the Annual Meeting of the American Academy of Child and Adolescent Psychiatry. Boston, October 23–28, 2007.
74. PDAC. Briefing document for psychopharmacologic drugs advisory committee (PDAC) meeting of June 9-10, 2009–Quetiapine. Efficacy and safety of Study 149 (D1441C00149). 2009. Available at: http://www.fda.gov/downloads/Advisory Committees/CommitteesMeetingMaterials/Drugs/PsychopharmacologicDrugs AdvisoryCommittee/UCM170736.pdf. Accessed June 15, 2012.
75. Barzman DH, DelBello MP, Kowatch RA, et al. The effectiveness and tolerability of aripiprazole for pediatric bipolar disorders: a retrospective chart review. J Child Adolesc Psychopharmacol 2004;14(4):593–600.
76. Biederman J, McDonnell MA, Wozniak J, et al. Aripiprazole in the treatment of pediatric bipolar disorder: a systematic chart review. CNS Spectr 2005;10(2):141–8.
77. Gibson AP, Crismon ML, Mican LM, et al. Effectiveness and tolerability of aripiprazole in child and adolescent inpatients: a retrospective evaluation. Int Clin Psychopharmacol 2007;22(2):101–5.
78. Biederman J, Mick E, Spencer T, et al. An open-label trial of aripiprazole monotherapy in children and adolescents with bipolar disorder. CNS Spectr 2007;12(9):683–9.
79. Findling RL, Nyilas M, Forbes RA, et al. Acute treatment of pediatric bipolar I disorder, manic or mixed episode, with aripiprazole: a randomized, double-blind, placebo-controlled study. J Clin Psychiatry 2009;70(10):1441–51.
80. Tramontina S, Zeni CP, Ketzer CR, et al. Aripiprazole in children and adolescents with bipolar disorder comorbid with attention-deficit/hyperactivity disorder: a pilot randomized clinical trial. J Clin Psychiatry 2009;70(5):756–64.
81. Barnett MS. Ziprasidone monotherapy in pediatric bipolar disorder. J Child Adolesc Psychopharmacol 2004;14(3):471–7.
82. Biederman J, Mick E, Spencer T, et al. A prospective open-label treatment trial of ziprasidone monotherapy in children and adolescents with bipolar disorder. Bipolar Disord 2007;9(8):888–94.

83. DelBello MP, Versavel M, Ice K, et al. Tolerability of oral ziprasidone in children and adolescents with bipolar mania, schizophrenia, or schizoaffective disorder. J Child Adolesc Psychopharmacol 2008;18(5):491–9.
84. Delbello M, Findling R, Wang P, et al. Safety and efficacy of ziprasidone in pediatric bipolar disorder. Presented at the Annual Meeting of the American Psychiatric Association. Washington, DC, May 3–8, 2008.
85. Cipriani A, Barbui C, Salanti G, et al. Comparative efficacy and acceptability of antimanic drugs in acute mania: a multiple-treatments meta-analysis. Lancet 2011;378(9799):1306–15.
86. Pavuluri MN, Henry DB, Findling RL, et al. Double-blind randomized trial of risperidone versus divalproex in pediatric bipolar disorder. Bipolar Disord 2010; 12(6):593–605.
87. DelBello MP, Kowatch RA, Adler CM, et al. A double-blind randomized pilot study comparing quetiapine and divalproex for adolescent mania. J Am Acad Child Adolesc Psychiatry 2006;45(3):305–13.
88. Bhangoo RK, Lowe CH, Myers FS, et al. Medication use in children and adolescents treated in the community for bipolar disorder. J Child Adolesc Psychopharmacol 2003;13(4):515–22.
89. Consoli A, Brunelle J, Bodeau N, et al. Medication use in adolescents treated in a French psychiatric setting for acute manic or mixed episode. J Can Acad Child Adolesc Psychiatry 2009;18(3):231–8.
90. Potter MP, Liu HY, Monuteaux MC, et al. Prescribing patterns for treatment of pediatric bipolar disorder in a specialty clinic. J Child Adolesc Psychopharmacol 2009;19(5):529–38.
91. Delbello MP, Schwiers ML, Rosenberg HL, et al. A double-blind, randomized, placebo-controlled study of quetiapine as adjunctive treatment for adolescent mania. J Am Acad Child Adolesc Psychiatry 2002;41(10):1216–23.
92. Pavuluri MN, Henry DB, Carbray JA, et al. A one-year open-label trial of risperidone augmentation in lithium nonresponder youth with preschool-onset bipolar disorder. J Child Adolesc Psychopharmacol 2006;16(3):336–50.
93. Pavuluri MN, Henry DB, Carbray JA, et al. Open-label prospective trial of risperidone in combination with lithium or divalproex sodium in pediatric mania. J Affect Disord 2004;82(Suppl 1):S103–11.
94. Wozniak J, Mick E, Waxmonsky J, et al. Comparison of open-label, 8-week trials of olanzapine monotherapy and topiramate augmentation of olanzapine for the treatment of pediatric bipolar disorder. J Child Adolesc Psychopharmacol 2009; 19(5):539–45.
95. Findling RL, McNamara NK, Gracious BL, et al. Combination lithium and divalproex sodium in pediatric bipolarity. J Am Acad Child Adolesc Psychiatry 2003; 42(8):895–901.
96. Findling RL, McNamara NK, Stansbrey R, et al. Combination lithium and divalproex sodium in pediatric bipolar symptom restabilization. J Am Acad Child Adolesc Psychiatry 2006;45(2):142–8.
97. Geller B, Tillman R, Craney JL, et al. Four-year prospective outcome and natural history of mania in children with a prepubertal and early adolescent bipolar disorder phenotype. Arch Gen Psychiatry 2004;61(5):459–67.
98. Karippot A. Pediatric bipolar depression. In: El-Mallakh RS, Ghaemi SN, editors. Bipolar depression: a comprehensive guide. Washington, DC: Amian Psychiatric Publishing, Inc; 2006. p. 101–15.
99. Chang K. Challenges in the diagnosis and treatment of pediatric bipolar depression. Dialogues Clin Neurosci 2009;11(1):73–80.

100. Ryan ND. Treatment of depression in children and adolescents [see comment]. Lancet 2005;366(9489):933–40.
101. Olfson M, Marcus SC, Shaffer D. Antidepressant drug therapy and suicide in severely depressed children and adults: a case-control study. Arch Gen Psychiatry 2006;63(8):865–72.
102. Faedda GL, Baldessarini RJ, Glovinsky IP, et al. Treatment-emergent mania in pediatric bipolar disorder: a retrospective case review. J Affect Disord 2004;82(1):149–58.
103. Biederman J, Mick E, Spencer TJ, et al. Therapeutic dilemmas in the pharmacotherapy of bipolar depression in the young. J Child Adolesc Psychopharmacol 2000;10(3):185–92.
104. Thase ME. Bipolar depression: issues in diagnosis and treatment. Harv Rev Psychiatry 2005;13(5):257–71.
105. American Psychiatric Association. Practice guideline for the treatment of patients with bipolar disorder (revision). Am J Psychiatry 2002;159(Suppl 4):1–50.
106. Nivoli AM, Colom F, Murru A, et al. New treatment guidelines for acute bipolar depression: a systematic review. J Affect Disord 2011;129(1–3):14–26.
107. Grunze H, Vieta E, Goodwin GM, et al. The World Federation of Societies of Biological Psychiatry (WFSBP) guidelines for the biological treatment of bipolar disorders: update 2010 on the treatment of acute bipolar depression. World J Biol Psychiatry 2010;11(2):81–109.
108. Yatham LN, Kennedy SH, Schaffer A, et al. Canadian Network for Mood and Anxiety Treatments (CANMAT) and International Society for Bipolar Disorders (ISBD) collaborative update of CANMAT guidelines for the management of patients with bipolar disorder: update 2009. Bipolar Disord 2009;11(3):225–55.
109. Kowatch RA, Fristad M, Birmaher B, et al. Treatment guidelines for children and adolescents with bipolar disorder. J Am Acad Child Adolesc Psychiatry 2005; 44(3):213–35.
110. Patel NC, DelBello MP, Bryan HS, et al. Open-label lithium for the treatment of adolescents with bipolar depression. J Am Acad Child Adolesc Psychiatry 2006;45(3):289–97.
111. Bildik T, Tamar M, Korkmaz S, et al. Lamotrigine add-on therapy to venlafaxine treatment in adolescent-onset bipolar II disorder: a case report covering an 8-month observation period. Int J Clin Pharmacol Ther 2006;44(5):198–206.
112. Soutullo CA, Diez-Suarez A, Figueroa-Quintana A. Adjunctive lamotrigine treatment for adolescents with bipolar disorder: retrospective report of five cases. J Child Adolesc Psychopharmacol 2006;16(3):357–64.
113. Pavuluri MN, Henry DB, Moss M, et al. Effectiveness of lamotrigine in maintaining symptom control in pediatric bipolar disorder. J Child Adolesc Psychopharmacol 2009;19(1):75–82.
114. Chang K, Saxena K, Howe M. An open-label study of lamotrigine adjunct or monotherapy for the treatment of adolescents with bipolar depression. J Am Acad Child Adolesc Psychiatry 2006;45(3):298–304.
115. DelBello MP, Chang K, Welge JA, et al. A double-blind, placebo-controlled pilot study of quetiapine for depressed adolescents with bipolar disorder. Bipolar Disord 2009;11(5):483–93.
116. Gijsman HJ, Geddes JR, Rendell JM, et al. Antidepressants for bipolar depression: a systematic review of randomized, controlled trials [see comment]. Am J Psychiatry 2004;161(9):1537–47.
117. Sidor MM, Macqueen GM. Antidepressants for the acute treatment of bipolar depression: a systematic review and meta-analysis. The J Clin Psychiatry 2011;72(2):156–67.

118. Bridge JA, Salary CB, Birmaher B, et al. The risks and benefits of antidepressant treatment for youth depression. Ann Med 2005;37(6):404–12.
119. Bridge JA, Iyengar S, Salary CB, et al. Clinical response and risk for reported suicidal ideation and suicide attempts in pediatric antidepressant treatment. JAMA 2007;297(15):1683–96.
120. Kowatch RA, Youngstrom EA, Danielyan A, et al. Review and meta-analysis of the phenomenology and clinical characteristics of mania in children and adolescents. Bipolar Disord 2005;7(6):483–96.
121. State RC, Frye MA, Altshuler LL, et al. Chart review of the impact of attention-deficit/hyperactivity disorder comorbidity on response to lithium or divalproex sodium in adolescent mania. J Clin Psychiatry 2004;65(8):1057–63.
122. Strober M, DeAntonio M, Schmidt-Lackner S, et al. Early childhood attention deficit hyperactivity disorder predicts poorer response to acute lithium therapy in adolescent mania. J Affect Disord 1998;51(2):145–51.
123. Consoli A, Bouzamondo A, Guile JM, et al. Comorbidity with ADHD decreases response to pharmacotherapy in children and adolescents with acute mania: evidence from a metaanalysis. Can J Psychiatry 2007;52(5):323–8.
124. Masi G, Perugi G, Millepiedi S, et al. Pharmacological response in juvenile bipolar disorder subtypes: a naturalistic retrospective examination. Psychiatry Res 2010;177(1–2):192–8.
125. Zeni CP, Tramontina S, Ketzer CR, et al. Methylphenidate combined with aripiprazole in children and adolescents with bipolar disorder and attention-deficit/hyperactivity disorder: a randomized crossover trial. J Child Adolesc Psychopharmacol 2009;19(5):553–61.
126. Findling RL, Short EJ, McNamara NK, et al. Methylphenidate in the treatment of children and adolescents with bipolar disorder and attention-deficit/hyperactivity disorder. J Am Acad Child Adolesc Psychiatry 2007;46(11):1445–53.
127. Scheffer RE, Kowatch RA, Carmody T, et al. Randomized, placebo-controlled trial of mixed amphetamine salts for symptoms of comorbid ADHD in pediatric bipolar disorder after mood stabilization with divalproex sodium. Am J Psychiatry 2005;162(1):58–64.
128. Chang K, Nayar D, Howe M, et al. Atomoxetine as an adjunct therapy in the treatment of co-morbid attention-deficit/hyperactivity disorder in children and adolescents with bipolar I or II disorder. J Child Adolesc Psychopharmacol 2009;19(5):547–51.
129. Hah M, Chang K. Atomoxetine for the treatment of attention-deficit/hyperactivity disorder in children and adolescents with bipolar disorders. J Child Adolesc Psychopharmacol 2005;15(6):996–1004.
130. Biederman J, Mick E, Prince J, et al. Systematic chart review of the pharmacologic treatment of comorbid attention deficit hyperactivity disorder in youth with bipolar disorder. J Child Adolesc Psychopharmacol 1999;9(4):247–56.
131. Axelson D, Birmaher B, Strober M, et al. Phenomenology of children and adolescents with bipolar spectrum disorders. Arch Gen Psychiatry 2006;63(10):1139–48.
132. Sala R, Axelson D, Castro-Fornieles J, et al. Comorbid anxiety in children and adolescents with bipolar spectrum disorders: prevalence and clinical correlates. J Clin Psychiatry 2010;71(10):1344–50.
133. Masi G, Toni C, Perugi G, et al. Anxiety disorders in children and adolescents with bipolar disorder: a neglected comorbidity. Can J Psychiatry 2001;46(9):797–802.

134. Joshi G, Mick E, Wozniak J, et al. Impact of obsessive-compulsive disorder on the antimanic response to olanzapine therapy in youth with bipolar disorder. Bipolar Disord 2010;12(2):196–204.
135. Walkup JT, Albano AM, Piacentini J, et al. Cognitive behavioral therapy, sertraline, or a combination in childhood anxiety. N Engl J Med 2008;359(26):2753–66 [Epub 2008 Oct 30].
136. Wilens TE, Biederman J, Kwon A, et al. Risk of substance use disorders in adolescents with bipolar disorder. J Am Acad Child Adolesc Psychiatry 2004; 43(11):1380–6.
137. Goldstein BI, Strober MA, Birmaher B, et al. Substance use disorders among adolescents with bipolar spectrum disorders. Bipolar Disord 2008;10(4):469–78.
138. DelBello MP, Welge J, Adler CM, et al. Topiramate for adolescents with co-occurring cannabis use and bipolar disorders. Presented at the Annual Meeting of the American Academy of Child and Adolescent Psychiatry. Toronto (Canada), October 18–23, 2011.
139. Frazier JA, Doyle R, Chiu S, et al. Treating a child with Asperger's disorder and comorbid bipolar disorder. Am J Psychiatry 2002;159(1):13–21.
140. Joshi G, Biederman J, Wozniak J, et al. Response to second generation antipsychotics in youth with comorbid bipolar disorder and autism spectrum disorder. CNS Neurosci Ther 2012;18(1):28–33.
141. Barzman DH, Delbello MP. Topiramate for co-occurring bipolar disorder and disruptive behavior disorders. Am J Psychiatry 2006;163(8):1451–2.
142. Barzman DH, DelBello MP, Adler CM, et al. The efficacy and tolerability of quetiapine versus divalproex for the treatment of impulsivity and reactive aggression in adolescents with co-occurring bipolar disorder and disruptive behavior disorder(s). J Child Adolesc Psychopharmacol 2006;16(6):665–70.
143. Strober M, Morrell W, Lampert C, et al. Relapse following discontinuation of lithium maintenance therapy in adolescents with bipolar I illness: a naturalistic study. Am J Psychiatry 1990;147(4):457–61.
144. Findling RL, McNamara NK, Youngstrom EA, et al. Double-Blind 18-Month Trial of Lithium Versus Divalproex Maintenance Treatment in Pediatric Bipolar Disorder. J Am Acad Child Adolesc Psychiatry 2005;44(5):409–17.
145. Geller B, Tillman R, Bolhofner K, et al. Pharmacological and non-drug treatment of child bipolar I disorder during prospective eight-year follow-up. Bipolar Disord 2010;12(2):164–71.
146. Henry CA, Zamvil LS, Lam C, et al. Long-term outcome with divalproex in children and adolescents with bipolar disorder. J Child Adolesc Psychopharmacol 2003;13(4):523–9.
147. Redden L, DelBello M, Wagner KD, et al. Long-term safety of divalproex sodium extended-release in children and adolescents with bipolar I disorder. J Child Adolesc Psychopharmacol 2009;19(1):83–9.
148. Duffy A, Milin R, Grof P. Maintenance treatment of adolescent bipolar disorder: open study of the effectiveness and tolerability of quetiapine. BMC Psychiatry 2009;9:4.
149. Calabrese JR, Keck PE Jr, Macfadden W, et al. A randomized, double-blind, placebo-controlled trial of quetiapine in the treatment of bipolar I or II depression. Am J Psychiatry 2005;162(7):1351–60.
150. Correll CU, Manu P, Olshanskiy V, et al. Cardiometabolic risk of second-generation antipsychotic medications during first-time use in children and adolescents. JAMA 2009;302(16):1765–73.
151. Grof P, Duffy A, Alda M, et al. Lithium response across generations. Acta Psychiatr Scand 2009;120(5):378–85.

Pharmacotherapy of Pediatric Attention-Deficit/Hyperactivity Disorder

Brigette Vaughan, MSN, APRN-BC, NP[a],
Christopher J. Kratochvil, MD[a,b],*

KEYWORDS

- ADHD • Pharmacotherapy • Methylphenidate • Amphetamine • Atomoxetine
- Guanfacine • Clonidine

KEY POINTS

- Pharmacotherapy for attention-deficit/hyperactivity disorder (ADHD) has a robust literature supporting its role as a first-line treatment.
- Methylphenidate, amphetamine, atomoxetine, clonidine, and guanfacine have all demonstrated acceptable risk/benefit profiles in the treatment of ADHD.
- The Multimodal Treatment Study of Children with ADHD (MTA) and Preschool ADHD Treatment Study (PATS) helped define the role of pharmacotherapy in the treatment of ADHD.
- Clinicians should be aware of potential growth and cardiovascular effects of the ADHD pharmacotherapies, educating patients and families as to these risks as well as assessing the risks before and throughout treatment.
- ADHD pharmacotherapy should be individualized for each patient, assessing the dose response and duration of action as well as tolerability when initiating and optimizing treatment.
- Due to the long-term nature of disorder for many individuals, it is important to engage the patients and families and involve them in the treatment plan while actively monitoring the effectiveness and tolerability of the treatment over time.

EMPIRIC EVIDENCE FOR ADHD PHARMACOTHERAPY

The role of pharmacotherapy as a first-line treatment of ADHD is strongly supported in the literature (**Table 1**).[1] The stimulant medications have decades of efficacy data from

Disclosure: Brigette Vaughan: Nothing to report. Christopher J. Kratochvil, MD: This past year received grant support from Eli Lilly, Shire, and the National Institutes of Health; been a consultant for Seaside, Quintiles, Otsuka, Pfizer, and the Food and Drug Administration; and received royalties from Oxford Press.
[a] Department of Psychiatry, University of Nebraska Medical Center, 985581 Nebraska Medical Center, Omaha, NE 68198-5581, USA; [b] Department of Pediatrics, University of Nebraska Medical Center, 987878 Nebraska Medical Center, Omaha, NE 68198-7878, USA
* Corresponding author. 985581 Nebraska Medical Center, Omaha, NE 68198-5581.
E-mail address: ckratoch@unmc.edu

Table 1
ADHD pharmacotherapies and FDA approval status

Medication	Age	FDA Approval Status	
		Mono- or Adjunctive Therapy	Maximum Dose
Short-acting stimulants			
• Methylphenidate (Ritalin)	Children ≥6 y	Monotherapy	60 mg QD
• Methylphenidate (Methylin)	Children ≥6 y	Monotherapy	Lesser of 2 mg/kg or 60 mg QD
• D-Methylphenidate (Focalin)	Children and adolescents 6–17	Monotherapy	Lesser of 1 mg/kg or 20 mg QD
• Mixed amphetamine salts (Adderall)	Children ≥3 y	Monotherapy	Lesser of 1 mg/kg or 40 mg
• Amphetamine (Dexedrine)	Children ≥3 y	Monotherapy	40 mg QD
• Amphetamine (Dextrostat)	Children ≥6 y	Monotherapy	40 mg QD
Long-acting stimulants			
• Methylphenidate (Ritalin SR; pulse)	Children ≥6 y	Monotherapy	60 mg QD
• Methylphenidate (Metadate ER; pulse)	Children ≥6 y	Monotherapy	Lesser of 2 mg/kg or 60 mg QD
• Methylphenidate (Methylin ER; pulse)	Children ≥6 y	Monotherapy	60 mg QD
• Methylphenidate (Metadate CD; pearls)	Children ≥6 y	Monotherapy	Lesser of 2 mg/kg or 60 mg
• Methylphenidate (Ritalin LA; pearls)	Children ≥6 y	Monotherapy	60 mg QD
• D-Methylphenidate (Focalin XR; pearls)	Children ≥6 y	Monotherapy	Lesser of 1 mg/kg or 30 mg QD
• Methylphenidate (Concerta; pump)	Children ≥6 y and adults	Monotherapy	Lesser of 2 mg/kg or 72 mg QD
• Methylphenidate (Daytrana; patch)	Children ≥6 y	Monotherapy	Lesser of 1 mg/kg or 30 mg
• Mixed amphetamine salts (pearls)	Children 6–12 y	Monotherapy	Lesser if 1 mg/kg or 30 mg
• Amphetamine (Dexedrine Spansule; pearls)	Children ≥6 y	Monotherapy	Lesser than 1 mg/kg or 40 mg
• Lisdexamfetamine (Vyvanse; prodrug)	Children ≥6 y	Monotherapy	Lesser than 1 mg/kg or 70 mg
	Children 6–12 y and Adults	Monotherapy	
Nonstimulants			
• Atomoxetine (Strattera)	Children ≥6 y Adolescents and adults	Monotherapy	Lesser of 1.4 mg/kg or 100 mg
• Guanfacine ER (Intuniv)	Children 6–17 y	Monotherapy and adjunctive	4 mg QD
• Clonidine ER (Kapvay)	Children 6–17 y	Monotherapy and adjunctive	0.2 mg BID

hundreds of controlled trials, with published information from as early as the 1930s. They have been well established as clinically effective treatments for ADHD since the 1970s. The pediatric safety and efficacy database on acute and long-term use of psychostimulants has expanded from an early focus on grade-school children to include data on children ranging from preschool age through adolescence[1–5] Nonstimulant pharmacotherapies for ADHD, including atomoxetine and α-adrenergic agents, have seen a more recent increase in supporting data over the past 10 years.[1–6] A meta-analysis of atomoxetine and stimulant studies revealed a robust effect size for both atomoxetine and the stimulants (atomoxetine 0.62, immediate-release stimulants 0.91, and long-acting stimulants 0.95).[7] The $α_2$-agonist, guanfacine extended release (ER), demonstrated similar effect sizes of 0.43 to 0.86 in 2 double-blind placebo-controlled (DBPC) trials.[8,9]

Stimulants

Two National Institute of Mental Health–funded studies have defined the role of stimulants in the treatment of ADHD and are the cornerstone of clinical practice guidelines for the American Academy of Pediatrics and the American Academy of Child and Adolescent Psychiatry (AACAP). The MTA randomized participants to intensive behavioral therapy, manualized pharmacotherapy using systematically dosed and titrated methylphenidate, a combination of the 2, or standard community care. Both the pharmacotherapy and combined treatment groups showed significant improvement in ADHD symptoms, and both were superior to behavioral therapy alone. The combined treatment group, however, did not have a significantly better response than the pharmacotherapy alone group, and, therefore, the MTA investigators concluded that medication seems to have the most significant acute impact on the treatment of core ADHD symptoms.[10] Combining behavioral intervention with pharmacotherapy did, however, increase the level of parent/caregiver and teacher satisfaction with treatment; led to greater improvement in children's social skills, internalizing symptoms, reading achievement, and management of comorbid conditions; and, on average, allowed for use of lower medication doses.[10] The PATS, including 3-year-old to 5.5-year-old children with moderate to severe ADHD, also demonstrated a less-than-optimal response to behavioral intervention alone, resulting in the majority of children in the study warranting the initiation of pharmacotherapy.[11]

MTA

The MTA demonstrated the tolerability and efficacy of immediate-release methylphenidate administered 3 times daily in a randomized trial of 579 7-year-old to 9.9-year-old children with the combined subtype of ADHD. Medication dose adjustments in the manualized pharmacotherapy arm were based on the overall effect of the medication as reported by parent and teacher rating scales and tolerability. Children in the methylphenidate monotherapy group had a mean final total daily methylphenidate dose of 32.1 ± 15.4 mg, and those assigned to combination treatment had a mean final dose of 28.9 ± 13.7 mg/d.[10]

PATS

Before the PATS, fewer than a dozen small placebo-controlled trials of immediate-release methylphenidate in preschoolers had been conducted.[12] Those studies used doses less than or equal to 0.6 mg/kg, below the range of up to 1.0 mg/kg used in trials involving older children[13,14] and used once-daily or twice-daily dosing schedules rather than the 3-times-a-day regimen often required for optimal effect. PATS included 165 3.5-year-old to 5-year-old children who were initially randomized to either placebo or immediate-release methylphenidate (1.25 mg, 2.5 mg, 5 mg, or 7.5 mg 3 times a day). Participants were treated with each dose for a week during the double-blind crossover titration phase of the trial. Nearly a quarter of subjects (22%) were identified as responding "best" to 7.5 mg 3 times a day. The mean final best dose in PATS was 14.22 ± 8.1 mg/d or 0.7 ± 0.4 mg/kg/d.[11]

MTA versus PATS

The efficacy of methylphenidate in preschoolers varies from that seen in older children[15] as does the adverse effect profile.[16] When comparing data between MTA and PATS, the younger children had lower optimal doses, by weight, of immediate-release methylphenidate (0.7 mg/kg/d compared with 1.0 mg/kg/d). Pharmacokinetic data also demonstrated that a single dose of methylphenidate had slower clearance in 4-year-old and 5-year-old children than in school-aged children.[17] Age-related variability was also seen when evaluating tolerability. Younger children tended to have more emotional adverse events (eg, crabbiness, irritability, and proneness to crying) than school-aged children. With these differences in mind, smaller doses of stimulants, slower titrations, and close monitoring are advised when treating young children.[18]

Methylphenidate and amphetamine

Current stimulant medications approved by the Food and Drug Administration (FDA) for the treatment of ADHD are all derivatives of either methylphenidate or amphetamine, both of which act by enhancing the neurotransmission of dopamine and norepinephrine.[1] DBPC studies in children, adolescents, and adults have demonstrated that 65% to 75% of subjects typically respond to treatment with a stimulant compared with only 4% to 30% with placebo.[3,18] With approximately three-quarters of patients responding to the first stimulant medication tried, and that number increasing to between 80% and 90% if 2 different stimulants are tried consecutively,[19] it is understandable why these medications have come to be viewed as first-line treatments for core ADHD symptoms.

Recent drug development has concentrated on improving stimulant delivery systems to extend the duration of action of these medications (**Table 2**). Although both MTA and PATS used immediate-release methylphenidate, the longer-acting ER preparations are now commonly used to simplify treatment, increase adherence, and improve the potential for full-day symptom management. To individualize treatment and optimally manage ADHD symptoms, short-release, intermediate-release, and ER preparations can be selected and titrated, sometimes in combination, according to tolerability and response.

A variety of administration options (eg, capsules, sprinkleable capsules, tablets, chewable tablets, oral solution, and transdermal patches) further facilitate a patient-specific tailored approach to pharmacotherapy. Most beaded capsules contain half the dose via immediate-release beads and half the dose in enteric-coated delayed-release beads, which release the medication approximately 4 hours later, essentially providing 2 doses in one capsule. For children who struggle with swallowing capsules whole, they can be opened and sprinkled on food while maintaining their delayed-release mechanism. An osmotic-release oral system (OROS) delivers methylphenidate in a unique way, via a tablet that is coated with immediate-release methylphenidate for the initial dose, and the remainder of the medication is gradually delivered via an osmotic pump over several hours. Children with reduced gastrointestinal absorption may not receive the full benefit of this type of delivery system, however, and because of the mechanism the tablet must be swallowed whole. The transdermal patch is an

Table 2
Delivery system and duration of effect

Name	Delivery System	Duration of Effect[20]
Methylphenidate		
Methylin	Solution	4 h
Methylin	Chewable tablet	4 h
Ritalin	Tablet	4 h
Ritalin SR	Sustained-release tablet	Up to 8 h
Metadate ER, Methyline ER	Beaded capsule	7–8 h
Ritalin LA	Beaded capsule	7–9 h
Metadate CD	Beaded capsule	8–9 h
Concerta	OROS capsule	Up to 12 h
Daytrana	Transdermal patch	12 h
d-Methylphenidate		
Focalin	Tablet	4 h
Focalin XR	Beaded capsule	Up to 12 h
Amphetamine		
Adderall	Tablet	6 h
Adderall XR	Beaded capsule	10 h
d-Amphetamine		
Dexedrine/dextrostat	Tablet	4 h
Dexedrine spansule	Spansule capsule	10 h
Lisdexamfetamine Vyvanse	Capsule	10 h
Atomoxetine		
Strattera	Capsule	24 h
Guanfacine ER		
Intuniv	Tablet	8–12 h

option that may be particularly useful for those who cannot swallow pills or who need flexibility in the duration of action, because the length of time the medication works is dependent on the duration the patch is worn. It is approved to be worn up to 9 hours, and the beneficial effect is predictably seen for 2 to 3 hours after the patch is removed. The patch commonly causes skin irritation, however, so children prone to contact dermatitis may not tolerate the patch.[20] The short-acting stimulants have their own particular benefits, including the ability to divide pills, which may be an advantage when treating young children, who may require smaller dose increments than allowed by sustained-release formulations, or as an addition in the afternoon to extend treatment coverage of school-time dosing. Additionally, several of the short-acting medications are available in inexpensive generic preparations.

General adverse effects
Methylphenidate and amphetamine-derived medications have similar adverse event profiles (**Table 3**).[3] Common side effects include insomnia, decreased appetite, weight loss, headache, stomach upset, and increases in heart rate and blood pressure. Additionally, as discussed previously, emotional outbursts and irritability have been frequently observed with stimulant use in younger children.[21]

Cardiovascular adverse effects
Concerns with the cardiovascular safety of stimulant medications have led to specific recommendations for pretreatment evaluation, treatment selection, and

Table 3
Adverse effects and ADHD pharmacotherapy

	Stimulants	Atomoxetine	α_2-Agonists
	Methylphenidate and amphetamine		Clonidine and guanfacine
Growth	Appetite suppression; weight loss; delays in growth (weight > height) which normalize over time[23]; effects likely dose dependent	Appetite suppression; weight loss; delays in growth, which normalize over time[62,63]; nausea and vomiting	————
Cardiovascular	Increased heart rate, blood pressure; ECG recommended if cardiac history/ physical warrants	Increased heart rate, blood pressure; ECG recommended if cardiac history/ physical warrants	Decreased blood pressure; bradycardia; dizziness; ECG recommended if cardiac history/ physical warrants
Sleep	Insomnia	Sedation	Sedation
Tics	May induce tics in some patients; some studies show decline in tics with stimulant treatment	Does not exacerbate tics	Combine with stimulant to treat tics in context of ADHD
Black box warnings	History of substance abuse/dependence; cardiac history; psychosis	Suicidality	

monitoring. Although medication-related changes in heart rate and blood pressure are commonly observed in healthy children treated with stimulants without incident, closer scrutiny should be given when considering use of these agents in children with known structural cardiac abnormalities.[22] Additionally, obtaining a cardiac-focused history to evaluate for the presence of heart disease, including palpitations; syncope; cardiomyopathy; arrhythmia; conduction abnormalities, such as long QT syndrome; and any familial history of early or sudden cardiac death as well as a physical examination is recommended by the American Academy of Pediatrics[23] as part of a premedication assessment. In cases of positive findings, an ECG and/or referral to cardiology may be warranted before starting pharmacotherapy. Cardiovascular risks may potentially be even more of an issue in the treatment of adults with ADHD, who are more likely to have concurrent hypertension and/or cardiovascular disease.

Growth
Swanson and colleagues[24] theorize that, in general, children with ADHD may display different growth trajectories than their peers without the disorder. They also observed, however, that children treated with stimulant medications grew more slowly and gained less weight than expected. Statistically significant effects on height and weight were also seen with stimulant treatment in a meta-analysis of 22 studies by Faraone and colleagues[25] with more significant weight deficits than height ($P = .002$). Faraone

and colleagues[25] also suggested that these growth effects may be dose related but were not unique to either methylphenidate or amphetamine.

Stopping the stimulant medication seemed to normalize growth, an effect observed in additional studies examining summer medication holidays or medication discontinuation.[26–29] MTA data,[30] however, showed that although discontinuation of methylphenidate treatment did not reverse losses in expected height, it did have a beneficial effect on weight gain.

The AACAP practice parameter for ADHD treatment specifically addresses monitoring height and weight, including serial plotting of growth parameters. A change in height or weight crossing 2 percentile lines suggests abnormal growth according to AACAP and potentially necessitates a medication holiday, dose adjustment, or even a medication change. Ultimately, reductions in growth must be balanced with benefits of treatment.[18]

Atomoxetine

Atomoxetine, which selectively blocks reuptake at the noradrenergic neuron, was the first FDA-approved nonstimulant medication for the treatment of ADHD. Two DBPC efficacy studies demonstrated significant improvement in ADHD symptoms with atomoxetine compared with placebo, with 64.1% and 58.7% of pediatric patients responding to atomoxetine,[31] and more than a dozen DBPC trials have subsequently added additional evidence supporting its safety and efficacy.[31–36] Two studies comparing atomoxetine with stimulants demonstrated both pharmacotherapeutic approaches to be efficacious in the treatment of ADHD, with a more robust response to the stimulants in both trials (**Table 4**). Atomoxetine was the first FDA-approved pharmacotherapy for adults with ADHD, based on 2 positive DBPC studies in that population.[37]

Atomoxetine is dosed by weight in the pediatric population, with a target therapeutic dose of 1.2 mg/kg/d, administered once daily or divided into twice-daily doses. Atomoxetine has a graded dose response, as observed in a dose-finding study, which demonstrated an improvement in ADHD symptoms with doses of 0.5 mg/kg/d, 1.2 mg/kg/d, and 1.8 mg/kg/d. The 0.5-mg/kg/d dose was associated with intermediate efficacy and with symptom reduction falling between that seen with placebo and the 2 higher doses, although no additional benefit on the core symptoms of ADHD by increasing the dose to 1.8 mg/kg/d. Additional improvements in psychosocial functioning were seen with the increase to the 1.8-mg/kg/d dose, without any significant difference in adverse events.[35]

Atomoxetine is not approved for use in children under 6 years of age; however, one DBPC trial examining the use of atomoxetine in 101 5-year-old and 6-year-old children demonstrated improvements on parent and teacher ADHD-IV (Attention Deficit Hyperactivity Disorder Rating Scale IV) ratings for children assigned to atomoxetine compared with those taking placebo ($P<.05$). The mean final daily dose of atomoxetine in this trial was 1.38 mg/kg/d. Despite statistically significant improvements in core ADHD symptoms and that the parents received concomitant education on ADHD and behavioral interventions as a part of the study, the children continued to display significant impairment on the ADHD-IV at study end.[38]

Adverse effects

Common adverse effects of atomoxetine include sedation, loss of appetite, nausea, vomiting, irritability, and headaches. No significant differences were noted in efficacy or tolerability of atomoxetine between young and older children.[39] Atomoxetine has additional warnings for hepatotoxicity and suicidality risk. Laboratory data analysis

Table 4
Atomoxetine and stimulant comparator trials

Study	Atomoxetine and OROS Methylphenidate[64]	Atomoxetine and Mixed-Amphetamine Salts[65]
Design	• DBPC comparator trial • 6 wk of ATMX up to 1.8 mg/kg/d or OROS methylphenidate up to 54 mg/d or placebo • Subjects initially assigned to OROS methylphenidate were switched to ATMX after 6 wk	• 3-Week laboratory school comparison
Age	6–16 y	6–12 y
Outcome	• ATMX and OROS were superior to placebo, with 45% ($P<.003$) and 56% ($P<.001$) responding, respectively. • Effect sizes: ATMX 0.6, OROS methylphenidate 0.8. • Stimulant-naïve patients response rates to ATMX (57%, $P = .004$) and OROS (64%, $P \leq .001$) were comparable ($P = .43$). • Subjects with prior stimulant exposure had better responses to OROS (51%, $P = .002$) than to ATMX (37%, $P = .09$) ($P = .03$). • Effect size for ATMX greater in stimulant-naïve patients (0.9) than in patients previously treated with stimulants (0.5). • OROS effect sizes in stimulant-naïve patients and those with prior exposure were 1.0 and 0.8, respectively. • 42% of ATMX nonresponders in the second phase of the study had previously responded to OROS during acute treatment. • 43% of Subjects who did not respond acutely to OROS went on to respond to ATMX.	• Improved attention and academic performance were noted with both treatments. • MAS-treated subjects had greater improvements than those who received ATMX ($P<.001$).
Adverse events	• Decreased appetite the only adverse event separating from placebo for both active treatments ($P<.05$). • Subjects receiving OROS methylphenidate reported experiencing insomnia, whereas those assigned to ATMX had more frequent complaints of somnolence. • Weight loss and increased diastolic blood pressure ($P<.05$) were noted as significant for both drugs compared with placebo, and an increased pulse rate was significant in the ATMX group compared with OROS and placebo ($P<.05$).	• The MAS group reported experiencing insomnia, decreased appetite, upper abdominal pain, anorexia, and headache. • The most common adverse events reported in the ATMX group were somnolence, appetite decrease, upper abdominal pain, vomiting, and headache. • Vital sign changes were similar for both groups and were not statistically significant.
Notes	A differential response to treatment for some patients may exist.	The short 3-week duration of the study may not have been sufficient to demonstrate the full effect of ATMX treatment.

Abbreviations: ATMX, atomoxetine; MAX, mixed-amphetamine salts.

from 7961 adult and pediatric subjects in clinical trials of atomoxetine revealed 41 instances of elevated aspartate aminotransferase and alanine aminotransferase. During its first 4 years on the market, there were 351 spontaneous reports of hepatic events, with only 3 suggesting atomoxetine as a probable cause. In all 3 cases, symptoms resolved when atomoxetine was discontinued; therefore, it is recommended that atomoxetine treatment be stopped if jaundice or elevations in liver enzymes occur.[40] An analysis of 14 studies of atomoxetine by Bangs and colleagues[41] in 2008 demonstrated that suicidal ideation was more common in subjects who received atomoxetine (0.37%, 5 of 1357 subjects) compared with those who were on placebo (0%, 0 of 851 subjects). No suicides occurred in any of the trials in the analysis.

α_2-Agonists

Clonidine (Catapres) and immediate-release guanfacine (Tenex), have been used commonly over the past decade as second-line or adjunctive treatments for ADHD. Immediate-release clonidine has been shown to reduce ADHD symptoms in patients with co-occurring tics, aggression, and conduct disorder; however, it is short acting and requires multiple divided doses throughout the day.[5] An ER formulation (Kapvay) was approved by the FDA in September 2010, for both monotherapy of ADHD in children and adolescents ages 6 to 17 years as well as in combination with a stimulant.

Guanfacine is a more selective α_2-adrenergic agonist with less sedation and a longer duration of action.[1] Immediate-release guanfacine showed improvements in hyperactivity and inattention in a small open-label study, with transient sedation the most common adverse event.[42] Additional studies have demonstrated its effectiveness and tolerability in treating ADHD with comorbid tic disorders and Tourette syndrome.[43,44] An ER form of guanfacine (Intuniv) was given FDA approval in 2009 as monotherapy for pediatric ADHD after 2 controlled trials in patients ages 6 to 17 years and then was approved for use in combination with stimulants based on an adjunctive study. The most common treatment-emergent adverse events were headache, somnolence, fatigue, sedation, and upper abdominal pain, and all seemed dose related. No clinically significant vital sign or ECG changes were seen in these studies[8,9]; however, bradycardia was reported in long-term studies.[45,46] Effect sizes and response rates for ER guanfacine also seemed dose related (effect size 0.43 to 0.86, with response rates 43% and 62% for doses of 3 mg once daily and 4 mg once daily, respectively).

Although the stimulants and atomoxetine can be abruptly discontinued, the ER α_2-adrenergics should be tapered gradually to avoid rebound hypertension. Clonidine ER should be decreased by 0.1 mg every 3 to 7 days[47] and guanfacine ER by 1 mg every 3 to 7 days.[48]

Non–FDA-Approved Pharmacotherapies

The evidence base for the non–FDA-approved pharmacotherapies, such as the immediate-release α_2-adrenergic agents, bupropion, and the tricyclics, is significantly less than for the FDA-approved medications, in particular the stimulants and atomoxetine.[49] Immediate-release guanfacine and clonidine do not have ADHD indications or significant research available, for example, so it is unknown if they would have similar efficacy as the long-acting formulations (discussed previously). Bupropion is an antidepressant with noradrenergic and dopaminergic properties that has been shown in one randomized controlled trial[50] to have a modest effect for ADHD and may seem of particular interest in treating individuals with ADHD and comorbid depression or tobacco use, but the few ADHD data limit enthusiasm.

The tricyclic antidepressants have some data supporting use; however, they are infrequently used due to their unfavorable side effect profile, which includes cardiovascular risks. Modafinil, a centrally acting agent, was shown in randomized controlled trials to be effective for ADHD[51,52]; however, FDA approval for the treatment of ADHD was not sought by its manufacturer after report of a suspected case of Stevens-Johnson syndrome.

Comorbidity

The presence of co-occurring learning, developmental, and other psychiatric disorders can affect response to treatment and/or complicate treatment planning. Nearly two-thirds of children diagnosed with ADHD also have at least one comorbid psychiatric disorder. The MTA sample included only 31% of participants who had ADHD alone, whereas 40% also met criteria for oppositional defiant disorder, 38% for anxiety/mood disorders, 14% for conduct disorder, and 11% for tic disorders.[10] If FDA-approved pharmacotherapies are not effective or are contraindicated, it may be necessary to consider a trial of combination therapy or a non–FDA-approved agent. Although clinically indicated, alternative therapy strategies or combination pharmacotherapies may elevate potential risks, which must be discussed with patients and caregivers and monitored closely.[18]

Longitudinal Course of Treatment

Epidemiologic data indicate that 2% to 6% of preschoolers meet diagnostic criteria for ADHD,[53,54] with prevalence rates in school-aged children conservatively estimated at between 3% and 7%.[55] The prevalence of ADHD decreases through adolescence and adulthood; however, significant adolescents and adults are estimated to be affected (3%–4% of adults).[56] Although the presentation of the disorder may vary from early childhood to adulthood, the impairment is not necessarily any less significant.[57] Although many patients experience a longitudinal course of ADHD, some patients outgrowing ADHD has led to the AACAP practice parameter recommendation reminding clinicians to periodically re-evaluate the need for ongoing pharmacotherapy. Follow-up clinic visits ensure that medication remains effective, dosing is optimized, and adverse events are minimized. The AACAP recommends that ADHD treatment be individualized and that the duration of treatment should continue as long as impairing symptoms are present.[18]

ADHD pharmacotherapy typically offers significant benefits in the reduction of the core ADHD symptoms of inattention, hyperactivity, and impulsivity. By reducing these, patients are better able to perform academically, socially, and occupationally. Long-term data from the MTA, however, demonstrated that the benefits of medication treatment were sustainable for up to 2 years for the majority of subjects and that, by year 3, only 1 in 3 subjects continued to demonstrate benefit with pharmacotherapy.[58] At 6-year and 8-year follow-ups, the MTA subjects as a group had poorer ratings of behavior and academic and overall functioning compared with normal controls despite having reduced ADHD symptoms.

Early treatment with methylphenidate does not seem to increase the risk for negative outcomes and may have beneficial effects in the long term.[59] Some longitudinal studies[60,61] found no evidence that stimulant treatment in childhood or adolescence either increases or decreases the risk for development of substance use disorders in young adulthood but that ADHD patients treated with stimulants were at significantly less risk of developing depressive and anxiety disorders, disruptive behavior, and repeating a grade in school than the ADHD patients who were not treated.

CLINICAL VIGNETTE: ADHD

A 7-year-old boy was diagnosed with ADHD, combined subtype, and oppositional defiant disorder. The ADHD was moderately severe, but his parents were reluctant to initiate pharmacotherapy at the time, so an 8-week trial of parent training was initiated.

Symptoms were tracked on a Vanderbilt rating scale and, although helpful for some of the ADHD and oppositional defiant disorder symptoms, impairing ADHD target symptoms at home, school, and socially persisted, so they decided to reconsider pharmacotherapy. He had no underlying cardiovascular history or other contraindications and was initiated on a 10-mg beaded methylphenidate product, which he tolerated well but he had inadequate response. He was titrated up to 20 mg per day, which he tolerated well with good results, as reflected by parent's and teacher's Vanderbilt scales.

Throughout the next 2 years, improvements in ADHD symptoms were well controlled, with sporadic behavioral therapy booster sessions used to address behavioral issues.

Throughout the fourth and fifth grades, his clinician noted a gradual increase in problematic behaviors on the annual rating scales from both parent and teacher. School symptoms had gradually increased and it was clear that coverage throughout the day was becoming inadequate and, with increasing homework demands, it was clear that the duration of action was inadequate as well. There were no identifiable psychosocial stressors, adherence to medication seemed adequate, and no new comorbidities evident, so a decision was made to change to an OROS-methylphenidate product, which would have a longer duration of action. The initial 36-mg dose was inadequate for schoolwork during the day. The dose was subsequently titrated up to 54 mg per day, which led to a robust response for schoolwork, but unfortunately initial insomnia was consistently 60 minutes per night and evening appetite was significantly diminished, with secondary weight loss. A switch back to the beaded methylphenidate, but dosed at 30 mg per day, led to an excellent response during the school day, which, when augmented with 10-mg short-acting methylphenidate at 3:00 PM, led to improved evenings with acceptable tolerability.

SUMMARY

ADHD is a common disorder, which can lead to significant morbidity when untreated. Fortunately, there are a significant number of pharmacotherapies with a long track record of safety and efficacy, in particular the stimulant medications. With improvements in the duration of action through sustained-release preparations and the more recent availability of nonstimulant ADHD treatments, available resources have rapidly expanded. Guided by the ever-expanding literature on ADHD pharmacotherapy, including the MTA and PATS, how to care for individuals with ADHD continues to be better understood.

As for the next generation of pharmacologic treatments for ADHD, the bar is set fairly high. The stimulants are one of the most robust treatments in psychiatry and in much of medicine. Although there are downsides to current medications, including abuse/diversion liability of stimulants, and tolerability issues of the specific ADHD pharmacotherapies, the efficacy, general tolerability, and clinician comfort with using these medications will require new treatments to be exceptional in some way.

REFERENCES

1. Biederman J, Spencer TJ. Psychopharmacological interventions. Child Adolesc Psychiatr Clin N Am 2008;17(2):439–58, xi.
2. American Academy of Pediatrics. Clinical practice guideline: treatment of the school-aged child with attention-deficit/hyperactivity disorder. J Pediatr 2001; 108(4):1033–44.

3. Greenhill LL, Pliszka S, Dulcan MK, et al. Practice parameter for the use of stimulant medications in the treatment of children, adolescents, and adults. J Am Acad Child Adolesc Psychiatry 2002;41(Suppl 2):26S–49S.

4. Pliszka SR, Liotti M, Bailey BY, et al. Electrophysiological effects of stimulant treatment on inhibitory control in children with attention-deficit/hyperactivity disorder. J Child Adolesc Psychopharmacol 2007;17(3):356–66.

5. Brown RT, Amler RW, Freeman WS, et al. Treatment of attention-deficit/hyperactivity disorder: overview of the evidence. Pediatrics 2005;115(6):e749–57.

6. Madaan V, Kinnan S, Daughton J, et al. Innovations and recent trends in the treatment of ADHD. Expert Rev Neurother 2006;6(9):1375–85.

7. Faraone S. Understanding the effect size of ADHD medications: implications for clinical care. Medsc Psychiatr Ment Health 2003;8(2).

8. Biederman J, Melmed RD, Patel A, et al. A randomized, double-blind, placebo-controlled study of guanfacine extended release in children and adolescents with attention-deficit/hyperactivity disorder. Pediatrics 2008;121(1):e73–84.

9. Sallee FR, McGough J, Wigal T, et al. Guanfacine extended release in children and adolescents with attention-deficit/hyperactivity disorder: a placebo-controlled trial. J Am Acad Child Adolesc Psychiatry 2009;48(2):155–65.

10. MTA Cooperative Group. A 14-month randomized clinical trial of treatment strategies for attention-deficit/hyperactivity disorder. The MTA cooperative group. Multimodal treatment study of children with ADHD. Arch Gen Psychiatry 1999;56(12):1073–86.

11. Greenhill L, Kollins S, Abikoff H, et al. Efficacy and safety of immediate-release methylphenidate treatment for preschoolers with ADHD. J Am Acad Child Adolesc Psychiatry 2006;45(11):1284–93.

12. Kratochvil CJ, Greenhill LL, March JS, et al. The role of stimulants in the treatment of preschool children with attention-deficit hyperactivity disorder. CNS Drugs 2004;18(14):957–66.

13. Arnold LE, Abikoff HB, Cantwell DP, et al. National Institute of Mental Health Collaborative Multimodal Treatment Study of Children with ADHD (the MTA). Design challenges and choices. Arch Gen Psychiatry 1997 Sep;54(9):865–70.

14. Arnold LE, Abikoff HB, Cantwell DP, et al. NIMH Collaborative Multimodal Treatment Study of Children with ADHD (the MTA). Design, methodology and protocol evolution. J Atten Disord 1997;2(3):141–58.

15. Connor DF. Preschool attention deficit hyperactivity disorder: a review of prevalence, diagnosis, neurobiology, and stimulant treatment. J Dev Behav Pediatr 2002;23(Suppl 1):S1–9.

16. Firestone P, Musten LM, Pisterman S, et al. Short-term side effects of stimulant medication are increased in preschool children with attention-deficit/hyperactivity disorder: a double-blind placebo-controlled study. J Child Adolesc Psychopharmacol 1998;8(1):13–25.

17. Wigal SB, Gupta S, Greenhill L, et al. Pharmacokinetics of methylphenidate in preschoolers with attention-deficit/hyperactivity disorder. J Child Adolesc Psychopharmacol 2007;17(2):153–64.

18. Pliszka S. Practice parameter for the assessment and treatment of children and adolescents with attention-deficit/hyperactivity disorder. J Am Acad Child Adolesc Psychiatry 2007;46(7):894–921.

19. Pliszka SR. Non-stimulant treatment of attention-deficit/hyperactivity disorder. CNS Spectr 2003;8(4):253–8.

20. Daughton JM, Kratochvil CJ. Review of ADHD pharmacotherapies: advantages, disadvantages, and clinical pearls. J Am Acad Child Adolesc Psychiatry 2009;48(3):240–8.

21. Wigal T, Greenhill L, Chuang S, et al. Safety and tolerability of methylphenidate in preschool children with ADHD. J Am Acad Child Adolesc Psychiatry 2006;45(11): 1294–303.
22. Winterstein AG, Gerhard T, Shuster J, et al. Cardiac safety of central nervous system stimulants in children and adolescents with attention-deficit/ hyperactivity disorder. Pediatrics 2007;120(6):e1494–501.
23. Perrin JM, Friedman RA, Knilans TK. Cardiovascular monitoring and stimulant drugs for attention-deficit/hyperactivity disorder. Pediatrics 2008;122(2):451–3.
24. Swanson JM, Ruff DD, Feldman PD, et al. Characterization of Growth in Children with ADHD. Paper presented at: Annual Meeting of the American Academy of Child and Adolescent Psychiatry. Toronto (Canada), October18–23, 2005.
25. Faraone SV, Biederman J, Morley CP, et al. Effect of stimulants on height and weight: a review of the literature. J Am Acad Child Adolesc Psychiatry 2008; 47(9):994–1009.
26. Klein RG, Mannuzza S. Hyperactive boys almost grown up. III. Methylphenidate effects on ultimate height. Arch Gen Psychiatry 1988;45(12):1131–4.
27. Safer D, Allen R, Barr E. Growth rebound after termination of stimulant drugs. J Pediatr 1975;86:113–6.
28. Gittelman R, Landa B, Mattes J, et al. Methylphenidate and growth in hyperactive children: a controlled withdrawal study. Arch Gen Psychiatry 1988;45:1127–30.
29. Kaffman M, Sher A, Bar-Sinai N. MBD children-variability in developmental patterns or growth inhibitory effects of stimulants? Isr Ann Psychiatr Relat Discip 1979;17:58–66.
30. National Institute of Mental Health Multimodal Treatment Study of ADHD follow-up. Changes in effectiveness and growth after the end of treatment. Pediatrics 2004;113(4):762–9.
31. Spencer T, Heiligenstein JH, Biederman J, et al. Results from 2 proof-of-concept, placebo-controlled studies of atomoxetine in children with attention-deficit/ hyperactivity disorder. J Clin Psychiatry 2002;63(12):1140–7.
32. Kelsey DK, Sumner CR, Casat CD, et al. Once-daily atomoxetine treatment for children with attention-deficit/hyperactivity disorder, including an assessment of evening and morning behavior: a double-blind, placebo-controlled trial. Pediatrics 2004;114(1):e1–8.
33. Michelson D, Adler L, Spencer T, et al. Atomoxetine in adults with ADHD: two randomized, placebo-controlled studies. Biol Psychiatry 2003;53(2):112–20.
34. Michelson D, Allen AJ, Busner J, et al. Once-daily atomoxetine treatment for children and adolescents with attention deficit hyperactivity disorder: a randomized, placebo-controlled study. Am J Psychiatry 2002;159(11):1896–901.
35. Michelson D, Faries D, Wernicke J, et al. Atomoxetine in the treatment of children and adolescents with attention-deficit/hyperactivity disorder: a randomized, placebo-controlled, dose-response study. Pediatrics 2001;108(5):E83.
36. Weiss M, Tannock R, Kratochvil C, et al. A randomized, placebo-controlled study of once-daily atomoxetine in the school setting in children with ADHD. J Am Acad Child Adolesc Psychiatry 2005;44(7):647–55.
37. Buitelaar JK, Michelson D, Danckaerts M, et al. A randomized, double-blind study of continuation treatment for attention-deficit/hyperactivity disorder after 1 year. Biol Psychiatry 2007;61(5):694–9.
38. Kratochvil CJ, Vaughan BS, Daughton JM, et al. Atomoxetine vs placebo for the treatment of ADHD in 5- and 6- year-old children. Paper presented at: Annual Meeting of the American Academy of Child and Adolescent Psychiatry. Chicago (IL), October 27–31, 2008.

39. Kratochvil CJ, Milton DR, Vaughan BS, et al. Acute atomoxetine treatment of younger and older children with ADHD: a meta-analysis of tolerability and efficacy. Child Adolesc Psychiatry Ment Health 2008;2(1):25.
40. Bangs ME, Jin L, Zhang S, et al. Hepatic events associated with atomoxetine treatment for attention-deficit hyperactivity disorder. Drug Saf 2008;31(4):345–54.
41. Bangs ME, Tauscher-Wisniewski S, Polzer J, et al. Meta-analysis of suicide-related behavior events in patients treated with atomoxetine. J Am Acad Child Adolesc Psychiatry 2008;47(2):209–18.
42. Hunt RD, Arnsten AF, Asbell MD. An open trial of guanfacine in the treatment of attention-deficit hyperactivity disorder. J Am Acad Child Adolesc Psychiatry 1995;34(1):50–4.
43. Chappell PB, Riddle MA, Scahill L, et al. Guanfacine treatment of comorbid attention-deficit hyperactivity disorder and Tourette's syndrome: preliminary clinical experience. J Am Acad Child Adolesc Psychiatry 1995;34(9):1140–6.
44. Scahill L, Chappell PB, Kim YS, et al. A placebo-controlled study of guanfacine in the treatment of children with tic disorders and attention deficit hyperactivity disorder. Am J Psychiatry 2001;158(7):1067–74.
45. Biederman J, Melmed RD, Patel A, et al. Long-term, open-label extension study of guanfacine extended release in children and adolescents with ADHD. CNS Spectr 2008;13(12):1047–55.
46. Sallee FR, Lyne A, Wigal T, et al. Long-term safety and efficacy of guanfacine extended release in children and adolescents with attention-deficit/hyperactivity disorder. J Child Adolesc Psychopharmacol 2009;19(3):215–26.
47. Kapvay [Package Insert]: Shionogi; 2010.
48. Intuniv [Package Insert]: Shire; 2011.
49. Hinshaw SP. Moderators and mediators of treatment outcome for youth with ADHD: understanding for whom and how interventions work. J Pediatr Psychol 2007;32(6):664–75.
50. Wilens TE, Spencer TJ, Biederman J, et al. A controlled clinical trial of bupropion for attention deficit hyperactivity disorder in adults. Am J Psychiatry 2001;158(2):282–8.
51. Biederman J, Swanson JM, Wigal SB, et al. A comparison of once-daily and divided doses of modafinil in children with attention-deficit/hyperactivity disorder: a randomized, double-blind, and placebo-controlled study. J Clin Psychiatry 2006;67(5):727–35.
52. Kahbazi M, Ghoreishi A, Rahiminejad F, et al. A randomized, double-blind and placebo-controlled trial of modafinil in children and adolescents with attention deficit and hyperactivity disorder. Psychiatry Res 2009;168(3):234–7.
53. Angold A, Erkanli A, Egger HL, et al. Stimulant treatment for children: a community perspective. J Am Acad Child Adolesc Psychiatry 2000;39(8):975–84 [discussion: 984–94].
54. Lavigne JV, Gibbons RD, Christoffel KK, et al. Prevalence rates and correlates of psychiatric disorders among preschool children. J Am Acad Child Adolesc Psychiatry 1996;35(2):204–14.
55. American Psychiatric Association. Diagnostic and statistical manual of mental disorders fourth edition text revision. Washington, DC: American Psychiatric Association; 2000.
56. Fayyad J, De Graaf R, Kessler R, et al. Cross-national prevalence and correlates of adult attention-deficit hyperactivity disorder. Br J Psychiatry 2007;190:402–9.
57. Kessler RC, Adler L, Barkley R, et al. The prevalence and correlates of adult ADHD in the United States: results from the national comorbidity survey replication. Am J Psychiatry 2006;163(4):716–23.

58. Swanson J, Arnold LE, Kraemer H, et al. Evidence, interpretation, and qualification from multiple reports of long-term outcomes in the multimodal treatment study of children with ADHD (MTA): part II: supporting details. J Atten Disord 2008;12(1):15–43.
59. Mannuzza S, Klein RG, Truong NL, et al. Age of methylphenidate treatment initiation in children with ADHD and later substance abuse: prospective follow-up into adulthood. Am J Psychiatry 2008;165(5):604–9.
60. Biederman J, Monuteaux MC, Spencer T, et al. Do stimulants protect against psychiatric disorders in youth with ADHD? a 10-year follow-up study. Pediatrics 2009;124(1):71–8.
61. Biederman J, Monuteaux MC, Spencer T, et al. Stimulant therapy and risk for subsequent substance use disorders in male adults with ADHD: a naturalistic controlled 10-year follow-up study. Am J Psychiatry 2008;165(5):597–603.
62. Spencer TJ, Newcorn JH, Kratochvil CJ, et al. Effects of atomoxetine on growth after 2-year treatment among pediatric patients with attention-deficit/hyperactivity disorder. Pediatrics 2005;116(1):e74–80.
63. Spencer TJ, Kratochvil CJ, Sangal RB, et al. Effects of atomoxetine on growth in children with attention-deficit/hyperactivity disorder following up to five years of treatment. J Child Adolesc Psychopharmacol 2007;17(5):689–700.
64. Newcorn JH, Kratochvil CJ, Allen AJ, et al. Atomoxetine and osmotically released methylphenidate for the treatment of attention deficit hyperactivity disorder: acute comparison and differential response. Am J Psychiatry 2008;165(6):721–30.
65. Wigal SB, McGough JJ, McCracken JT, et al. A laboratory school comparison of mixed amphetamine salts extended release (Adderall XR) and atomoxetine (Strattera) in school-aged children with attention deficit/hyperactivity disorder. J Atten Disord 2005;9(1):275–89.

Psychopharmacology of Autism Spectrum Disorder: Evidence and Practice

Matthew Siegel, MD[a,b,c],*

KEYWORDS

- Autism spectrum disorder • Comorbid psychopathology • Psychopharmacology
- Symptom-specific treatment

KEY POINTS

- Children with autism spectrum disorder (ASD) present with high rates of behavioral symptoms and comorbid psychopathology.
- No medications have shown efficacy for the core symptoms of ASD.
- Successful treatment depends on careful dissection of etiologic factors, only some of which may be responsive to psychopharmacologic intervention.
- The controlled evidence base provides important guidance for pharmacologic treatment choices.

INTRODUCTION

The ASDs—autistic disorder, Asperger syndrome, and pervasive developmental disorder not otherwise specified (PDD-NOS)—share core impairments in the domains of social communication and restricted, repetitive interests and behaviors. Increased identification of children with ASD, now estimated at 1 in 88 by the Centers for Disease Control and Prevention,[1] and the prevalence of comorbid psychiatric and behavioral disorders in the population have contributed to increased exposure of children with ASD to psychotropic medication.

Over the past 3 decades the number and quality of randomized controlled trials (RCTs) of psychotropic medications in children with ASD have increased substantially (**Fig. 1**). Despite this burgeoning evidence base, it remains the case that there is no medication that has shown efficacy for treating the core impairments of ASD. Psychotropic treatment approaches, therefore, currently center on the amelioration of associated symptoms or identifiable comorbid psychiatric disorders.

Dr Siegel has no financial disclosures or conflicts of interest.
^a Department of Psychiatry, Tufts University School of Medicine, 800 Washington Street, Boston, MA 02111, USA; ^b Developmental Disorders Program, Spring Harbor Hospital, 123 Andover Road, Westbrook, ME 04092, USA; ^c Center for Outcomes Research and Evaluation, Maine Medical Center Research Institute, 509 Forest Avenue, Portland, Maine 04103, USA
* Developmental Disorders Program, Spring Harbor Hospital, 123 Andover Road, Westbrook, ME 04092.
E-mail address: siegem@springharbor.org

Child Adolesc Psychiatric Clin N Am 21 (2012) 957–973
http://dx.doi.org/10.1016/j.chc.2012.07.006
1056-4993/12/$ – see front matter © 2012 Elsevier Inc. All rights reserved.

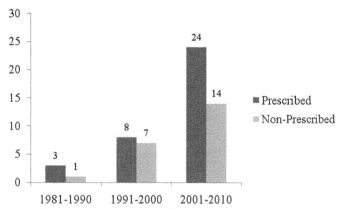

Fig. 1. RCTs of medications in children with ASD.

Two recent systematic reviews graded the controlled evidence base for medications in ASD. The first review included antipsychotics, serotonin reuptake inhibitors, and stimulants in children under 12 years.[2] The second review included those medication classes as well as α_2-agonists, mood stabilizers, norepinephrine reuptake inhibitors, opioid receptor antagonists, and other medications in children up to 18 years old.[3] Both studies found moderate to strong/established evidence for risperidone and aripiprazole for challenging and repetitive behaviors, and the Siegel and Beaulieu[3] study also found established evidence for haloperidol for hyperactivity and stereotypy, promising evidence for methylphenidate for hyperactivity, and preliminary evidence for atomoxetine and naltrexone for hyperactivity.

This article focuses on the controlled evidence base, discussing uncontrolled data when necessary. Because the evidence for psychopharmacology is limited and the presenting problems typically have a multifactorial cause, successful treatment of children with ASD requires a broad differential diagnostic approach, incorporation of multidisciplinary interventions, and the use of targeted psychopharmacology based on the best evidence for treatment of specific symptoms or syndromes. Symptom specific approaches are presented.

CURRENT USE OF PSYCHOTROPICS IN THE ASD POPULATION

Studies of local and nationally representative populations in the United States in the past decade have consistently reported that 30% to 60% of children with ASD use at least 1 psychotropic medication.[4–7] In several studies,[8] more severe autistic symptoms and older age have been associated with greater likelihood of prescription medication use. In a Medicaid-enrolled sample, Mandell and colleagues[6] examined more than 60,000 claims and found that increasing age, Asperger syndrome as opposed to autistic disorder, presence of a comorbid psychiatric condition, and greater intellectual disability were correlated with psychotropic medication use. Among the children in the sample, 58% were prescribed at least 1 psychotropic medication. As a Medicaid sample, however, the findings may reflect a disproportionately poor and severely affected group.

In a study of more than 5000 children with ASD with varying insurance status enrolled in a voluntary Web-based parent report registry, 35% used at least 1 psychotropic medication and almost 10% reported 3 or more concurrent psychotropic medications. Those who were insured by Medicaid were more likely to use 3 or more psychotropic medications.[9] The most common medication classes were stimulants, antipsychotics, and antidepressants. The majority of children received psychotropic prescriptions from psychiatrists (48%) and neurologists (20%), followed by developmental pediatricians (12%) and pediatricians (10%); 39% of respondents reported 1 or more psychiatric comorbidities. As the study showed that insurance status and prescriber specialty affect medication use, it suggests that non-clinical factors may contribute to exposure to psychotropic medications.

The economic impact of medication use is ASD is large. The global market for autism therapeutics has been estimated at $2.2 billion to $3.5 billion.[10] Children with ASD incurred 8 to 9 times higher medication costs than children without ASD in a large group-model health plan, accounting for 27% of annual health care expenditures for these children.[11]

COMORBID PSYCHOPATHOLOGY IN ASD

A strong predictor of medication use in children with ASD is the presence of comorbid psychopathology. Diagnosing comorbid psychopathology in children with ASD, particularly in children at a minimal or non-verbal communication level, is a complex endeavor. Assessments must take into account whether children's symptoms are typical of ASD, normal for their developmental age, serve a specified adaptive function, and/or are modeled or reinforced in their environment, among other considerations. An additional complexity is that most epidemiologic samples of children with ASD report the presence of intellectual disability in at least 50% of subjects.

Children with ASD usually perform in an aberrant fashion on standard psychiatric diagnostic instruments that are designed for the neurotypical population. This can lead to overidentification of comorbid psychiatric disorders. For example, a 2001 study revealed that half of the individuals with ASD assessed with the Structured Clinical Interview met criteria for schizophrenia.[12] Similarly, De Bruin and colleagues[13] used the Diagnostic Interview Schedule for Children Version IV[14] to diagnose comorbidity in 94 children with PDD-NOS and reported that more than 80% of the sample had a comorbid psychiatric disorder, including 61% with a disruptive behavior disorder and 55% with an anxiety disorder. Even higher rates were reported among children with ASD who were referred to a pediatric psychopharmacology clinic and diagnosed using the Schedule for Affective Disorders and Schizophrenia for School-Age Children.[15] This study identified an average of 6.4 comorbid diagnoses in each child, and 95% of the sample met criteria for 3 or more comorbid diagnoses.[16]

Less dramatic findings were obtained by Simonoff and colleagues,[17] who used the Child and Adolescent Psychiatric Assessment to diagnose a population-derived sample of 112 children (ages 10–14 years) with PDD-NOS or autistic disorder identified by parent interview. They found at least 1 comorbid psychiatric disorder in 70% of the sample and 2 or more in 41% of the sample. Most common were social phobia, attention-deficit/hyperactivity disorder (ADHD), and oppositional defiant disorder. Although it likely over-identified psychopathology, the strength of this study was the use of a population-derived sample, suggesting that comorbid disorders occur with some frequency in the general ASD population, not just in clinically referred samples.

Several investigators have worked to develop diagnostic measures of psychopathology specific to children with ASD. Leyfer and colleagues[18] modified the Schedule for Affective Disorders and Schizophrenia for School-Age Children[19] to account for symptoms typical of autism and for how psychiatric symptoms may present in children with ASD, producing the Autism Co-morbidity Interview—Present and Lifetime Version. The instrument was piloted in a sample of 109 children who had at least some spoken language and a performance IQ greater than 65 who were diagnosed with an ASD using the Autism Diagnostic Observation Schedule[20] and the Autism Diagnostic Interview–Revised.[21] The sample was 94% male, and 72% of participants were diagnosed with at least 1 comorbid *DSM-IV* disorder. The most common disorders included

- Specific phobia: 44% (one-third of which were fear of needles or crowds)
- Obsessive-compulsive disorder (OCD): 37%
- ADHD: 31% (two-thirds inattentive type)
- Separation anxiety disorder: 12%
- Major depressive episode: 10%

The study was limited by a sample that was mostly male, verbal, and higher functioning as well as by the use of parental reports as the sole data source.

Sukholdolsky[22] modified the 26-item Child and Adolescent Symptom Inventory[23] to create a 20-item parent-rated screening tool to detect symptoms across 8 anxiety disorders, attempting to take into account typical ASD and ADHD symptoms. At least 10 of the items required children to provide verbal evidence. A total of 172 medication-free children with ASD (ages 5–17 years) with either high levels of aggression, tantrums, and self-injury or high levels of hyperactivity were screened. The sample included a full range of cognitive ability, from average intelligence to profound intellectual disability. Screening items included statements, such as "has difficulty controlling worries" and "has nightmares about being separated from parents." In this pilot study, 43% of subjects met the screening criteria for at least 1 anxiety disorder, twice the estimated rate for the neurotypical child population. The specific disorders that screened positive differed by level of intellectual disability, with those reliant on verbal articulation by the patients of their internal experience—generalized anxiety disorder, somatization disorder, separation anxiety disorder, and panic disorder—detected at significantly lower rates in the group with IQ less than 70. Because the instrument was likely somewhat insensitive to the sample with lower cognitive ability or verbal limitations, it is possible that the reported rate of anxiety disorders is an underestimate for that group.

Several investigators have provided evidence that psychiatric comorbidity is common in children with ASD, in particular anxiety and attention/impulsivity disorders. At this time, ASD-specific comorbidity measures have been confined primarily to the higher functioning, verbal population and have yet to develop into a scale brief enough for clinical practice. The absence of a gold standard diagnostic tool for psychiatric comorbidity in ASD has been a barrier to clinical efficacy, targeted research trials, and the ability to rationally extend the large literature on psychopharmacology in neurotypical children to those with ASD. In this context, clinicians are best served by accumulating experience with typical presentations of different subpopulations of children with ASD and taking a broad approach to presenting problems.

DIFFERENTIAL DIAGNOSIS OF PROBLEM BEHAVIORS: DEVELOPING THE WHOLE FROM A PART

Psychiatric comorbidity is just one of the potential causes of the problem behaviors that are prevalent in the general population of children with ASD. Using the Nisonger Child Behavior Rating Form,[24] an instrument developed for assessing young people with developmental disabilities, LeCavalier[25] conducted a survey of the parents and teachers of 487 school children receiving educational services for ASD. This survey of a non-clinically referred community sample revealed high rates of

- Easy frustration: 60%
- Inattention: 50%
- Hyperactivity: 40%
- Temper tantrums: 30%

Other symptoms included

- Irritability: 20%
- Fearfulness/anxiety: 13%
- Harming self: 11%
- Destroying property: 11%
- Physical fighting: 5%

Success in treating problem behaviors is likely to increase if a broad differential diagnostic approach is used based on a multidisciplinary consideration of causes. In the broadest sense, symptoms should be analyzed in terms of whether environmental (operant) conditions or intrinsic factors are responsible for maintenance of the presentation. Whether the symptoms are best explained by environmental reinforcement, such as the removal of task demands when a child strikes an educational aide, or as neurobiologically mediated, such as aggression that arises when a severely anxious child experiences stimuli flooding, can be considered.

For any given symptom or symptom constellation, clinicians should consider etiologic domains that include

- Medical: pain, seizure, nutrition
- Genetic: fragile X syndrome
- Communication
- Sensory-related
- Psychological: family dynamics, individuation
- Psychopathologic: anxiety, depression, ADHD
- Behavioral operant
- Iatrogenic: polypharmacy, sedation
- And others (**Tables 1** and **2**)

Only a few of these causes are likely to be responsive to psychotropic medication.

Table 1
ASD presenting problem differential diagnosis

Etiologic Domains	Examples of Potential Factors
Medical	Pain Seizure Nutrition Constipation
Genetic	Fragile X, 22q11.2 deletion syndrome
Communication	Absence of functional communication system
Sensory-related	Hypersensitivities or hyposensitivities
Cognitive	Intellectual disability
Psychological	Family dynamics Individuation
Psychopathologic	Anxiety Depression ADHD
Behavioral operant	Environmental maintenance
Iatrogenic	Polypharmacy Sedation Prompt dependence
Others	

Table 2
Evidence for medication by target symptom/disorder

Target Symptom	Agent	Dosing Studied	Level of Evidence
Aggression/ irritability	Aripiprazole	5–15 mg/d	Established evidence
	Risperidone	0.5–3.5 mg/d (mean dose 1.8 mg/d)	Established evidence
	Haloperidol	0.25–4 mg/d	Established evidence (in 2–7 y olds)
	Divalproex sodium	Mean level of 75–90 μg/mL	Insufficient evidence (conflicting results)
	Levitiracetam	20–30 mg/kg/d	Insufficient evidence
	Olanzapine	10 mg/d average	Insufficient evidence
	Lamotrigine	5 mg/kg/d	Evidence of no effect
Anxiety/OCD	Buspirone	15–45 mg qd	Insufficient evidence
	Sertraline	25–50 mg qd	Insufficient evidence
Hyperactivity	Methylphenidate	0.25–0.30 mg/kg/dose best response	Promising evidence
	Aripiprazole	5–15 mg/d	Promising evidence
	Risperidone	0.5–3.5 mg/d (mean dose 1.8 mg/d)	Promising evidence
	Haloperidol	0.25–4 mg qd	Promising evidence (in 2–7 y olds)
	Atomoxetine HCl	20–100 mg divided bid (mean 44 mg/d)	Preliminary evidence
	Naltrexone	0.5–1 mg/kg/d	Preliminary evidence
	Clomipramine	100–150 mg/d (mean 128.4 mg/d)	Insufficient evidence
	Clonidine	0.15–0.20 mg/d	Insufficient evidence
	Guanfacine	1–3 mg/d divided tid	Insufficient evidence
Insomnia	Melatonin	1–3 mg/d	Preliminary evidence
Repetitive behavior/stereotypy	Risperidone	0.5–3.5 mg/d (mean dose 1.8 mg/d)	Established evidence
	Haloperidol	0.25–4 mg/d	Established evidence (in 2–7 y olds)
	Aripiprazole	5–15 mg/d	Established evidence
	Divalproex Sodium	500–1500 mg/d	Insufficient evidence
	Fluoxetine	9.9 mg/d mean	Insufficient evidence
	Clomipramine	100–150 mg/d (mean 128.4 mg/d)	Evidence of no effect
	Citalopram	16.5 mg/d mean	Evidence of no effect
Self-injury	Naltrexone	Approximately 1 mg/kg/d	Insufficient evidence (conflicting results)
Social communication/ emotional regulation	Methylphenidate	0.25–0.30 mg/kg/dose best response	Insufficient evidence
	Risperidone	0.5–3.5 mg/d (mean dose 1.8 mg/d)	Insufficient evidence

Data from Siegel M, Beaulieu A. Psychotropic medications in children with autism spectrum disorders: a systematic review and synthesis for evidence-based practice. J Autism Dev Disord 2012;42:1592–605.

MEASURING CHANGE DURING PHARMACOTHERAPY

Because many children with ASD exhibit variations in symptom severity on a daily to weekly basis, reflecting the multifactorial etiology of most problem behaviors, it is vital to use behavioral data or rating instruments in a longitudinal fashion to drive treatment decision making. Relying solely on parent report, which may reflect only the most recent or most severe data, contributes to abbreviated treatment trials and increases the risk of polypharmacy.

The most widely used standardized outcome measure for children with ASD is the Aberrant Behavior Checklist (ABC).[26] The ABC is a 58-item parent or teacher-rated measure validated for children with developmental disabilities that produces 5 subscale scores in the domains of

1. Irritability
2. Lethargy/Social Withdrawal
3. Stereotypy
4. Hyperactivity
5. Inappropriate speech

The Irritability subscale comprises items that primarily reflect aggression, self-injury, and tantrums and has been used in multiple RCTs. Significant decreases in the irritability subscale contributed to the FDA approval for risperidone and aripiprazole in the treatment of irritability in ASD. Caution is advised, however, in applying the term, *irritability*, too freely to presenting symptoms, because 1 study found that only 20% of children with ASD were rated by parents and teachers as irritable.[25]

The Children's Yale-Brown Obsessive Compulsive Scale (CYBOCS) modified for PDDs[27] is an adaptation of the CYBOCS, designed to better characterize compulsions in the setting of ASD. The symptom checklist was expanded to include spinning objects, twirling, staring, and repetitive communications, and the informant was changed from the child to the parent. Whether the repetitive behaviors commonly seen in ASD represent obsessive-compulsive phenomena, which are typically egodystonic, or are better conceptualized as self-stimulatory actions that maintain sensorial equilibrium or provide self-reinforcing pleasurable feedback has not been established. Finally, several measures designed to assist in diagnosing autism have been used to evaluate response to treatment, including the Childhood Autism Rating Scale (CARS),[28] Gilliam Autism Rating Scale (GARS),[29] Autism Diagnostic Observation Schedule, though the validity of their use for this purpose has not been well established.

At this point there is no comprehensive scale for assessing change in the full range of maladaptive behaviors seen in children with ASD. Definition and recording of target behavior occurrences in educational and home treatment settings has become more common, providing an important source of data.

EVIDENCE BASE FOR PSYCHOTROPIC TREATMENT
Aggression and Irritability

Aggression, irritability, and self-injury are prevalent in the ASD population and treatments for some of these symptoms have the strongest evidence in ASD psychopharmacology. The most common outcome measure for this symptom cluster, the ABC Irritability subscale, contains 15 items that individually probe physical aggression toward others, self-injurious behavior, and irritability of mood or tantrum behaviors. Because the individual irritability subscale item data are not typically presented in published reports, further parsing of the symptom cluster has been limited.

In a recent report, the author of the instrument performed a line-item analysis of the irritability subscale data from 2 RCTs of aripiprazole in children with ASD. The ABC Irritability score was significantly improved, but individual item improvement was confined to the aggression and tantrum behavior items – self-injury items did not show statistically significant improvement.[30] For maximal clinical utility, this article groups aggression and irritability together and separately examines the few trials that have specifically targeted self-injury.

Risperidone and aripiprazole have the best evidence for reducing irritability and aggression, as shown in multiple RCTs. In the groundbreaking Research Units on Pediatric Psychopharmacology (RUPP)[31] RCT in 101 children ages 5 to 17 with ASD, risperidone (at an average of 1.8 mg/d) produced a significant improvement. In the treatment group, there was a 57% decrease in the ABC Irritability score compared with a 14% reduction in the placebo group. Responders in the blinded portion of the trial were enrolled in an open-label continuation phase for an additional 16 weeks, followed by an 8-week randomized, double-blinded discontinuation phase. In the open-label continuation, 51 of 63 initial responders remained stable, and of the 32 individuals who participated in the discontinuation study, 10 (62.5%) in the placebo group relapsed versus 2 (12.5%) in the medication group. A second RCT, performed by a separate investigative group, produced results largely similar to the treatment phase.[32]

In the preschool population, 2 RCTs of risperidone have been conducted. Luby and colleagues[33] performed an RCT in 24 children, ages 2.5 to 6 years, who received concurrent applied behavior analysis. At doses of 0.5 mg/d to 1.5 mg/d, the most common adverse events were sedation, sialorrhea, and increased appetite. Because the CARS and GARS diagnostic measures were the primary outcome measures, results are difficult to interpret but showed no effect on core symptom domains — although effects may have been muted by the lack of symptomatic entry criteria. A second RCT in preschoolers demonstrated some efficacy at 1 mg/d on the Children's Global Assessment Scale and the CARS.[34]

The RCTs of risperidone in school-aged children have shown mean weight gain in the medication group of 2.7 kg to 2.8 kg more than in the placebo group. Somnolence was the most common side effect, and the risperidone group had more extrapyramidal symptoms (EPS) reported than the placebo group. Cognitive effects of risperidone were assessed in the RUPP study and no significant adverse changes were detected.

Two pharmaceutical industry–sponsored large RCTs of aripiprazole showed efficacy for reduction of irritability. The first trial enrolled 98 children ages 6 to 17 years[35] and the second examined 218 children.[36] ABC Irritability subscale scores decreased 12.4 to 14.4 points in the medication group, compared with 5 to 8.4 points in the placebo group; 52.2% to 55.8% of subjects were considered responders. As with risperidone, somnolence was the most common side effect, EPSs were more common in the medication group than the placebo group, and 10.6% of the aripiprazole group discontinued the medication. Weight gain was less dramatic than in the risperidone studies but subjects taking aripiprazole did have a mean increase of 1.3 kg to 2 kg compared with 0.3 kg to 0.8 kg in the placebo group.

Haloperidol was reported as equivalent to risperidone in a study with methodologic and reporting issues.[37] An earlier crossover design RCT that included 24 children ages 10 to 18 years; however, found no difference on the ABC Irritability subscale between the placebo group and those treated with haloperidol at an average of 1.3 mg/d.[38] Results from the latter study need to be interpreted in light of a sample not selected for aggression or irritability, possible carryover effects between groups, and a low dosing scheme. Two older RCTs of haloperidol by Anderson[39,40] reported reduction in aggression, among several other symptoms, in mid-sized samples of 2-year-old to 7-year-old children with ASD. Despite the evidence for efficacy, use of haloperidol is best reserved for treatment of refractory cases due to the side-effect profile, which includes risks of dyskinesia and dystonia.

Mood stabilizers have been studied in several RCTs for reducing irritability/aggression and have yet to produce consistent evidence of benefit. Two RCTs of divalproex sodium targeting global clinical irritability or ABC-defined irritability have produced conflicting results. In 30 individuals with ASD, ages 6 to 20 years, Hellings and colleagues[41] found no significant difference on the ABC Irritability subscale between medication and placebo groups, with a mean trough level of 77.8 μg/mL. The study also described high intersubject variability and a large placebo effect. Hollander and colleagues[42] used more severe symptom entry criteria to reduce intersubject variability and showed a significant difference between divalproex sodium and placebo in favor of divalproex, particularly for those who obtained serum levels of 87 μg/mL to 110 μg/mL.

RCTs on lamotrigine and levitirecetam produced no significant effect on irritability.[43,44] There is insufficient evidence for olanzapine based on 1 small RCT, which showed improvement confined to the CGI,[45] and both ziprasidone and quetiapine have only uncontrolled data thus far. In addition, there is marginal evidence that methylphenidate can be helpful for reducing aggression in children with ASD and high degrees of impulsivity.[46,47]

Given the multifactorial etiology of most presenting problems, recent studies have begun to examine the efficacy of combining medication with behavioral management. The first enrolled 124 children with ASD (4–13 years old) and demonstrated greater reduction in the ABC Irritability score for patients who received an average dose of risperidone of 1.98 mg/d and 10.9 parent training sessions than the group who received risperidone at a mean dose of 2.26/d without parent training.[48] A recently published secondary analysis of adaptive behavior outcomes in this study demonstrated modestly greater gains (effect size [ES] = 0.14–0.35) in the socialization and communication domains for the risperidone plus parent training group.[49] Although early, these results are intriguing given the small investment required in providing 11 parent training sessions and the currently widespread use of behavioral management strategies in educational and treatment settings.

Anxiety/OCD

Despite multiple diagnostic surveys reporting anxiety disorders as the most common psychiatric comorbidity in children with ASD, there have been no controlled trials of pharmacologic treatment targeting anxiety in the population. The most frequently reported anxiety disorders are simple phobias, generalized anxiety disorder, separation anxiety disorder, and OCD.[50] Because anxiety is prevalent across the range of functioning in ASD, the need for better assessment tools of anxiety in both verbal and minimal or non-verbal children is urgent.

Perhaps related to the lack of assessment tools, studies targeting anxiety are restricted to small, uncontrolled trials and scattered case reports. Sertraline was studied in an uncontrolled trial of 9 children, 6 to 12 years old, with transition-induced behavioral deterioration, which was interpreted as related to transition anxiety.[51] Eight of the 9 subjects were reported to experience clinically significant improvement at 25 mg/d to 50 mg/d, based on parent report without standardized outcome measures. This pilot report has not been followed-up with a controlled trial.

Buspirone was the subject of an open label, uncontrolled trial in 22 children with ASD ages 6 to 17 years who were given 15–45 mg/d.[52] The investigators reported qualitative reduction of "overwhelming anxiety," although the primary outcome measure was only the CGI, which was reported as much/very much improved in 16 of 22 subjects. Side effects included oral-buccal movements in 1 subject.

Little is known about treating anxiety and OCD with riluzole, a compound that has complex effects on glutamate activity. There is currently a double-blind, placebo-controlled trial of riluzole being conducted by the National Institute of Mental Health in which riluzole or placebo is being given to youths ages 7 to 17 years who have treatment refractory moderate to severe OCD. Half of the enrolled subjects can also have ASD.

Hyperactivity-Impulsivity and Inattention

Symptoms of inattention, hyperactivity, or impulsivity are common in children with ASD. Concerns based on smaller uncontrolled studies regarding poor response or high rates of adverse events for the developmental disorders population have not been fully supported by controlled studies.

One large RCT has been performed targeting hyperactivity in children with ASD. Low (0.125 mg/kg), medium (0.25 mg/kg), and high (0.5 mg/kg) doses of methylphenidate were given twice a day, with a smaller third dose in the late afternoon, to 72 children (ages 5–14 years) with ASD (65% autistic disorder) and significant hyperactivity-impulsivity scores on the SNAP-IV ADHD scale.[49] A few subjects (8.3% of the sample) did not proceed beyond a test dose. Based on parent ratings, 49% of children were responders on the ABC hyperactivity subscale, with the greatest ES (.54) seen at the medium dose. 18% of subjects exited the study due to side effects. A smaller RCT was performed by Handen and colleagues on 13 children with ASD (69% autistic disorder) and ADHD symptoms, ages 5 to 11 years.[48] The study compared low (0.3 mg/kg/d) and high (0.6 mg/kg/d) doses of methylphenidate divided 2 or 3 times a day. On the ABC hyperactivity subscale, the high dose outperformed placebo, and both doses out-performed placebo on the Conners' Abbreviated Symptom Questionnaire, as rated by teachers. The most common adverse events across the 2 studies included irritability, emotional outbursts, social withdrawal, sadness, or dullness. A recent small RCT of methylphenidate in 12 preschoolers with ASD and ADHD showed a 50% response rate (ES = 0.97) on the Conners' Parent Rating Scale (CPRS)–Revised ADHD subscale but also demonstrated higher side-effect rates than in studies of methylphenidate in older children.[53]

Atomoxetine has been subjected to 1 small, double-blind RCT in 16 children ages 5 to 15 years with ASD and ADHD symptoms.[54] Atomoxetine produced an ES of 0.90 on the primary outcome measure, the ABC hyperactivity subscale, and 56% of subjects were considered responders. As with methylphenidate, the primary gains were in hyperactivity and impulsivity rather than inattentive symptoms; 18% of the sample exited the study and side effects were primarily gastrointestinal.

Risperidone has also been shown to reduce hyperactivity in children with ASD in at least 3 RCTs, the strongest of which is the RUPP 2002 study,[29] which showed 69% of subjects as responders on the ABC hyperactivity subscale (ES = 1.0) at the 8-week endpoint. Aripiprazole was tested in 2 large RCTs and demonstrated efficacy in reducing the ABC hyperactivity score of children with ASD by 12.7 to 16.3 points compared with a mean decrease of 2.8 to 7.7 points in the placebo group.

Naltrexone has been evaluated in 5 RCTs in children with ASD, primarily to test efficacy for reducing self-injury, but was found to have significant effects on hyperactivity. The largest of these studies produced significant reductions in the CPRS hyperactivity factor among 41 children 3 to 8 years old given 0.5 mg/kg/d to 1 mg/kg/d of naltrexone, and reported side effects of sedation, decreased appetite, and vomiting in the medication group.[55] Other treatments have included haloperidol, which demonstrated efficacy in reducing hyperactivity on the CPRS in 2 medium-sized RCTs in 40 to 45 children ages 2 to 7 years old.[39,40] Because sedation, irritability, and EPS were significant side effects, haloperidol is not a preferred choice for treatment of ADHD symptoms.

Guanfacine and clonidine have undergone small controlled studies targeting ADHD symptoms in ASD. Handen and colleagues[56] performed the only published RCT of guanfacine, targeting inattention and hyperactivity in 11 children with ASD ages 5 to

9 years; 45% of the sample showed more than a 50% reduction in the ABC hyperactivity score and approximately 45% of participants exhibited drowsiness. Approximately 27% of participants, experienced a level of drowsiness, irritability, or enuresis that prevented titration to the maximum dosage. A few open-label studies have been performed and a large RCT of long-acting guanfacine is currently under way. Two small RCTs of clonidine have been performed, each of which showed mixed results based on the reporter, and significant rates of sedation and hypotension.[57,58]

Clomipramine and desipramine seemed to show some efficacy in reducing hyperactivity in children with ASD.[59] A later RCT on clomipramine, however, evaluated 31 children and found no significant difference between clomipramine and placebo on the ABC hyperactivity subscale. In addition, twice as many participants receiving clomipramine stopped the study medication due to side effects or lack of efficacy than those on placebo.[39]

Based on these data, methylphenidate produces a somewhat lower response rate in children with ASD and ADHD symptoms (50%–60%) than it does in the neurotypical population (70%–90%). The evidence for methylphenidate is significantly stronger than that for atomoxetine, with best average results seen at a methylphenidate dose of approximately 0.25 mg/kg to 0.30 mg/kg given 2 to 3 times a day. Naltrexone has shown some efficacy in reducing hyperactivity. Risperidone and airpiprazole also appear efficacious for reducing hyperactivity, although their side-effect profile makes them a second-line choice for targeting hyperactivity.

Repetitive Behavior/Stereotypy

The domain of repetitive/stereotypic behaviors can be a treatment target when these symptoms interfere with educational programming or family life.

Risperidone has the best evidence for reducing repetitive behaviors, as shown in the large RUPP RCT[31] (discussed previously). In this trial, risperidone, at an average of 1.8 mg/d, produced a decrease in mean ABC stereotypy subscale scores from a baseline of 10.6 to an endpoint of 5.8 at 8 weeks of treatment. A decrease was also found in a modified, parent-rated Ritvo-Freeman Real Life Rating Scale sensory-motor subscale that included many repetitive behaviors. Decreased repetitive behavior was further evidenced by decreases in a modified CYBOCS, altered to better capture repetitive behaviors in nonverbal children, with a change from 15.51 at baseline to 11.65 at the 8-week endpoint (ES = 0.55). The RCTs of aripiprazole have also demonstrated significant reductions in the ABC stereotypy subscale.[36,37] Haloperidol demonstrated strong evidence for efficacy in reducing stereotypy on the CPRS in 2 moderately sized RCTs in 40 to 45 children ages 2 to 7 years old.[40,41] Sedation, irritability, and EPS were significant side effects and relegate haloperidol to being a second-line agent for use in stereotypy.

SRIs have proved disappointing when subjected to rigorous RCTs to evaluate effects on repetitive behavior. King and colleagues[10] demonstrated no significant difference between placebo and citalopram at a mean dose of 16.5 mg/d in 145 children with ASD (ages 5–17) on the CYBOCS-PDD. Side effects seen in the citalopram group included increased energy levels, impulsiveness, decreased concentration, hyperactivity, and stereotypy, among others. An RCT of fluoxetine in 39 children 5 to 17 years old used a crossover design and showed a 1.3-point, clinically insignificant, decrease on the 20-point CYBOCS.[60] The crossover design for an ultra–long-acting compound and the relatively low dosing scheme may have affected results. Clomipramine was initially reported to have positive effects on repetitive behavior in open-label and small controlled studies, whereas a medium-sized RCT of clomipramine showed no separation from placebo on the ABC stereotypy subscale.[39]

Finally, a small RCT of divalproex sodium in 13 children with ASD showed no clinically significant effect on repetitive behaviors as measured by an approximately 1-point decrease in the 20-point CYBOCS with a mean dilvalproex level of 58.[61]

Self-Injury

Naltrexone has been the subject of at least 5 RCTs examining self-injury, which have produced conflicting results and have suffered from methodologic problems. Initially, it was hoped that naltrexone would be efficacious in children with self-injurious behavior (SIB) based on the theory that the SIB is maintained through endogenous opioid release. The largest study was of 41 children with ASD ages 3 to 8 years, who were given naltrexone (1 mg/kg for 2 weeks) and found no significant difference between medication and placebo groups for self-injury or aggression.[54] Another RCT was performed on 20 children with ASD (ages 3–7 years) using a single higher dose (mean 1.96 mg/kg) in a crossover design.[62] This study produced a significant reduction in the ABC Irritability subscale score in the medication group. The same investigator then performed an RCT with an 8-week crossover design (4 weeks in each arm) with an average daily dose of 0.98 mg/kg/d.[63] Parent and teacher ratings on the ABC Irritability subscale, which includes aggression and self-injury, were conflicting, although the study sample was not selected for children with significant SIB. Despite the generally disappointing results, some investigators reported impressive effects in several subjects and noted that the selected populations were heterogeneous. In practice, when faced with a child with moderate to severe self-injury for whom behavioral and other interventions have failed, a trial of naltrexone is likely warranted.

Sleep Disturbance

Insomnia is reported to be highly prevalent in children with ASD, occurring in 44% to 86%.[64] Other sleep disturbances may include irregular sleep-wake patterns, early awakening, and poor sleep routines. The evaluation and treatment of sleep disturbance is multifactorial. In the author's clinical experience admitting many children with ASD to a specialized inpatient psychiatric unit, parent-reported sleep difficulties that are observed in the home frequently cease on entry to the hospital, suggesting that environmental factors are prominent.

Melatonin is the only compound that has been subjected to controlled study for use in sleep disturbance in children with ASD. At least 2 small RCTs have been performed, showing modest efficacy for melatonin in the population. An RCT of controlled-release melatonin (5 mg) included 16 children with ASD who had not responded to sleep hygiene interventions. The study reported a significant reduction in sleep latency and longer nighttime sleep in the children with ASD.[65] A small RCT of immediate release melatonin in 7 children with ASD showed reduction in sleep latency of 0.85 hours and increase in total sleep time of 1.09 hours compared with the placebo group.[66] Other potential sleep enhancing options, such as trazodone, mirtazapine, clonazepam, or diphenhydramine, have not been studied for this indication in ASD.

Social Communication, Hyperarousal, and Self-Regulation

Deficits in social communication and emotional regulatory mechanisms are persistent features in individuals across the ASD spectrum. Evidence from controlled trials of compounds targeting these areas is currently limited to secondary outcome analyses.

Jahromi and colleagues[67] performed a secondary analysis of the RUPP methylphenidate sample to examine a subgroup of 33 children with ASD and hyperactivity between the ages of 5 and 13 years, with mental ages less than 9 years. Using a validated procedure to assess joint attention initiations, response to bids for joint attention, self-regulation, and affective state, significant improvements were seen in the methylphenidate group. Parameters were measured repeatedly by blinded observer ratings of video recordings of both a scripted, semi-structured social communication task and a parent-child interaction. The investigators describe this as a pilot investigation, because it is a secondary analysis using a novel assessment strategy.

Risperidone demonstrated possible evidence for improvements in social communication in a secondary analysis of the RUPP 2002[29] data, which revealed significant improvement on the Ritvo-Freeman Real Life Rating Scale-affective reactions subscale, although there were no significant changes on the relationship to people or language subscales.[68] Other marginal evidence comes from an RCT of risperidone that showed a 63% decrease in the ABC social withdrawal subscale versus a 40% reduction for the placebo group.[30] One or more RCTs of secretin,[69] naltrexone,[61] and donepezil[70] have refuted earlier uncontrolled reports that suggested improved social interaction or significant cognitive enhancement could be seen with these agents.

The secondary analyses discussed raise the intriguing question as to whether methylphenidate's well-described effects on executive functioning or risperidone's effects on the dopaminergic reward system and other areas may lead directly or indirectly to improved social communication and emotional regulation in children with ASD.

SUMMARY

Children with ASD have high rates of problem behaviors and comorbid psychiatric disorders, which are associated with use of psychotropic medications. Accurate assessment of presenting symptoms requires a broad differential diagnostic approach and recognition of the multitude of factors that may pertain, only some of which are likely responsive to psychotropic medication. Psychopharmacology should be based on the best evidence for efficacy in ameliorating the target symptom or syndrome, balanced against the risk and severity of side effects.

ACKNOWLEDGMENTS

The author is thankful to Benjamin Handen, PhD, BCBA, for his thoughtful input on the manuscript.

REFERENCES

1. Autism and developmental disabilities monitoring network prevalence of autism spectrum disorders—autism and developmental disabilities monitoring network, 14 Sites, United States, 2012. MMWR Surveill Summ 2012;61(3):1–19. Available at: www.cdc.gov/mmwr/pdf/ss/ss6103.pdf. Accessed April 1, 2012.
2. Mcpheeters ML, Warren Z, Sathe N, et al. A systematic review of medical treatments for children with autism spectrum disorders. Pediatrics 2011;127:e1312.
3. Siegel M, Beaulieu A. Psychotropic medications in children with autism spectrum disorders: a systematic review and synthesis for evidence based practice. J Autism Dev Disord 2012;42(8):1592–605.
4. Aman MG, Lam KS, Van Bourgondien ME. Medication patterns in patients with autism: temporal, regional, and demographic influences. J Child Adolesc Psychopharmacol 2005;15(1):116–26.

5. Green VA, Pituch KA, Itchon J, et al. Internet survey of treatments used by parents of children with autism. Res Dev Disabil 2006;27(1):70–84.
6. Mandell DS. Psychiatric hospitalization among children with autism spectrum disorders. J Autism Dev Disord 2008;38:1059–65.
7. Witwer A, Lecavalier L. Treatment incidence and patterns in children and adolescents with autism spectrum disorders. J Child Adolesc Psychopharmacol 2005; 15(4):671–81.
8. Oswald DP, Sonenklar NA. Medication use among children with autism spectrum disorders. J Child Adolesc Psychopharmacol 2007;17(3):348–55.
9. Rosenberg RE, Mandell DS, Farmer JE, et al. Psychotropic medication use among children with autism spectrum disorders enrolled in a national registry, 2007-2008. J Autism Dev Disord 2010;40(3):342–51.
10. King BH, Hollander E, Sikich L, et al. Lack of efficacy of citalopram in children with autism spectrum disorders and high levels of repetitive behavior. Arch Gen Psychiatry 2009;66(6):583–90.
11. Croen LA, Najjar DV, Ray GT, et al. A comparison of health care utilization and costs of children with and without autism spectrum disorders in a large group-model health plan. Pediatrics 2006;118(4):1203–11.
12. Konstantareas MM, Hewitt T. Autistic disorder and schizophrenia: diagnostic overlaps. J Autism Dev Disord 2001;31(1):19–28.
13. De Bruin EI, Ferdinand RF, Meester S, et al. High rates of psychiatric co-morbidity in PDD-NOS. J Autism Dev Disord 2007;37:877–86.
14. Ferdinand RF, Van der Ende J. Diagnostic interview schedule for children IV. Parent-version. Rotterdam (The Netherlands): Erasmus University, Department of Child and Adolescent Psychiatry; 1998.
15. Ovraschel H. Schedule for affective disorder and schizophrenia for school-age children epidemiologic version. Fort Lauderdale (FL): Nova Southeastern University, Center for Psychological Studies; 1994.
16. Joshi G, Petty C, Wozniak J, et al. The heavy burden of psychiatric co-morbidity in youth with autism spectrum disorders: a large comparative study of a psychiatrically referred population. J Autism Dev Disord 2010;40:1361–70. http://dx.doi.org/10.1007/s10803-010-0996-9.
17. Simonoff E, Pickles A, Charman T, et al. Psychiatric disorders in children with autism spectrum disorders: prevalence, co-morbidity, and associated factors in a population-derived sample. J Am Acad Child Adolesc Psychiatry 2008;47:921–9.
18. Leyfer OT, Folstein SE, Bacalman S, et al. Comorbid psychiatric disorders in children with autism: Interview development and rates of disorders. J Autism Dev Disord 2006;36:849–61.
19. Kaufman J, Birmaher B, Brent D, et al. Schedule for affective disorders and schizophrenia for school-age children-present and lifetime version (K-SADS-PL): initial reliability and validity data. J Am Acad Child Adolesc Psychiatry 1997;36:980–8.
20. Lord C, Risi S, Lambrecht L, et al. The autism diagnostic observation schedule-generic: a standard measure of social and communication deficits associated with the spectrum of autism. J Autism Dev Disord 2000;30:205–23.
21. Lord C, Rutter M, LeCouteur AL. Autism diagnostic interview-revised: a revised version of the diagnostic interview for caregivers of individuals with possible pervasive developmental disorders. J Autism Dev Disord 1994;24:659–85.
22. Sukhodolsky DG, Scahill L, Gadow KD, et al. Parent-rated anxiety symptoms in children with pervasive developmental disorders: frequency and association with core autism symptoms and cognitive functioning. J Abnorm Child Psychol 2008;36(1):117–28.

23. Gadow, Sprafkin. Child symptom inventory-4. Stony Brook (NY): Checkmate Plus; 1998.
24. Aman MG, Tassé MJ, Rojahn J, et al. The nisonger CBRF: a child behavior rating form for children with developmental disabilities. Res Dev Disabil 1996; 17:41–57.
25. LeCavalier L. Behavioral and emotional problems in young people with pervasive developmental disorders: relative prevalence, effects of subject characteristics, and empirical classification. J Autism Dev Disord 2006;36:1101–14.
26. Aman M, Singh N, Stewart A, et al. The aberrant behavior checklist: a behavior rating scale for the assessment of treatment effects. Am J Ment Defic 1985;89:485–91.
27. Scahill L, McDougle CJ, Williams SK, et al, Research Units on Pediatric Psychopharmacology Autism Network. Children's Yale-Brown obsessive compulsive scale modified for pervasive developmental disorders. J Am Acad Child Adolesc Psychiatry 2006;45(9):1114–23.
28. Schopler E, Reichler RJ, Renner BR. The Childhood Autism Rating Scale (CARS), for diagnostic screening and classification in autism. New York: Irvington; 1986.
29. Gilliam JE. Gilliam autism rating scale. Austin (TX): PRO-ED; 1995.
30. Aman MG, Kasper W, Manos G, et al. Line-item analysis of the Aberrant Behavior Checklist: results from two studies of aripiprazole in the treatment of irritability associated with autistic disorder. J Child Adolesc Psychopharmacol 2010;20(5): 415–22.
31. Research Units on Pediatric Psychopharmacology Autism Network. Risperidone in children with autism and serious behavioral problems. N Engl J Med 2002; 347(5):314–21.
32. Shea S, Turgay A, Carroll A, et al. Risperidone in the treatment of disruptive behavioral symptoms in children with autistic and other pervasive developmental disorders. Pediatrics 2004;114:e634–41.
33. Luby J, Mrakotsky C, Stalets MM, et al. Risperidone in preschool children with autistic spectrum disorders: an investigation of safety and efficacy. J Child Adolesc Psychopharmacol 2006;16(5):575–87.
34. Nagaraj R, Singhi P, Malhi P. Risperidone in children with autism: randomized, placebo-controlled, double-blind study. J Child Neurol 2006;21(6):450–5.
35. Owen R, Sikich L, Marcus RN, et al. Aripiprazole in the treatment of irritability in children and adolescents with autistic disorder. Pediatrics 2009;124:1533–40.
36. Marcus RN, Owen R, Kamen L, et al. A placebo-controlled, fixed-dose study of aripiprazole in children and adolescents with irritability associated with autistic disorder. J Am Acad Child Adolesc Psychiatry 2009;48(11):1110–9.
37. Miral S, Gencer O, Inal-Emiroglu FN, et al. Risperidone versus haloperidol in children and adolescents with AD: a randomized, controlled, double-blind trial. Eur Child Adolesc Psychiatry 2008;17(1):1–8.
38. Remington G, Sloman L, Konstantareas M, et al. Clomipramine versus haloperidol in the treatment of autistic disorder: a double-blind, placebo-controlled, crossover study. J Clin Psychopharmacol 2001;4:440–4.
39. Anderson LT, Campbell M, Adams P, et al. The effects of haloperidol on discrimination learning and behavioral symptoms in autistic children. J Autism Dev Disord 1989;19(2):227–39.
40. Anderson LT, Campbell M, Grega DM, et al. Haloperidol in infantile autism: Effects on learning and behavioral symptoms. Am J Psychiatry 1984;141(10):195–202.
41. Hellings JA, Weckbaugh M, Nickel EJ, et al. A double-blind, placebo controlled study of valproate for aggression in youth with pervasive developmental disorders. J Child Adolesc Psychopharmacol 2005;15(4):682–92.

42. Hollander E, Chaplin W, Soorya L, et al. Divalproex sodium vs. placebo for the treatment of irritability in children and adolescents with autism spectrum disorders. Neuropsychopharmacology 2010;35(4):990–8.
43. Belsito L, Law P, Kirk K, et al. Lamotrigine therapy for autistic disorder: a randomized double-blind placebo-controlled trial. J Autism Dev Disord 2001;31(2):175–81.
44. Wasserman S, Iyengar R, Chaplin WF, et al. Levetiracetam versus placebo in childhood and adolescent autism: a double-blind placebo-controlled study. Int Clin Psychopharmacol 2006;21(6):363–7.
45. Hollander E, Wasserman S, Swanson EN, et al. A double-blind placebo-controlled pilot study of olanzapine in childhood/adolescent pervasive developmental disorder. J Child Adolesc Psychopharmacol 2006;16:541–8.
46. Quintana H, Birmaher B, Stedge D, et al. Use of methylphenidate in the treatment of children with autistic disorder. J Autism Dev Disord 1995;25(3):283–94.
47. Handen BL, Johnson CR, Lubetsky M. Efficacy of methylphenidate among children with autism and symptoms of attention-deficit hyperactivity disorder. J Autism Dev Disord 2000;30(3):245–55.
48. Research Units on Pediatric Psychopharmacology Autism Network. A randomized, double-blind, placebo-controlled, crossover trial of methylphenidate in children with hyperactivity associated with pervasive developmental disorders. Arch Gen Psychiatry 2005;62:1266–74.
49. Scahill L, McDougle CJ, Aman MG, et al, Research Units on Pediatric Psychopharmacology Autism Network. Effects of risperidone and parent training on adaptive functioning in children with pervasive developmental disorders and serious behavioral problems. J Am Acad Child Adolesc Psychiatry 2012;51(2):136–46.
50. White SW, Oswald D, Ollendick T, et al. Anxiety in children and adolescents with autism spectrum disorders. Clin Psychol Rev 2009;29(3):216–29.
51. Steingard RJ, Zimnitzky B, DeMaso DR, et al. Sertraline treatment of transition-associated anxiety and agitation in children with autistic disorder. J Child Adolesc Psychopharmacol 1997;7(1):9–15.
52. Buitelaar JK, van der Gaag RJ, van der Hoeven J. Buspirone in the management of anxiety and irritability in children with pervasive developmental disorders: results of an open-label study. J Clin Psychiatry 1998;59(2):56–9.
53. Ghuman JK, Aman MG, Lecavalier L, et al. Randomized, placebo-controlled, crossover study of methylphenidate for attention-deficit/hyperactivity disorder symptoms in preschoolers with developmental disorders. J Child Adolesc Psychopharmacol 2009;19(4):329–39.
54. Arnold LE, Aman MG, Cook AM, et al. Atomoxetine for hyperactivity in autism spectrum disorders: placebo-controlled crossover pilot trial. J Am Acad Child Adolesc Psychiatry 2006;45(10):1196–205.
55. Campbell M, Anderson LT, Small AM, et al. Naltrexone in autistic children: Behavioral symptoms and attentional learning. J Am Acad Child Adolesc Psychiatry 1993;32(6):1283–91.
56. Handen BL, Sahl R, Harden A. Guanfacine in children with autism and/or intellectual disabilities. J Dev Behav Pediatr 2008;29(4):303–8.
57. Fankhauser MP, Karumanchi VC, German ML, et al. A double-blind, placebo-controlled study of the efficacy of transdermal clonidine in autism. J Clin Psychiatry 1998;53(3):77–82.
58. Jaselskis CA, Cook EH, Fletcher KE, et al. Clonidine treatment of hyperactive and impulsive children with autistic disorder. J Clin Psychopharmacol 1992;12(5):322–7.

59. Gordon CT, State RC, Nelson JF, et al. A double-blind comparison of clomipramine, deipramine, and placebo in the treatment of autistic disorder. Arch Gen Psychiatry 1993;50:441–7.
60. Hollander E, Phillips A, Chaplin W, et al. A placebo controlled crossover trial of liquid fluoxetine on repetitive behaviors in childhood and adolescent autism. Neuropsychopharmacology 2005;30(3):582–9.
61. Hollander E, Soorya L, Wasserman S, et al. Divalproex sodium vs. placebo in the treatment of repetitive behaviours in autism spectrum disorder. Int J Neuropsychopharmacol 2006;9(2):209–13.
62. Willemsen-Swinkels SH, Buitelaar JK, Weijnen FG, et al. Placebo-controlled acute dosage naltrexone study in young autistic children. Psychiatry Res 1995;58(3): 203–15.
63. Willemsen-Swinkels SH, Buitelaar JK, van Engeland H. The effects of chronic naltrexone treatment in young autistic children: a double-blind placebo-controlled crossover study. Biol Psychiatry 1996;39(12):1023–31.
64. Johnson KP, Malow BA. Assessment and pharmacologic treatment of sleep disturbance in Autism. Child Adolesc Psychiatr Clin N Am 2008;17:773–85.
65. Wasdell MB, Jan JE, Bomben MM, et al. A randomized, placebo-controlled trial of controlled release melatonin treatment of delayed sleep phase syndrome and impaired sleep maintenance in children with neurodevelopmental disabilities. J Pineal Res 2008;44(1):57–64.
66. Garstang J, Wallis M. Randomized controlled trial of melatonin for children with autistic spectrum disorders and sleep problems. Child Care Health Dev 2006; 32(5):585–9.
67. Jahromi LB, Kasari CL, McCracken JT, et al. Positive effects of methylphenidate on social communication and self-regulation in children with pervasive developmental disorders and hyperactivity. J Autism Dev Disord 2009;39(3):395–404.
68. McDougle CJ, Scahill L, Aman MG, et al. Risperidone for the core symptom domains of autism: results from the study by the autism network of the research units on pediatric psychopharmacology. Am J Psychiatry 2005;162(6):1142–8.
69. Williams KJ, Wray JJ, Wheeler DM. Intravenous secretin for autism spectrum disorder. Cochrane Database Syst Rev 2005;(3):CD003495. http://dx.doi.org/10.1002/14651858.CD003495.pub2.
70. Handen BL, Johnson CR, McAuliffe-Bellin S, et al. Safety and efficacy of donepezil in children and adolescents with autism: neuropsychological measures. J Child Adolesc Psychopharmacol 2011;21(1):43–50.

Index

Note: Page numbers of article titles are in **boldface** type.

Child Adolesc Psychiatric Clin N Am 21 (2012) 975–992
http://dx.doi.org/10.1016/S1056-4993(12)00105-8
1056-4993/12/$ – see front matter © 2012 Elsevier Inc. All rights reserved.

United States Postal Service
Statement of Ownership, Management, and Circulation
(All Periodicals Publications Except Requestor Publications)

1. Publication Title	2. Publication Number								3. Filing Date
Child and Adolescent Psychiatric Clinics of North America	0	1	1	-	3	6	8	8	9/14/12

4. Issue Frequency	5. Number of Issues Published Annually	6. Annual Subscription Price
Jan, Apr, Jul, Oct	4	$297.00

7. Complete Mailing Address of Known Office of Publication (Not printer) (Street, city, county, state, and ZIP+4®)

Elsevier Inc.
360 Park Avenue South
New York, NY 10010-1710

Contact Person: Stephen R. Bushing
Telephone (Include area code): 215-239-3688

8. Complete Mailing Address of Headquarters or General Business Office of Publisher (Not printer)

Elsevier Inc., 360 Park Avenue South, New York, NY 10010-1710

9. Full Names and Complete Mailing Addresses of Publisher, Editor, and Managing Editor (Do not leave blank)

Publisher (Name and complete mailing address)

Kim Murphy, Elsevier, Inc., 1600 John F. Kennedy Blvd. Suite 1800, Philadelphia, PA 19103-2899

Editor (Name and complete mailing address)

Joanne Husovski, Elsevier, Inc., 1600 John F. Kennedy Blvd. Suite 1800, Philadelphia, PA 19103-2899

Managing Editor (Name and complete mailing address)

Barbara Cohen-Kligerman, Elsevier, Inc., 1600 John F. Kennedy Blvd. Suite 1800, Philadelphia, PA 19103-2899

10. Owner (Do not leave blank. If the publication is owned by a corporation, give the name and address of the corporation immediately followed by the names and addresses of all stockholders owning or holding 1 percent or more of the total amount of stock. If not owned by a corporation, give the names and addresses of the individual owners. If owned by a partnership or other unincorporated firm, give its name and address as well as those of each individual owner. If the publication is published by a nonprofit organization, give its name and address.)

Full Name	Complete Mailing Address
Wholly owned subsidiary of	1600 John F. Kennedy Blvd. Ste. 1800
Reed/Elsevier, US holdings	Philadelphia, PA 19103-2899

11. Known Bondholders, Mortgagees, and Other Security Holders Owning or Holding 1 Percent or More of Total Amount of Bonds, Mortgages, or Other Securities. If none, check box ☐ None

Full Name	Complete Mailing Address
N/A	

12. Tax Status (For completion by nonprofit organizations authorized to mail at nonprofit rates) (Check one)
The purpose, function, and nonprofit status of this organization and the exempt status for federal income tax purposes:
- ☐ Has Not Changed During Preceding 12 Months
- ☐ Has Changed During Preceding 12 Months (Publisher must submit explanation of change with this statement)

PS Form 3526, September 2007 (Page 1 of 3 (Instructions Page 3)) PSN 7530-01-000-9931 PRIVACY NOTICE: See our Privacy policy in www.usps.com

---

13. Publication Title	14. Issue Date for Circulation Data Below
Child and Adolescent Psychiatric Clinics of North America	July 2012

15. Extent and Nature of Circulation		Average No. Copies Each Issue During Preceding 12 Months	No. Copies of Single Issue Published Nearest to Filing Date
a. Total Number of Copies (Net press run)		654	557
b. Paid Circulation (By Mail and Outside the Mail)	(1) Mailed Outside-County Paid Subscriptions Stated on PS Form 3541. (Include paid distribution above nominal rate, advertiser's proof copies, and exchange copies)	404	365
	(2) Mailed In-County Paid Subscriptions Stated on PS Form 3541 (Include paid distribution above nominal rate, advertiser's proof copies, and exchange copies)		
	(3) Paid Distribution Outside the Mails Including Sales Through Dealers and Carriers, Street Vendors, Counter Sales, and Other Paid Distribution Outside USPS®	73	82
	(4) Paid Distribution by Other Classes Mailed Through the USPS (e.g. First-Class Mail®)		
c. Total Paid Distribution (Sum of 15b (1), (2), (3), and (4))	▲	477	447
d. Free or Nominal Rate Distribution (By Mail and Outside the Mail)	(1) Free or Nominal Rate Outside-County Copies Included on PS Form 3541	67	61
	(2) Free or Nominal Rate In-County Copies Included on PS Form 3541		
	(3) Free or Nominal Rate Copies Mailed at Other Classes Through the USPS (e.g. First-Class Mail)		
	(4) Free or Nominal Rate Distribution Outside the Mail (Carriers or other means)		
e. Total Free or Nominal Rate Distribution (Sum of 15d (1), (2), (3) and (4))	▲	67	61
f. Total Distribution (Sum of 15c and 15e)	▲	544	508
g. Copies not Distributed (See instructions to publishers #4 (page #3))	▲	110	49
h. Total (Sum of 15f and g)	▲	654	557
i. Percent Paid (15c divided by 15f times 100)		87.68%	87.99%

16. Publication of Statement of Ownership

☐ If the publication is a general publication, publication of this statement is required. Will be printed in the October 2012 issue of this publication. ☐ Publication not required.

17. Signature and Title of Editor, Publisher, Business Manager, or Owner

Stephen R. Bushing – Inventory Distribution Coordinator

Date: September 14, 2012

I certify that all information furnished on this form is true and complete. I understand that anyone who furnishes false or misleading information on this form or who omits material or information requested on the form may be subject to criminal sanctions (including fines and imprisonment) and/or civil sanctions (including civil penalties).

PS Form 3526, September 2007 (Page 2 of 3)

Moving?

Make sure your subscription moves with you!

To notify us of your new address, find your **Clinics Account Number** (located on your mailing label above your name), and contact customer service at:

Email: journalscustomerservice-usa@elsevier.com

800-654-2452 (subscribers in the U.S. & Canada)
314-447-8871 (subscribers outside of the U.S. & Canada)

Fax number: 314-447-8029

**Elsevier Health Sciences Division
Subscription Customer Service
3251 Riverport Lane
Maryland Heights, MO 63043**

*To ensure uninterrupted delivery of your subscription, please notify us at least 4 weeks in advance of move.

Printed and bound by CPI Group (UK) Ltd, Croydon, CR0 4YY

03/10/2024

01040447-0009